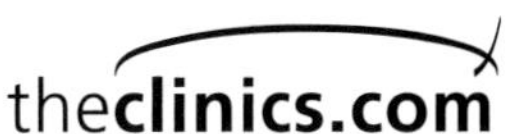

theclinics.com

NEUROSURGERY CLINICS OF NORTH AMERICA

Neuroendovascular Surgery

GUEST EDITORS
Elad I. Levy, MD
Lee R. Guterman, PhD, MD
L. Nelson Hopkins, MD

CONSULTING EDITORS
Andrew T. Parsa, MD, PhD
Paul C. McCormick, MD, MPH

April 2005 • Volume 16 • Number 2

SAUNDERS
An Imprint of Elsevier, Inc.
PHILADELPHIA LONDON TORONTO MONTREAL SYDNEY TOKYO

W.B. SAUNDERS COMPANY
A Division of Elsevier Inc.

The Curtis Center • Independence Square West • Philadelphia, Pennsylvania 19106

http://www.theclinics.com

NEUROSURGERY CLINICS OF NORTH AMERICA **Volume 16, Number 2**
April 2005 **ISSN 1042-3680**
Editor: Molly Jay **ISBN 1-4160-2853-6**

Neurosurgery Clinics of North America (ISSN 1042-3680) is published quarterly by Elsevier Inc. Corporate and editorial offices: 170 S Independence Mall W 300 E, Philadelphia, PA 19106-3399. Accounting and circulation offices: 6277 Sea Harbor Drive, Orlando, FL 32887-4800. Periodicals postage paid at Orlando, FL 32862, and additional mailing offices. Subscription prices are $205.00 per year (US individuals), $315.00 per year (US institutions), $225.00 per year (Canadian individuals), $380.00 per year (Canadian institutions), $265.00 per year (international individuals), $380.00 per year (international institutions), $133.00 per year (US students), and $133.00 per year (international students). International air speed delivery is included in all *Clinics* subscription prices. All prices are subject to change without notice. POSTMASTER: Send address changes to *Neurosurgery Clinics of North America*, W.B. Saunders Company, Periodicals Fulfillment, Orlando, FL 32887-4800. **Customer Service: 1-800-654-2452 (US). From outside of the US, call 1-407-345-4000.** E-mail: hhspcs@harcourt.com.

Neurosurgery Clinics of North America is covered in *Index Medicus, EMBASE/Excerpta Medica,* and *Current Contents/Clinical Medicine (CC/CM).*

Printed in the United States of America.

CONSULTING EDITORS

PAUL C. MCCORMICK, MD, MPH, Professor of Clinical Neurosurgery, Columbia University College of Physicians and Surgeons, New York, New York

ANDREW T. PARSA, MD, PhD, Assistant Professor, Department of Neurological Surgery, Neurospinal Research Center and The Brain Tumor Research Center, University of California San Francisco, San Francisco, California

GUEST EDITORS

ELAD I. LEVY, MD, Associate Professor, Departments of Neurosurgery and Radiology, and Toshiba Stroke Research Center, School of Medicine and Biomedical Sciences, University at Buffalo, State University of New York, Buffalo, New York

LEE R. GUTERMAN, PhD, MD, Associate Professor, Departments of Neurosurgery and Radiology, and Toshiba Stroke Research Center, School of Medicine and Biomedical Sciences, University at Buffalo, State University of New York, Buffalo, New York

L. NELSON HOPKINS, MD, FACS, Professor and Chairman, Department of Neurosurgery, Toshiba Stroke Research Center; and Professor, Department of Radiology, School of Medicine and Biomedical Sciences, University at Buffalo, State University of New York, Buffalo, New York

CONTRIBUTORS

FELIPE C. ALBUQUERQUE, MD, Division of Neurological Surgery, Barrow Neurological Institute, St. Joseph's Hospital and Medical Center, Phoenix, Arizona

ISSAM A. AWAD, MD, Professor, Department of Neurological Surgery, Feinberg School of Medicine, Northwestern University, Chicago, Illinois

JEFFREY BALZER, PhD, Associate Professor, Department of Neurological Surgery, University of Pittsburgh, Pittsburgh, Pennsylvania

H. HUNT BATJER, MD, Professor and Chair, Department of Neurological Surgery, Feinberg School of Medicine, Northwestern University, Chicago, Illinois

BERNARD R. BENDOK, MD, Assistant Professor, Departments of Neurological Surgery and Radiology, Feinberg School of Medicine, Northwestern University, Chicago, Illinois

BRETT CAMPANELLA, RN, Interventional Neuroradiology Nurse, Department of Neurosurgery, State University of New York at Buffalo, Buffalo, New York

KEVIN M. COCKROFT, MD, MSc, FACS, Assistant Professor, Departments of Radiology and Neurosurgery, Milton S. Hershey Medical Center, Pennsylvania State University, Hershey, Pennsylvania

VIVEK R. DESHMUKH, MD, Division of Neurological Surgery, Barrow Neurological Institute, St. Joseph's Hospital and Medical Center, Phoenix, Arizona

JOHNATHAN A. ENGH, MD, Resident, Department of Neurosurgery, University of Pittsburgh, Pittsburgh, Pennsylvania

DAVID J. FIORELLA, MD, Division of Neurological Surgery, Barrow Neurological Institute, St. Joseph's Hospital and Medical Center, Phoenix, Arizona

KENNETH FRASER, MD, Departments of Neurosurgery and Radiology, Neurovascular Center, Illinois Neurological Institute, University of Illinois College of Medicine at Peoria, Peoria, Illinois

CHRISTOPHER C. GETCH, MD, Assistant Professor, Department of Neurological Surgery, Feinberg School of Medicine, Northwestern University, Chicago, Illinois

WILLIAM A. GRAY, MD, Director, Department of Endovascular Care, Swedish Cardiovascular Research, Swedish Medical Center, Seattle, Washington

CHARLES A. GUIDOT, MD, Clinical Assistant Professor, Department of Neurosurgery, State University of New York at Buffalo, Buffalo, New York

LEE R. GUTERMAN, PhD, MD, Associate Professor, Departments of Neurosurgery and Radiology, and Toshiba Stroke Research Center, School of Medicine and Biomedical Sciences, University at Buffalo, State University of New York, Buffalo, New York

RICARDO A. HANEL, MD, Clinical Assistant Professor, Department of Neurosurgery and Toshiba Stroke Research Center, School of Medicine and Biomedical Sciences, University at Buffalo, State University of New York, Buffalo, New York

ROBERT E. HARBAUGH, MD, Professor and Chairman, Department of Neurosurgery, Penn State University College of Medicine, Milton S. Hershey Medical Center, Hershey, Pennsylvania

MARK R. HARRIGAN, MD, Assistant Professor, Division of Neurosurgery, Department of Surgery, The University of Alabama at Birmingham, Birmingham, Alabama

L. NELSON HOPKINS, MD, FACS, Professor and Chairman, Department of Neurosurgery, Toshiba Stroke Research Center; and Professor, Department of Radiology, School of Medicine and Biomedical Sciences, University at Buffalo, State University of New York, Buffalo, New York

JAY U. HOWINGTON, MD, Associate Clinical Professor of Surgery, Neurological Institute of Savannah, Memorial Health University Hospital, Savannah, Georgia

SUNG-KYUN HWANG, MD, Assistant Professor, Department of Neurosurgery, Ewha Women's University School of Medicine; and Department of Neurosurgery, Thomas Jefferson University Hospital, Philadelphia, Pennsylvania

BRIAN JANKOWITZ, MD, Clinical Assistant Instructor, Department of Neurological Surgery, University of Pittsburgh Medical Center, Pittsburgh, Pennsylvania

CHARLES W. KERBER, MD, Professor, Departments of Radiology and Neurological Surgery, University of California at San Diego, San Diego, California

CHRISTOPHER J. KOEBBE, MD, Resident, Department of Neurological Surgery, Thomas Jefferson University Hospital, Pittsburgh, Pennsylvania

GIUSEPPE LANZINO, MD, Departments of Neurosurgery and Radiology, Neurovascular Center, Illinois Neurological Institute, University of Illinois College of Medicine at Peoria, Peoria, Illinois

ELAD I. LEVY, MD, Associate Professor, Departments of Neurosurgery and Radiology, and Toshiba Stroke Research Center, School of Medicine and Biomedical Sciences, University at Buffalo, State University of New York, Buffalo, New York

CHRISTOPHER M. LOFTUS, MD, Professor and Chairman, Department of Neurosurgery, Temple University School of Medicine, Philadelphia, Pennsylvania

DEMETRIUS K. LOPES, MD, Assistant Professor, Departments of Neurosurgery and Radiology, Rush-Presbyterian—St. Luke's Hospital, Chicago, Illinois

THOMAS J. MASARYK, MD, Section Head of Neuroradiology, Section of Cerebrovascular and Endovascular Neurosurgery, Departments of Neurosurgery and Radiology, The Cleveland Clinic Foundation, Cleveland, Ohio

CAMERON G. MCDOUGALL, MD, Division of Neurological Surgery, Barrow Neurological Institute, St. Joseph's Hospital and Medical Center, Phoenix, Arizona

ANDREW J. MOLYNEUX, MB, BChir, FRCR, Honorary Senior Clinical Lecturer, Department of Neuroradiology, University of Oxford, Neurovascular Research Unit, Radcliffe Infirmary, University of Oxford, Oxford, United Kingdom

PETER NAKAJI, MD, Attending Physician, Division of Neurological Surgery, Barrow Neurological Institute, St. Joseph's Hospital and Medical Center, Phoenix, Arizona

BRIAN A. O'SHAUGHNESSY, MD, Resident, Department of Neurological Surgery, Feinberg School of Medicine, Northwestern University, Chicago, Illinois

RICHARD J. PARKINSON, MD, Cerebrovascular Fellow, Department of Neurological Surgery, Feinberg School of Medicine, Northwestern University, Chicago, Illinois

DAVID G. PIEPGRAS, MD, Professor, Department of Neurologic Surgery, Mayo Clinic, Rochester, Minnesota

PETER A. RASMUSSEN, MD, Associate Staff, Section of Cerebrovascular and Endovascular Neurosurgery, Departments of Neurosurgery and Radiology, The Cleveland Clinic Foundation, Cleveland, Ohio

ANDREW J. RINGER, MD, Neurosurgeon, Departments of Neurosurgery and Neuroradiology, The Neuroscience Institute; Assistant Professor, University of Cincinnati College of Medicine, Cincinnati; and Neurosurgeon, Mayfield Clinic, Cincinnati, Ohio

ROBERT H. ROSENWASSER, MD, FACS, Professor and Chairman, Department of Neurosurgery, and Director, Division of Cerebrovascular Surgery and Interventional Neuroradiology, Thomas Jefferson University Hospital, Philadelphia, Pennsylvania

ERIC J. RUSSELL, MD, Professor and Chair, Department of Radiology, Feinberg School of Medicine, Northwestern University, Chicago, Illinois

LEO SALUD, MD, Department of Neurosurgery, University of Cincinnati College of Medicine, Cincinnati, Ohio

ERIC SAUVAGEAU, MD, Clinical Assistant Instructor, Neuroendovascular Fellow, Department of Neurosurgery and Toshiba Stroke Research Center, School of Medicine and Biomedical Sciences, University at Buffalo, State University of New York, Buffalo, New York

ALI SHAIBANI, MD, Assistant Professor, Department of Radiology, Feinberg School of Medicine, Northwestern University, Chicago, Illinois

BRIAN E. SNELL, MD, Fellow in Spinal Surgery, Department of Neurological Surgery, Medical College of Wisconsin, Milwaukee, Wisconsin

ROBERT F. SPETZLER, MD, Division of Neurological Surgery, Barrow Neurological Institute, St. Joseph's Hospital and Medical Center, Phoenix, Arizona

THOMAS A. TOMSICK, MD, Department of Neuroradiology, The Neuroscience Institute; and University of Cincinnati College of Medicine, Cincinnati, Ohio

DAVID WANG, DO, Department of Neurology, Neurovascular Center, Illinois Neurological Institute, University of Illinois College of Medicine at Peoria, Peoria, Illinois

HUAN WANG, MD, Department of Neurosurgery, Neurovascular Center, Illinois Neurological Institute, University of Illinois College of Medicine at Peoria, Peoria, Illinois

J. CHRISTOPHER WEHMAN, MD, Clinical Assistant Instructor, Neuroendovascular Fellow, Department of Neurosurgery and Toshiba Stroke Research Center, School of Medicine and Biomedical Sciences, University at Buffalo, State University of New York, Buffalo, New York

DAVID O. WIEBERS, MD, Professor, Department of Neurology, Mayo Medical School, Mayo Clinic, Rochester, Minnesota

HENRY H. WOO, MD, Associate Staff, Section of Cerebrovascular and Endovascular Neurosurgery, Departments of Neurosurgery and Radiology, The Cleveland Clinic Foundation, Cleveland, Ohio

CONTENTS

Intracranial atherosclerosis is the third leading cause of ischemic stroke, and patients with known intracranial stenoses seem to be at high risk for the development of a stroke. Despite the high prevalence of this disease process, intracranial atherosclerosis remains tremendously difficult to treat, and failure rates associated with the best medical therapy are unacceptably high. An emerging alternative therapy for patients with intracranial atherosclerosis is intracranial angioplasty with or without stenting. Endovascular techniques have already been shown to be feasible for patients with medically refractory disease. The authors demonstrate the risks and benefits of endovascular therapy for intracranial stenosis as well as the newer directions of the field, including drug-eluting stents and staged stenting.

This article discusses the implications of natural history and treatment morbidity and mortality for decision making regarding patient management of unruptured intracranial aneurysms.

This article reviews the evidence and indications for endovascular coil treatment of intracranial aneurysms and the potential role of the new devices that are becoming available.

Dramatic advances occurring over the past decade in endovascular technology and techniques have revolutionized the field of cerebrovascular neurosurgery. The goal of this article is to review the evidence supporting endovascular approaches for the treatment of intracranial aneurysms and to discuss basic treatment techniques, complication avoidance, and the management and treatment of vasospasm from the perspective of "hybrid" cerebrovascular neurosurgeons who perform open and catheter-based interventions.

The endovascular treatment of cerebral arteriovenous malformations (AVMs) has advanced greatly in the four decades since Luessenhop and Spence first described the use of silastic spheres to embolize an AVM. The innovations have been in the agents used to embolize as well as in the devices used to deliver the agent to the AVM. Endovascular therapies have helped to decrease operative morbidity by making it easier for the surgeon to resect the AVM and, in some cases, by eliminating the need for surgery

FORTHCOMING ISSUES

July 2005

Intervential Neuroradiology
Arun Paul Amar, MD, and Sean Lavine, MD
Guest Editors

October 2005

Motion Sparing Surgery
Dean Chou, MD, and Christopher Ames, MD,
Guest Editors

RECENT ISSUES

April 2004

Peripheral Nerve Tumors: Diagnosis and Management
Eric L. Zager, MD, and Jason H. Huang, MD
Guest Editors

July 2004

Pain Treatment
Gary Heit, MD, PhD, *Guest Editor*

October 2004

Metastatic Spine Disease
Meic H. Schmidt, MD,
Daryl R. Fourney, MD, FRCSC, and
Ziya L. Gokaslan, MD, FACS, *Guest Editors*

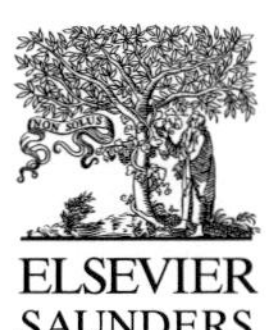

ELSEVIER
SAUNDERS

Neurosurg Clin N Am 16 (2005) xiii–xv

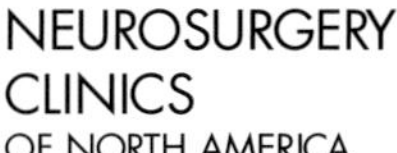

NEUROSURGERY
CLINICS
OF NORTH AMERICA

Preface

Neuroendovascular Surgery: Techniques, Indications, and Patient Selection

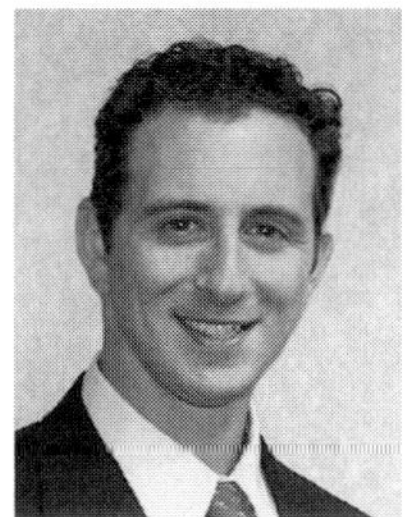

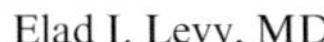

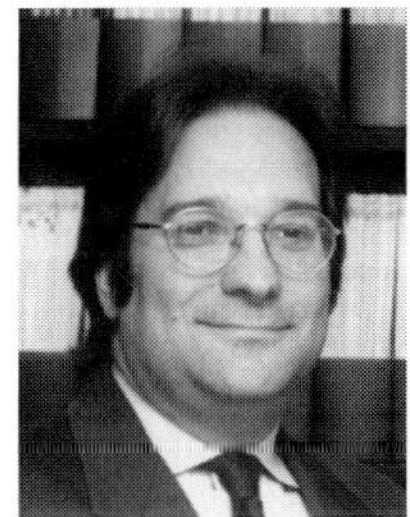

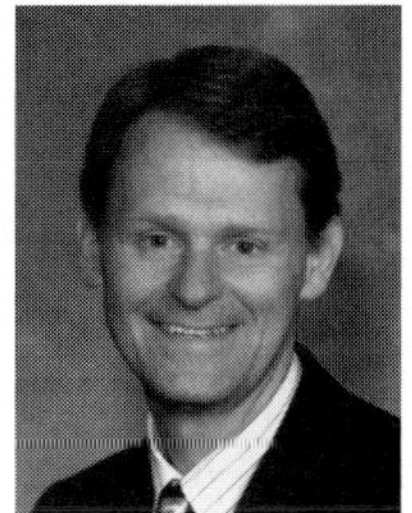

Elad I. Levy, MD   Lee R. Guterman, PhD, MD   L. Nelson Hopkins, MD, FACS
Guest Editors

Catheter-based treatments for cerebrovascular disease are displacing open surgical techniques at a rapid pace. The impetus for this is fueled by the medical consumer's appetite for minimally invasive solutions for complex surgical problems. A technologic revolution has occurred over the past 10 years based on the introduction of percutaneous catheter-based vascular devices. The interventional cardiology community has provided a framework for technology development and clinical trial design that has laid the foundation for the use of catheter-based treatments in the intracranial and extracranial cerebrovascular circulation.

Until recently, prospective randomized clinical trial data have not been the primary driver of practice habits for cerebrovascular disease. Historically, the Extracranial-to-Intracranial (EC-IC) Bypass Study [1], the North American Symptomatic Carotid Endarterectomy Trial (NASCET) [2], and the Asymptomatic Carotid Atherosclerosis Study (ACAS) [3] represented the entire body of the level 1 data on cerebrovascular disease. With the completion of the International Subarachnoid Aneurysm Trial (ISAT) [4], it became clear that coil occlusion of ruptured aneurysms had become established as an alternative to open surgical ligation based on a randomized prospective trial of more than 2000 patients. Recent results in the control arms of large aneurysm trials indicate that coils may be superior to open surgery for unruptured intracranial aneurysms (Congress of Neurological Surgeons Annual Meeting, San Francisco, October 16–21, 2004, personal communication).

Medical device manufacturers have driven the adoption of endovascular techniques for treating intracranial aneurysms. There are now at least six different detachable coil manufacturers competing for aneurysm patients worldwide. In the United States, the percentage of aneurysms treated with interventional techniques has increased to almost 50%. In some countries, aneurysms are treated with coils as a primary therapy. Surgery is reserved for aneurysms that cannot be coiled.

The evolution of the development of detachable coils for cerebral aneurysms has been rapid. Presently, biologic coatings made of suture material, hydrogels, and other substances claim to improve healing at the aneurysm neck. Clinical evidence of the biologic healing has been limited, but randomized trials are underway. The future should see new devices for treating wide-necked aneurysms increase the percentage of unruptured and ruptured aneurysms that can be treated by endovascular techniques.

1042-3680/05/$ - see front matter
doi:10.1016/j.nec.2004.12.001

The treatment of cerebral arteriovenous malformations (AVMs) pairs embolization with stereotactic radiosurgery or open resection. Embolization of these lesions with N-butyl-cyanoacrylate (NBCA; histoacryl) alone did not produce a significant number of permanent occlusions. Recent approval of Onyx (Micro Therapeutics, Irvine, California), a dimethyl sulfoxide–based liquid embolic precipitate, has increased the likelihood of embolic material penetrating the AVM nidus. Embolization with Onyx forms a cast of the malformation and may lead to an increase in the number of permanent occlusions using embolization therapy in cerebral AVMs.

Dural arteriovenous fistulae still present a challenge for open surgery and catheter-based therapy. It seems that the most successful catheter-based treatments occlude the fistulae by filling the proximal venous vasculature with embolic material. Transvenous access plays an important role in treating these inoperable lesions. Improved embolic materials should see the eradication of these lesions using endovascular therapy.

Standard surgical techniques for extracranial carotid artery stenosis have been challenged by angioplasty and stent techniques. Large clinical trials comparing patients with symptomatic and asymptomatic carotid stenosis have defined a role for stent-assisted angioplasty in patients with high-risk characteristics, including excessive medical comorbidities, unstable angina, carotid restenosis, laryngeal nerve palsy, and radiation-induced stenosis. The Carotid Revascularization Endarterectomy versus Stent Trial (CREST) [5,6], a randomized trial for symptomatic patients with carotid stenosis, is well underway; the final results should be available sometime during the latter part of this decade.

An increasing incidence of intracranial stenosis has been identified as a result of the availability of minimally invasive imaging techniques, such as computed tomographic and magnetic resonance angiography. The results of the Warfarin-Aspirin Symptomatic Intracranial Disease (WASID) trial indicate that warfarin may not provide adequate stroke protection [7–9]. As a result, high-grade symptomatic intracranial stenosis is being treated with stent-assisted angioplasty. Although drug-eluting stents have reduced the incidence of in-stent stenosis in coronary arteries, these stents have not been widely used in the intracranial circulation. Presently available drug-coated stents tend to be difficult to track into the intracranial circulation. More flexible stent designs are being developed for intracranial atherosclerotic lesions and should become available over the next few years.

Acute ischemic stroke patients comprise a population that is at least one order of magnitude larger in number than that of cerebral aneurysm patients. Ischemic cerebrovascular disease accounts for 80% of all strokes in the United States. Although thrombolytic agents have been the first line of treatment for acute ischemic stroke, atherosclerotic cerebrovascular disease may be more effectively treated using stent-assisted angioplasty in combination with multiagent drug administration. A combination of antiplatelet, thrombolytic, and anticoagulation agents may help to keep mechanically recanalized vessels open.

The application of high-resolution noninvasive neuroimaging techniques to the cerebral vasculature is identifying an increasing number of patients with asymptomatic stenosis. The results of the WASID trial indicate that warfarin provides suboptimal stroke protection in patients with symptomatic intracranial atherosclerotic disease. The role of stent-assisted angioplasty in this patient population remains to be seen.

The ever-increasing role of catheter-based treatments for cerebrovascular disease mandates that future cerebrovascular surgeons have the skills to perform open surgery and catheter-based interventions. The successful treatment of cerebrovascular disease represents a final frontier in medicine. Treatment of patients with cerebrovascular disease represents an exciting challenge that should reward those who accept it with dedication and enthusiasm.

Elad I. Levy, MD
Toshiba Stroke Research Center
School of Medicine and Biomedical Sciences
University at Buffalo
State University of New York
3 Gates Circle
Buffalo, NY 14209, USA

E-mail address: elevy@buffns.com

Lee R. Guterman, PhD, MD
Toshiba Stroke Research Center
School of Medicine and Biomedical Sciences
University at Buffalo
State University of New York
3 Gates Circle
Buffalo, NY 14209, USA

L. Nelson Hopkins, MD, FACS
Toshiba Stroke Research Center
School of Medicine and Biomedical Sciences
University at Buffalo
State University of New York
3 Gates Circle
Buffalo, NY 14209, USA

References

[1] EC/IC Bypass Study Group. Failure of extracranial-intracranial arterial bypass to reduce the risk of ischemic stroke. Results of an international randomized trial. N Engl J Med 1985;313:1191–200.

[2] North American Symptomatic Carotid Endarterectomy Trial Collaborators. Beneficial effect of carotid endarterectomy in symptomatic patients with high-grade carotid stenosis. N Engl J Med 1991;325: 445–53.

[3] Executive Committee for the Asymptomatic Carotid Atherosclerosis Study. Endarterectomy for asymptomatic carotid artery stenosis. JAMA 1995;273:1421–8.

[4] Molyneux A, Kerr R, Stratton I, et al. International Subarachnoid Aneurysm Trial (ISAT) of neurosurgical clipping versus endovascular coiling in 2143 patients with ruptured intracranial aneurysms: a randomised trial. Lancet 2002;360:1267–74.

[5] Hobson RW II. CREST (Carotid Revascularization Endarterectomy versus Stent Trial): background, design, and current status. Semin Vasc Surg 2000;13: 139–43.

[6] Hobson RW II, Brott T, Ferguson R, et al. CREST: Carotid Revascularization Endarterectomy versus Stent Trial. Cardiovasc Surg 1997;5:457–8.

[7] Chimowitz MI. WASID trial. Neurosurgery Grand Rounds: Millard Fillmore Gates Circle Hospital, Buffalo, NY, August 5, 2004.

[8] Chimowitz MI, Kokkinos J, Strong J, et al. The Warfarin-Aspirin Symptomatic Intracranial Disease Study. Neurology 1995;45:1488–93.

[9] Yarab N. Warfarin-Aspirin Symptomatic Intracranial Disease (WASID) study. Presented at the American Stroke Association 28th International Conference. Phoenix, Arizona, February 13–15, 2003. Available at: http://www.strokeconference.org/sc_includes/pdfs/CTP10.pdf.

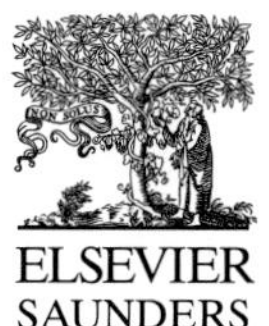

ELSEVIER
SAUNDERS

Neurosurg Clin N Am 16 (2005) 223–229

NEUROSURGERY
CLINICS
OF NORTH AMERICA

The Evolution of Endovascular Therapy for Neurosurgical Disease

Huan Wang, MD[a], Kenneth Fraser, MD[a,b], David Wang, DO[c], Giuseppe Lanzino, MD[a,b,*]

[a]*Department of Neurosurgery, Neurovascular Center, Illinois Neurological Institute, University of Illinois College of Medicine at Peoria, PO Box 1649, One Illini Drive, Peoria, IL 61656, USA*

[b]*Department of Radiology, Neurovascular Center, Illinois Neurological Institute, University of Illinois College of Medicine at Peoria, PO Box 1649, One Illini Drive, Peoria, IL 61656, USA*

[c]*Department of Neurology, Neurovascular Center, Illinois Neurological Institute, University of Illinois College of Medicine at Peoria, PO Box 1649, One Illini Drive, Peoria, IL 61656, USA*

The field of endovascular neurosurgery has evolved rapidly and successfully over the past few decades. This dynamic evolution has resulted in numerous new and effective endovascular therapies for the management of intracranial aneurysms; arteriovenous malformations (AVMs); dural arteriovenous fistulae; acute stroke; carotid-cavernous fistulae (CCFs); carotid artery disease; vasospasm; and vascular tumors of the head, neck, and spine. The rapidly advancing technologies as well as our constantly enlarging body of knowledge about the central nervous system are catalyzing this evolution. Although we anticipate the future of endovascular neurosurgery with great enthusiasm, it is important to review its history to gain a sense of direction and discover the renewed pertinence of past ideas.

Cerebral angiography

Cerebral angiography is the foundation of neuroendovascular therapies. Antonio Egas Moniz (Fig. 1), a Portuguese neurologist and the recipient of the Nobel Prize in Physiology and Medicine in 1949, was the first to develop and describe cerebral angiography in 1927 [1]. Moniz exemplified personal traits common to other endovascular pioneers: vision and perseverance despite almost insurmountable obstacles. After successfully obtaining cerebral angiograms in dogs, he transported cadaveric specimens obtained from the pathology department in his limousine to a radiology laboratory in another part of the city to develop the technique further. The first successful cerebral angiogram performed in a living person was obtained in a 48-year-old patient with Parkinson's disease. Moniz ligated the internal carotid artery (ICA) temporarily for 2 minutes and injected a 70% solution of strontium bromide into the ICA at a dose of 13 to 14 mL. The first film showed contrast filling of the middle and posterior cerebral arteries. Unfortunately, the patient died 8 hours later from thrombophlebitis. Thereafter, angiography passed through many phases of development to evolve from a one-time hazardous technique to a simple and safe procedure.

Intracranial aneurysms

Beginnings

Although attempts to induce thrombosis of peripheral aneurysms by introducing foreign bodies or applying local electrical or thermal energy date back to the early 1800s [2], it was not until 1941 that Werner et al [3] reported the first successful electrothermic thrombosis of an intracranial aneurysm (Fig. 2). With a transorbital

* Corresponding author.
E-mail address: Lanzino@uic.edu (G. Lanzino).

1042-3680/05/$ - see front matter
doi:10.1016/j.nec.2004.08.006

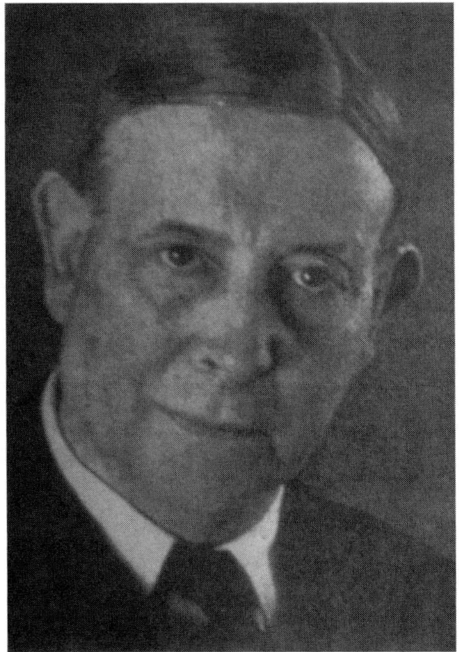

Fig. 1. Antonio Egas Moniz, a Portuguese neurologist who won the Nobel Prize in Physiology and Medicine in 1949, developed and described cerebral angiography in 1927.

approach, "thirty feet of No. 34 gauge coin silver enameled wire was introduced into the aneurysm through a special needle" and "the wire was heated to an average temperature of 80°C for a total of 40 seconds. The aneurysm no longer bled when the needle was cleared at the conclusion of the operation" [3].

1960s and 1970s

In 1964, while attempting to occlude a supraclinoid aneurysm by advancing a silicone balloon, Luessenhop (Fig. 3) and Velasquez made the first endovascular attempt to treat an aneurysm [4]. In 1964 and 1965, Mullan (Fig. 4) et al [5,6] reported their clinical experience with inducing aneurysm thrombosis by applying an electrical current after direct and stereotactic insertion of needles and copper wires transfundally into ruptured and unruptured aneurysms. They acknowledged that controlling the degree of thrombosis was exceedingly difficult. In 1969, Alksne and Fingerhut [7] published their clinical results relating to metallic thrombosis of aneurysms. They embolized aneurysms with iron particles introduced through a needle intravascularly and maintained within the aneurysmal sac by stereotactic application of a magnetic probe against the sac.

After observing how easily helium-filled balloons were maneuvered by simple manipulations of their tether lines, Serbinenko (Fig. 5) developed a balloon-tipped microcatheter with flow-directional capabilities to allow for more effective intracranial catheterization [8]. In the 1970s, he further revolutionized endovascular neurosurgery by developing nondetachable and detachable balloon catheters to allow for direct aneurysmal obliteration or parent artery sacrifice and to make temporary balloon occlusion easy, safe, and

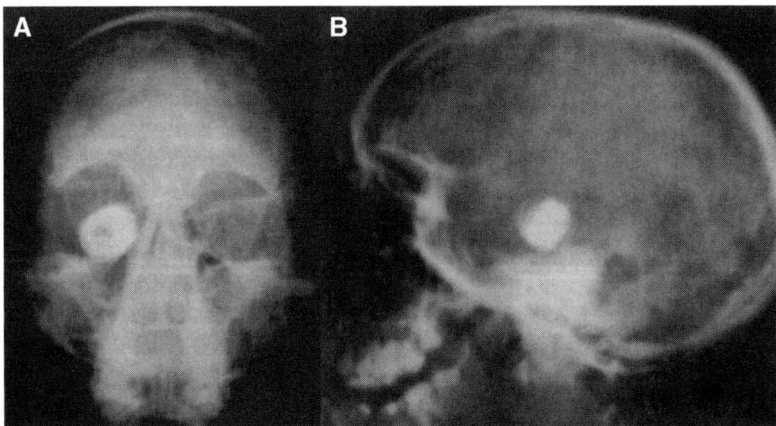

Fig. 2. Anteroposterior (*A*) and lateral (*B*) follow-up cranial radiographs of the patient whose aneurysm was successfully treated with a silver wire inserted through the orbit. (*From* Werner SC, Blakemore AH, King BG. Aneurysm of the internal carotid artery within the skull: wiring and electrothermic coagulation. JAMA 1941;116:578–82; with permission.)

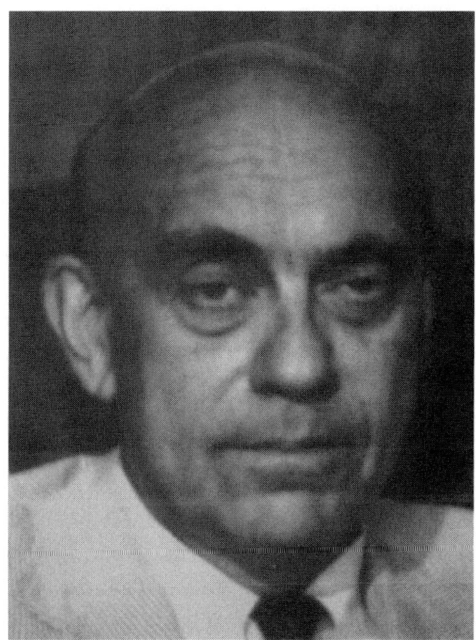

Fig. 3. In 1964, neurosurgeon Alfred J. Luessenhop (along with his colleague A.C. Velasquez) made the first endovascular attempt to treat an intracranial aneurysm. To recognize his invaluable pioneering contributions, a lecture in his name is offered each year at the joint cerebrovascular meeting of the American Association of Neurological Surgeons/Congress of Neurological Surgeons/American Society of Interventional and Therapeutic Neuroradiology.

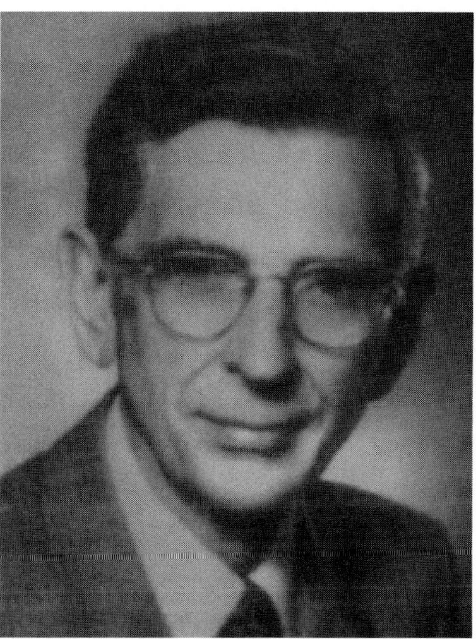

Fig. 4. In 1964, neurosurgeon Sean F. Mullan pioneered the technique of using electrical current to induce aneurysm thrombosis.

reliable. His seminal innovations gave birth to the modern era of endovascular neurosurgery [8].

1970s and 1980s

Balloon occlusion techniques were further developed and refined in the 1970s and 1980s, during which time, a vast amount of clinical experience was accumulated. In 1982, Romodanov and Shcheglov reported 137 intravascular occlusions of saccular aneurysms using detachable balloons [9]. In 1990, Higashida et al [10] reported the use of balloons for endovascular therapy of 87 cavernous carotid artery aneurysms between 1981 and 1989. In 1991, Moret et al [11] reported their results with balloon treatment of 128 aneurysms. Other large reports from these two decades regarding the use of detachable balloons included those by Shcheglov et al (725 cases), Serbinenko et al (267 cases), and George et al (92 cases) [9]. As more experience was acquired, several major disadvantages of this technique became apparent. Catheterization of the aneurysm was difficult, because no guidewire could be used. The preformed shape of the balloon often prevented it from adequately filling a geometrically complex aneurysm without leaving the fundus unprotected or creating a ball-valve system of aneurysmal refilling. Subsequently, the focus of endovascular therapy shifted from balloon occlusion to platinum coil occlusion. Several authors, including Hilal and Solomon, Dowd, Arnaud, and Higashida, reported the occlusion of intracranial aneurysms with "pushable" platinum coils [2]. Coiling for intracranial aneurysms remained a dangerous procedure, however, primarily because of the inability to retrieve the advanced coils as well as the often inadvertent migration of these highly thrombogenic coils into the distal intracranial vasculature.

1990s and 2000s

The invention of detachable coils by the Italian neurosurgeon Guido Guglielmi in the early 1990s ushered in a new era in the endovascular treatment of aneurysms [12]. The design of the Guglielmi detachable coil (GDC) permitted the position and effectiveness of the coil to be examined before the coil was released electrolytically from its tether. In addition, the flexibility and softness of the coil enabled the satisfactory

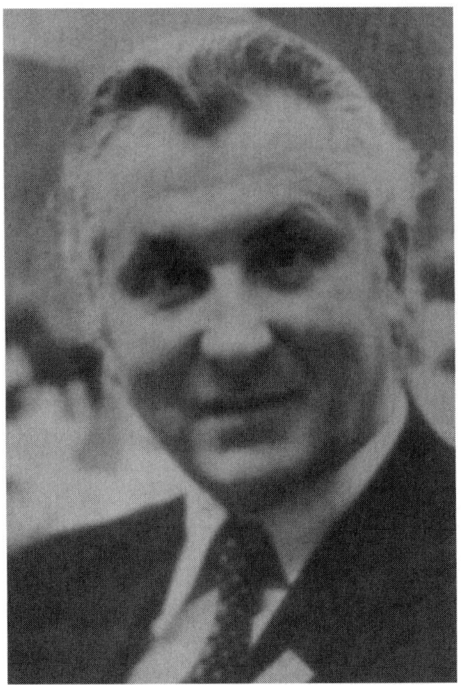

Fig. 5. Neurosurgeon Fedor A. Serbinenko revolutionized endovascular neurosurgery by inventing and developing the technique of balloon embolization for catheterization and occlusion of major cerebral vessels.

filling of a geometrically complex aneurysm with minimal procedural risk of rupture. On April 12, 1990, the first intracranial aneurysm was treated using this new technology [12]. In 1992, Guglielmi et al [13] published the results of the first multicenter GDC clinical trial. Small-necked and wide-necked lesions showed 81% and 15% immediate complete occlusion, respectively. Procedure-related morbidity and mortality rates were 4.8% and 2.4%, respectively. The GDC system immediately achieved worldwide acceptance and became the focus of most published work on endovascular aneurysm therapy [2].

Despite the newly acquired advantages from the GDC system, larger aneurysms or wide-necked lesions remained difficult to manage. New techniques were clearly required to keep the coils within the aneurysmal sac after deployment. Moret et al [14] pioneered and popularized the balloon-remodeling technique using a balloon as a mechanical barrier to prevent coil herniation into the parent vessel during its delivery. This technique also facilitated a better conformation of the coil mass to the complex geometry of an aneurysm. In 1997, Moret et al [14] published their results with use of the balloon-remodeling technique for the treatment of 56 cases of previously untreatable wide-necked intracranial aneurysms. Their reported morbidity and mortality rates were no higher than rates associated with routine GDC treatment. After some early experimental work done by Wakhloo et al [15] and Geremia et al [16], an alternative approach to advance coils through a stent to treat aneurysms was proposed by several authors [2]. The stent maintained a patent lumen and provided a buttress to prevent coil herniation. Since its introduction, this stent-assistance technique has been further explored and expanded by an increasing number of neuroendovascular surgeons [2].

With the rapidly advancing knowledge of basic science, the new millennium holds exciting promises for the advent of coils coated with various biologic agents, leading to the improved formation of neointima across the aneurysm neck and thus a much reduced risk of coil compaction and aneurysmal recanalization. Additionally, the potential use of liquid embolization agents to treat aneurysms is being evaluated in a clinical setting.

Arteriovenous malformations

Since the successful introduction of cerebral angiography by Egas Moniz in 1927, much progress has been made in the diagnosis and evaluation of AVMs. The modern-day detailed radiographic study of the malformation involves evaluating the hemodynamic and anatomic characteristics of the lesion, including examination of the feeding arteries, the nidus itself, and venous drainage of the lesion. Exponential advances in catheter technology and refinements of embolic agents have greatly facilitated the rapid evolution of AVM embolization.

In 1930, Brooks [17] reported successful closure of a CCF with a muscle embolus introduced surgically into the carotid artery. Three decades later, Luessenhop and Spence [18] expanded this strategy and performed the first embolization procedure on an intracerebral AVM by surgically introducing silastic spheres made of methyl methacrylate into the ICA. Thereafter, in the search for the ideal embolic agent, various materials, including silk sutures, porcelain beads, Gelfoam, steel balls, Teflon-coated spheres, and polyvinyl alcohol, were explored with varying degrees of efficacy [2]. Without the technologies and devices for direct nidus embolization, use of these flow-directed emboli was associated with a high complication rate secondary to inadvertent embolization of a normal cerebral vessel.

In 1976, Kerber [19] developed the first calibrated-leak balloon that allowed the direct embolization of an AVM nidus through the use of a rapidly solidifying polymer. This new system for catheter therapy, in combination with advances in imaging techniques and delivery devices, ushered in the modern era of AVM embolization. Calibrated-leak balloon catheters, however, were associated with a high incidence of arterial perforation. The development of flow-guided and wire-guided microcatheters allowed for superselective catheterization with great improvements in precision and safety. With the introduction of road-mapping techniques, a microcatheter can now be successfully navigated into a small distal vessel while an image generated from a previous contrast injection is superimposed on a negative map of the vascular tree.

Embolization of AVMs has evolved immensely over the last few decades to become a highly valuable adjunct, and even an alternative in some cases, to surgery or stereotactic radiosurgery. Embolization can be used to occlude deep feeding arteries or intranidal arterial aneurysms to reduce venous hypertension and the volume of an AVM before radiosurgery. Endovascular cure of parenchymal AVMs is possible only in some small lesions that possess a limited number of arterial feeders and draining veins and a compact nidus, however. In addition, the morbidity associated with endovascular embolization of parenchymal AVMs is still significant.

Stroke prevention and acute management

As early as 1969, 5 years after introducing percutaneous transluminal angioplasty, Charles Dotter published a new technique to percutaneously place endovascular spiral stents [20]. The revival of interest in the early 1980s contributed to the development of several important stent designs, such as the balloon-expanded stents and Palmaz stents [21]. Since the publication of reports of the successful performance of angioplasty [22] and the placement of stents in the coronary arteries [23], both techniques have become well established, with large, well-organized, multi-institutional trials in the coronary and other peripheral vessels [2]. Concerns about the potentially catastrophic consequences of small distal emboli delayed the development of angioplasty and stenting in diseased carotid and vertebral arteries for stroke prevention [2]. Reports of carotid angioplasty in the 1980s and more recent studies of angioplasty or stenting of extracranial carotid artery disease [2] have suggested that procedural safety and complication rates are comparable with those for carotid endarterectomy (CEA). Although CEA remains the "gold standard" for the treatment of atherosclerotic carotid disease, the rapidly evolving nature of endovascular therapy—with new technologies and devices being developed almost on a monthly basis—begs the question as to whether endoluminal revascularization should be proposed as the true alternative to CEA. Large, prospective, randomized trials are in progress.

The development of new angioplasty balloon catheters and flexible stents has redefined the management strategy for symptomatic intracranial stenosis. A growing number of studies have reported a low complication profile and satisfactory rates of angiographic patency at follow-up [2]. The answer to the question of whether angioplasty or stenting should be the first line of treatment for patients with symptomatic intracranial stenosis requires data obtained from well-designed, prospective, multicenter studies.

The concept of intra-arterial thrombolysis for acute stroke management dates back to 1958, when Sussmann and Fitch reported successful recanalization of an acute ICA occlusion with intra-arterial fibrinolysis using plasmin [24]. After further clinical trials failed to show convincing benefits, this concept of treating acute stroke with pharmacologic revascularization was essentially abandoned [2]. Before 1995, stroke therapy consisted exclusively of supportive management and efforts to prevent recurrence [2]. The development of safer thrombolytic agents and an improved understanding of the pathophysiology of ischemic stroke rekindled the interest in pharmacologic thrombolysis, however. In 1995, the National Institute of Neurological Disorders and Stroke reported that early intravenous thrombolysis using tissue plasminogen activator was more effective than placebo [25]. The concept of intra-arterial pharmacologic thrombolysis was further expanded and solidified in 1999 with the completion of the Prolyse in Acute Cerebral Thromboembolism study [26]. This study clearly showed that intra-arterial injection of the thrombolytic agent into the immediate proximity of or within the thrombus within 6 hours of stroke onset significantly improved patient outcome, despite an increased incidence of early symptomatic intracranial hemorrhage. Intravenous thrombolysis and intra-arterial thrombolysis have received widespread acceptance and truly revolutionized the management of acute stroke.

Summary

The exponential evolution of endovascular neurosurgery over the past few decades has redefined the treatment strategies for cerebrovascular diseases. Entering the new millennium, one must have the mindset to embrace and nurture the progress and technologic advances. Thomas Fogarty eloquently stated: "When envisioning the technologic process, we must think young' and consider the impossible. The mindset is best achieved in an environment where innovators consider the unachievable as being possible" [27]. Indeed, the pioneers of endovascular neurosurgery considered the impossible and tenaciously stood by their dreams. Their revolutionary ideas and inventions truly reflected their courage, faith, and determination. With a better understanding of the molecular basis of diseases and further advancements in gene therapy, the future is ideal and holds exciting promise for endovascular neurosurgery to deliver biologic factors with minimal risk and high precision and to develop effective therapies for the entire spectrum of neurologic diseases.

References

[1] Lobo-Antunes J. Egas Moniz and cerebral angiography. J Neurosurg 1974;40:427–32.

[2] Hopkins LN, Lanzino G, Guterman LR. Treating complex nervous system vascular disorders through a "needle stick": origins, evolution, and future of neuroendovascular therapy. Neurosurgery 2001; 48(3):463–75.

[3] Werner SC, Blakemore AH, King BG. Aneurysm of the internal carotid artery within the skull: wiring and electrothermic coagulation. JAMA 1941;116: 578–82.

[4] Luessenhop AJ, Velasquez AC. Observations on the tolerance of intracranial arteries to catheterization. J Neurosurg 1964;21:85–91.

[5] Mullan S, Bechkman F, Vailati G. An experimental approach to the problem of cerebral aneurysms. J Neurosurg 1964;21:838–45.

[6] Mullan S, Raimondi AJ, Dobben G, Vailati G, Hekmatpanah J. Electrically induced thrombosis in intracranial aneurysms. J Neurosurg 1965;22:539–47.

[7] Alksne JF, Fingerhut AG. Magnetically controlled metallic thrombosis of intracranial aneurysms: a preliminary report. Bull LA Neurol Soc 1965;3:154–5.

[8] Teitelbaum GP, Larsen DW, Zelman V, Lysachev AG, Likhterman LB. A tribute to Dr. Fedor A. Serbinenko, founder of endovascular neurosurgery. Neurosurgery 2000;46(2):462–70.

[9] Horowitz MB, Levy E, Kassam A, Purdy PD. Endovascular therapy for intracranial aneurysms: a historical and present status review. Surg Neurol 2002;57:147–59.

[10] Higashida RT, Halbach VV, Dowd C, Barnwell SL, Dormandy B, Bell J, et al. Endovascular detachable balloon embolization therapy of cavernous carotid artery aneurysms: results in 87 cases. J Neurosurg 1990;72:857–63.

[11] Moret J, Boulin A, Mawad M, Castaings L. Endovascular treatment of berry aneurysms by endosaccular balloon occlusion. Neuroradiology 1991; 33(Suppl):135–6.

[12] Guglielmi G, Vinuela F, Dion J, Duckwiler G. Electrothrombosis of saccular aneurysms via endovascular approach. Part 2: preliminary clinical experience. J Neurosurg 1991;75:8–14.

[13] Guglielmi G, Vinuela F, Duckwiler G. Endovascular treatment of posterior circulation aneurysms by electrothrombosis using electrically detachable coils. J Neurosurg 1992;77:515–24.

[14] Moret J, Cognard C, Weill A, Castaings L, Rey A. The "remodeling technique" in the treatment of wide neck intracranial aneurysms: angiographic results and clinical follow-up in 56 cases. Intervent Neuroradiol 1997;21:838–45.

[15] Wakhloo AK, Schellhammer F, de Vries J, Haberstroh J, Schumacher M. Self-expanding and balloon-expandable stents in the treatment of carotid aneurysms: an experimental study in a canine model. AJNR Am J Neuroradiol 1994;15(3):493–502.

[16] Geremia G, Haklin M, Brennecke L. Embolization of experimentally created aneurysms with intravascular stent devices. AJNR Am J Neuroradiol 1994; 15(3):1223–31.

[17] Brooks B. Discussion of paper by Noland L, Taylor AS. Trans South Surg Assoc 1931;43:176–7.

[18] Luessenhop AJ, Spence WT. Artificial embolization of cerebral arteries: report of use in a case of arteriovenous malformation. JAMA 1960;172:1153–5.

[19] Kerber C. Balloon catheter with a calibrated leak: a new system for superselective angiography and occlusive catheter therapy. Radiology 1976;120: 547–50.

[20] Dotter CT. Transluminally placed coilspring endarterial tube grafts: long-term patency in canine popliteal artery. Invest Radiol 1969;4:327–32.

[21] Zollikofer CL, Antonucci F, Stuckmann G, Mattias P, Salomonowitz EK. Historical overview on the development and characteristics of stents and future outlooks. Cardiovasc Intervent Radiol 1992;15: 272–8.

[22] Gruntzig AR, Stenning A, Siegenthaler WE. Nonoperative dilatation of coronary-artery stenosis: percutaneous transluminal coronary angioplasty. N Engl J Med 1979;301:61–8.

[23] Sigwart U, Puel J, Mirkovitch V, Joffre F, Kappenberger L. Intravascular stents to prevent occlusion and restenosis after transluminal angioplasty. N Engl J Med 1987;316:701–6.

[24] Sussmann BJ, Fitch TSP. Thrombolysis with fibrinolysis in cerebral arterial occlusion. JAMA 1958; 167:1705–9.

[25] National Institute of Neurological Disorders and Stroke rt-PA Stroke Study Group. Tissue plasminogen activator for acute ischemic stroke: the National Institute of Neurological Disorders and Stroke rt-PA Stroke Study Group. N Engl J Med 1995;333: 1581–7.

[26] Furlan A, Higashida R, Wechsler L, Gent M, Rowley H, Kase C, et al. Intra-arterial prourokinase for acute ischemic stroke: the PROACT II study—a randomized controlled trial. Prolyse in Acute Cerebral Thromboembolism. JAMA 1999; 282:2003–11.

[27] Fogarty TJ. Vision of relevant technologic progress for the next two decades. J Vasc Surg 1996;24: 291–6.

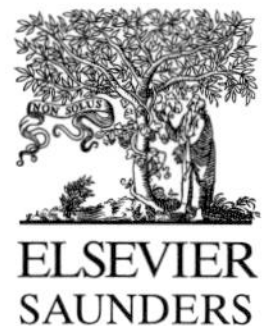

ELSEVIER
SAUNDERS

Neurosurg Clin N Am 16 (2005) 231–239

NEUROSURGERY
CLINICS
OF NORTH AMERICA

Preparation of the Interventional Suite for Treatment of Neurovascular Diseases and Emergencies

Christopher J. Koebbe, MD[a,*], Charles A. Guidot, MD[b], Brett Campanella, RN[b], Jeffrey Balzer, PhD[a], Elad I. Levy, MD[a,b]

[a]*Department of Neurosurgery, University of Pittsburgh, 1312 Pocono Street, Pittsburgh, PA 15218, USA*
[b]*Department of Neurosurgery, State University of New York at Buffalo, 3 Gates Circle, Buffalo, NY 14209–1194, USA*

The current scope of endovascular technology and associated clinical applications has led to the need to modify the angiography suite to have more of an operating room type of environment so as to perform the full range of elective and emergent neurovascular procedures. This conversion is a complex task given the wide spectrum of disorders, equipment, and personnel involved. As the "captain of the ship," the neurointerventionist must have a good understanding of the pathophysiology of the patient's disease and be able to use the skills of all team members to provide optimal patient care. This article provides an overview of the physiology and pharmacology encountered in the neurointerventional suite and the necessary room or equipment setup and personnel roles required to treat neurovascular disease successfully. Patients presenting to the neurointerventional suite may need elective (eg, unruptured aneurysm or arteriovenous malformation [AVM], carotid or intracranial stenosis, tumor embolization, radiosurgery, angiography, petrosal sinus sampling) or emergent (eg, hemorrhage caused by ruptured aneurysm or AVM, vasospasm, thromboembolic stroke, vein of Galen malformations, epistaxis) care (Table 1).

Before the procedure begins

Many patients treated by endovascular techniques are poor surgical candidates because of multiple medical comorbidities that require special consideration during preprocedural evaluation. A thorough review of systems should be performed to identify cardiopulmonary dysfunction, any abnormality that might increase the risk of anesthesia, renal disease, peripheral vascular disease that might affect vascular access, recent fever or infections that might limit the use of implanted devices, hematologic disorders that might affect hemostasis, and contrast allergies. Patients with intracranial hemorrhage (ICH) must be evaluated for hydrocephalus, because it is preferable to perform procedures like placement of a ventriculostomy before using the anticoagulants that are needed during endovascular procedures. The neurologic examination, when possible, should document any preexisting deficits and should evaluate mental status as well as cranial nerve, motor, sensory, and cerebellar function. Laboratory analysis, including a complete blood cell count as well as electrolyte, blood urea nitrogen, and creatinine levels, should be obtained. Informed consent for an endovascular procedure includes a thorough discussion of the risks and benefits of the planned procedure, the potential for surgical intervention (ventriculostomy, carotid endarterectomy, or craniotomy) in the face of a complication, and alternative therapies. A discussion between the neurointerventionist and the treatment team (nursing staff, technical staff, anesthesia staff, and, if available, the neurophysiologist) regarding the patient's condition and the planned procedures allows for preparation of the proper pharmacologic agents and endovascular devices. The decision to use general

* Corresponding author.
E-mail address: chriskoebbe@hotmail.com (C.J. Koebbe).

1042-3680/05/$ - see front matter
doi:10.1016/j.nec.2004.08.007

Table 1
Neurovascular diseases within the neurointerventional suite

Condition	Treatment goal/devices	Potential complications/need for emergent intervention
Aneurysm	Detachable coils, intracranial stents, liquid embolic agents, balloon occlusion	SAH with hydrocephalus: ICP control Procedure-related vascular rupture: complete the embolization, ventriculostomy, control BP, reverse heparin Thromboembolic event: antiplatelet agents, thrombolysis, angioplasty/stent
Thrombo-occlusive disease/stroke intervention	Thrombolytic agents, angioplasty balloons, mechanical thrombolytic devices, intracranial stents	Cerebral ischemia: increase MAP and oxygenation, anticoagulate Vessel perforation: occlude/stent bleeding site, ventriculostomy, craniotomy
Vascular malformations	Embolic agents (NBCA, coils, PVA, liquid agents) radiosurgical angiography, surgical exposure for venous access (SOV cutdown)	Hemorrhage: ICP control, ventriculostomy, decrease MAP Thromboembolic events
Carotid stenosis	Angioplasty balloons, stents	Prepare for complications related to comorbidities, including cardiac disease and peripheral vascular disease Angioplasty-induced bradycardia: atropine, fluids, vasopressors or pacing device if necessary
Medically intractable vasospasm	Angioplasty balloons, intra-arterial vasodilatation agents	Prevent further ischemia: increase MAP, barbiturates, CSF drainage Vessel perforation (see above)
Tumors/epistaxis	Embolic agents (coils, liquid agents, PVA)	Thromboembolic event: attempt to identify and avoid all potential anastomoses Tumor swelling: steroids, be ready to resect tumor if necessary

Abbreviations: BP, blood pressure; CSF, cerebrospinal fluid; ICP, intracranial pressure; MAP, mean arterial pressure; NBCA, N-butyl cyanoacrylate; PVA, polyvinyl alcohol; SAH, subarachnoid hemorrhage; SOV, superior ophthalmic vein.

anesthesia on noncomatose patients in the neurointerventional suite remains controversial, because the advantages of a real-time neurologic assessment in the awake patient must be weighed against the added control over patient cooperation and physiologic variables in the anesthetized patient.

Developing the surgical plan

When possible, the neurointerventionist should develop a comprehensive plan of attack so that each member of the team understands his or her role and is ready to perform his or her duties as required. A preoperative strategy should include contingency plans to use in the case of a complication so that the team can quickly attempt to stabilize the patient. The technical staff should attempt to have potentially necessary endovascular devices readily available so as to avoid delays in the case of an emergency. The nursing staff must be aware of any critical care issues that require their attention, including monitoring vital signs, respiratory status, and intracranial pressure (ICP). This includes preparing medications that may be needed during the procedure. The anesthesia staff should be aware of the treatment goals and should be prepared to intervene as needed, such as to administer protamine to reverse the effect of heparin in the face of a hemorrhagic complication.

The key to a successful surgical plan is establishing a clear treatment goal leading to a safe and effective end result. The neurointerventionist may be tempted to stray from this goal to produce a better angiographic result, but this may compromise the patient's outcome with no additional clinical benefit. One example is intracranial angioplasty and stenting for atherosclerotic disease. Poiseuille's law states that flow through a cylindric pipe is directly proportional to the radius to the fourth power. This suggests that the slightest increase in vessel diameter might produce a clinically significant improvement in blood flow even if the angiogram documents some degree of residual stenosis. This same concept should guide the surgical plan during coiling of a broad-based ruptured aneurysm in a poor-grade subarachnoid hemorrhage (SAH) patient. It may be safer and more efficient to coil only the dome of the aneurysm to temporarily protect against rerupture until the patient recovers and can better tolerate a longer and more definitive stent-assisted coiling procedure or surgical procedure. The rapid expansion of endovascular techniques and technology is not an indication for their immediate use. New techniques and devices must be closely scrutinized to ensure that their use adds a clinical benefit.

Physiology and pharmacology

The neurointerventionist should attempt to understand the patient's underlying disease state before beginning treatment. The basic concepts of cerebral physiology are paramount to appropriate preprocedural evaluation and management. The brain constitutes only 2% of body weight but receives almost 15% of cardiac output. This disproportionate amount of blood flow to the brain is necessary to meet the high rate of oxygen metabolism (cerebral metabolic rate of oxygen [$CMRO_2$] = 3.5 mL of oxygen per minute per 100 g of brain tissue) [1]. Cerebral blood flow (CBF) averages 50 mL per 100 g/min, and when CBF falls below 10 mL per 100 g/min, irreversible neuronal cell death occurs [2]. CBF is autoregulated by a dynamic cerebrovascular resistance mechanism that maintains CBF over a systemic perfusion pressure of 50 to 150 mm Hg [3]. Blood pressure (BP), oxygen/carbon dioxide tensions, and temperature affect CBF, and these variables can be manipulated to increase the brain's ischemic tolerance. Every 1–mm Hg change in partial pressure of carbon dioxide (Pco_2), when Pco_2 is between 20 and 80 mm Hg, linearly alters the rate of CBF by 1 mL per 100 g. In the face of ischemia, this mechanism causes vasodilatation, thus augmenting flow to oxygen-deprived brain. Profound hypothermia (<17°C) reduces $CMRO_2$ to 8% of normal and subsequently decreases CBF. These concepts can be used not only to improve ischemic tolerance in the brain but to reduce ICP.

ICP is determined by the presence of brain tissue (84% or 1100 mL), cerebrospinal fluid (CSF, 12% or 150 mL), and blood volume (4% or 50 mL) within the confines of the fixed intracranial vault [4]. ICP is maintained within a normal range when the volume of one component increases so long as a compensatory decrease in the other components occurs. When the compensation mechanisms fail and ICP increases, the brain attempts to maintain adequate cerebral perfusion pressure (CPP = mean arterial pressure [MAP] − ICP) by driving up systemic BP. Although many devices exist to monitor ICP (eg, epidural or subdural transducer lead, intraparenchymal monitor), a ventriculostomy catheter provides reliable ICP readings and treatment of elevated ICP with CSF drainage. Intracranial hypertension can be treated in the neurointerventional suite with CSF drainage, mild hyperventilation, and pharmacologic agents. Reduction of brain interstitial fluid with mannitol (an osmotic diuretic) or Lasix (a loop diuretic) provides rapid but short-term ICP control. Barbiturates are a powerful tool to reduce ICP and prolong cerebral ischemic tolerance by reducing $CMRO_2$ to 50% of normal and decreasing cerebral blood volume by vasoconstriction (Table 2).

Although a nurse anesthetist or anesthesiologist is present in the neurointerventional suite during the induction and initial administration of general anesthesia, the neurointerventionist should have a basic understanding of the cerebral and systemic effects of the anesthetic agents selected. Isoflurane is the preferred inhaled anesthetic for neurosurgical patients because it causes less vasodilatation or CBF increase than halothane and enflurane while reducing $CMRO_2$ to a greater extent. Sevoflurane provides effects similar to those seen with isoflurane and may have additional cerebral protective effects [5,6]. Certain inhaled agents are avoided when elevated ICP is a concern; these include enflurane (seizure risk), desflurane (increases ICP), and nitrous oxide (increases ICP and CBF). Intravenous anesthetics (eg, propofol, barbiturates) reduce $CMRO_2$ with cerebral vasoconstriction but also cause cardiovascular depression. Benzodiazepines (midazolam) and opioids (fentanyl) can be combined to provide adequate conscious sedation by providing rapid-onset anxiolytic effects and reducing sympathetic responses [7]. Nondepolarizing muscle relaxants (eg, vecuronium) are preferred over succinylcholine (increases ICP and causes hyperkalemia) when rapid-sequence induction is not needed (see Table 2).

Table 2
Pharmacologic agents used in the neurointerventional suite

	Class/mechanism	Dosage, time to effect	Relevant side effects
Diuretics (ICP control)			
Mannitol	Plasma expansion, osmotic diuresis	0.25–1.0-mg/kg bolus Onset: 1–5 minutes Peak: 30–60 minutes	Increases serum osmolarity, hypotension
Furosemide	Loop diuretic	10–20-mg bolus Peak effect: minutes	Hypokalemia
Neuroprotectives/sedatives			
Midazolam (Versed)	Benzodiazepine	1–2-mg initial bolus with total up to 0.1–0.15 mg/kg Onset: 15 minutes Peak: 30 minutes	Respiratory arrest (reverse with flumazenil)
Fentanyl	Narcotic	25–100-μg bolus, repeat as needed Peak: 10–20 minutes	Respiratory arrest (reverse with naloxone)
Propofol (Diprivan)	Hypnotic, mild neuroprotection	5–10-μg/kg/min, titrate to maximum of 50 μg/kg/min Onset: 30–60 seconds	Respiratory depression, hypotension
Pentobarbital	Hypnotic, improved neuroprotection	100-mg bolus, maximum dose of 500 mg Onset: minutes	Respiratory depression, hypotension
Paralytics			
Vecuronium	Nondepolarizing neuromuscular blockade	0.1-mg/kg bolus Onset: 3 minutes Duration: 30 minutes	Prolonged effect in renal failure
Succinylcholine	Depolarizing neuromuscular blockade	1-mg/kg bolus Onset: 30–60 seconds	Hyperkalemia with neuronal damage
Anticoagulants/thrombolytic agents			
Heparin	Inactivates/blocks thrombin, preventing clotting cascade	Dosage is weight based, titrate to goal ACT >250 seconds	Does not lyse formed clot, hemorrhage risk, thrombocytopenia, platelet aggregation
t-PA (Activase)	Fibrinolysis	Intra-arterial dosage is variable	Hemorrhage risk
Integrilin	GPIIb-IIIa receptor block, preventing platelet aggregation	180-μg/kg bolus, then weight-based infusion dosage	Hemorrhage risk, thrombocytopenia
Abciximab (ReoPro)	GPIIb-IIIa receptor block, preventing platelet aggregation	Intravenous bolus of 0.25 mg/kg, then infusion of 10 μg/min Intra-arterial dosage varies	Hemorrhage risk, neutropenia
Clopidogrel (Plavix)	Inhibits ADP-induced platelet aggregation	300-mg oral load, then 75 mg daily with aspirin, 325 mg Peak effect: 5 days	Hemorrhage risk
Bivalirudin	Direct thrombin inhibitor	Dose is variable	Hemorrhage risk

Abbreviations: ACT, activated coagulation time; ADP, adenosine diphosphate; GP, glycoprotein; ICP, intracranial pressure; t-PA, tissue plasminogen activator.

Adapted from PDR.net.

The use of neurophysiologic monitoring is equally controversial to the use of general anesthesia on noncomatose patients. In patients undergoing procedures with general anesthesia, this form of continuous real-time evaluation serves as an early warning detection system compelling the endovascular surgeon to address and treat arterial compromise or injury. Early and rapid intervention or technique adjustment can then be instituted and is believed to translate into improved clinical outcomes. Persistent changes in or the disappearance of electroencephalography, brainstem auditory evoked potential, and somatosensory evoked potential recordings often correlate with development of new neurologic deficits after cerebral vascular procedures. As with open cerebral aneurysm surgery, the impetus for simultaneously using these various neurophysiologic techniques during endovascular treatment of aneurysms stems from the correlation that has been demonstrated between electrophysiologic change and alterations in CBF [8–10]. Circumstances encountered during endovascular treatment of cerebral aneurysms (eg, emboli, parent vessel or aneurysm rupture, vasospasm, temporary occlusion with balloon remodeling) can result in cerebral ischemia, which is easily detectable using neurophysiologic monitoring modalities. Neurophysiologic monitoring has proven to be useful in many potentially adverse situations encountered during endovascular coiling of cerebral aneurysms in the anesthetized patient. Benefits include adding a level of confidence regarding the occlusion time that can be tolerated while the aneurysm is treated by use of the balloon-remodeling technique, providing the interventionist with important physiologic information when aneurysm rupture occurs, recognition of distal embolic events not necessarily observed during the coiling procedure itself, and detection of reduced cerebral perfusion secondary to vasospasm in proximal vessels through which the catheter has been passed.

Designing the ideal neurointerventional suite

Given the wide array of neurovascular disorders treated in the neurointerventional suite, the room space must be efficiently allocated to each team member so as to provide an environment for implementing the coordinated treatment plan. When determining the size and layout of the room, it is important to consider storage area requirements for devices and drugs while minimizing unusable floor space as a result of mobile imaging equipment, doors, and monitoring devices. A clear path must be maintained in the room for movement of anesthesia and neuromonitoring equipment and the largest bed used by the facility. Mobile ceiling-mounted monitors allow visualization of the fluoroscopic and angiographic images as well as the patient's physiologic data from either side of the operating table while reducing floor space needs. Additional monitors are necessary in the control room. Focused lighting for the angiographic table and accessory tables should be available, because many of the devices used during neurointerventional procedures are small and difficult to see in low light settings. Electrical outlets and the various gas and suction connections should be unobstructed and available wherever they would be needed, because extension cords and tubing can also represent a hazard. Uninterruptible power supplies with emergency backup circuits and a dedicated telephone line inside the procedure room are necessary. Special ventilation may be necessary, such as when mixing bone cement. With the increasing complexity of endovascular procedures being performed, often using implanted devices, the importance of performing these procedures in a sterile environment is more apparent. Not only is there presumed to be an advantage to the patient when physicians and other staff use gowns, gloves, hats, and masks, but this same equipment, when combined with eye protection, reduces the risk of exposure of the staff to the patient's body fluids. In most cases, new endovascular suites should be designed to be operating room compatible, and the alterations necessary to achieve this state should be considered when renovating an existing suite. Some of the engineering issues that need to be considered include room air flow; lighting; scrub sink placement; restricted-access corridors; wall, ceiling, and floor materials; and the placement of electrical outlets and gas and suction connections.

Imaging equipment

Diagnostic studies, such as cerebral angiograms, can be obtained using single- or biplane angiography. Advantages of biplane angiography include superior visualization of the anatomy and pathologic findings as well as reduced radiation and contrast doses. Therapeutic procedures, such as aneurysm or AVM embolization, can be performed more efficiently and safely with the use of biplane angiography and fluoroscopy, because different views may be appreciated simultaneously. For neurointerventional procedures, simultaneous biplane fluoroscopy and road mapping are useful, as is rotational angiography. On new equipment, three-dimensional angiography should be available. Because of the increasing incidence of obesity, patients weighing more than 150 kg are being treated more frequently; thus, the capacity of the angiographic table should be carefully considered. Angiographic tables that can tilt and rotate are helpful for certain studies, such as for imaging the hand during radial artery access.

Twelve- to 13-in image intensifiers are currently the size most commonly installed in new neurointerventional rooms. Image intensifiers used for angiography usually have three to five modes. When using a larger diameter image intensifier in magnification mode, the radiation dose to the patient increases somewhat; it takes more radiation to generate enough light within the image intensifier for it to function properly. This is one of the disadvantages of using larger than necessary image intensifiers. Another disadvantage associated with larger image intensifiers is that it is often more difficult to position the image intensifier close to the patient; steeply angulated views may not be possible, because the image intensifier will collide with the patient or the table. Biplane flat-panel angiographic equipment will likely be available from the major manufacturers soon. Flat-panel technology is currently more expensive than standard image intensifiers. One advantage of flat-panel technology is its greater latitude or dynamic range. In the future, it is likely that the use of flat-panel technology will be associated with lower radiation doses and increased resolution.

It is important to be able to acquire, process, and review the image data quickly and easily. User-friendly image acquisition and processing hardware and software should be a primary consideration when purchasing new angiographic equipment. Consider how easy it is to magnify images, adjust their brightness and contrast (window/level), add or subtract bone detail, view entire runs or save and recall single images, and add or subtract images from different phases of a run. The operators should be able to calibrate the system accurately and quickly to measure vessels or other structures. Postprocedure image storage, recall, and manipulation should also be easy and fast.

The neurointerventional suite, whether new or a renovation of an existing room, is a major investment. This room will likely be used for many years before being updated or replaced. Therefore, it is important that the construction of this room be carefully planned and executed. Not only should the room be designed to accommodate the procedures performed today, but the designers should attempt to determine how else the room might be used during its lifetime.

Function of the neurovascular team during routine and emergent cases

The endovascular management of the following disorders is discussed in greater detail elsewhere in this issue. The discussion below provides a summary of the role that each team member plays before, during, and after the procedure, with emphasis on the neurointerventionist as the captain of the ship responsible for all actions in the neurointerventional suite.

Thrombo-occlusive disease/stroke intervention

For elective stenting and angioplasty procedures to treat carotid, vertebrobasilar, or intracranial lesions, a thorough evaluation of coexistent peripheral vascular and coronary disease should be obtained. General anesthesia and neuromonitoring provide a safe environment for the procedure, although some interventionists prefer the patient be awake, allowing for real-time neurologic assessment and eliminating the risk of general anesthesia. Given the narrow time window for intra-arterial thrombolysis and clot disruption to produce a favorable outcome, the efforts of each team member must be coordinated during an emergent stroke intervention. The patient is placed under general anesthesia with neuromonitoring, when available, without delay. The designated team member gains arterial access while the nursing team and technician prepare the catheters, thrombolytics, or antiplatelets for microcatheter infusion. The anesthesia team and critical care nurse should work on volume expansion and increasing the MAP to improve collateral flow. Patients may be pretreated with an antiplatelet agent and often receive heparin for anticoagulation during the procedure (see Table 2). Given the risk of hemorrhagic complications with these agents, when possible, all anticipated invasive procedures, such as central line placement and Foley catheterization, should be performed before heparinization. For carotid stenting, premedication with atropine reduces the bradycardic response associated with balloon dilatation of the carotid bulb [11]. Intravenous fluid and vasopressors, such as dopamine or phenylephrine, must be readily available to treat hypotension and thus reduce the risk of myocardial and cerebral ischemia.

Aneurysm

Patients with intracranial aneurysms present to the neurointerventional suite with elective unruptured aneurysms or SAH after aneurysmal rupture requiring emergent treatment. Special considerations present in the latter group include medical comorbidities, such as aspiration pneumonia or myocardial damage, risk of rerupture and vasospasm, and hydrocephalus requiring ventriculostomy. Ventriculostomy should be performed before the interventional procedure not only to allow ICP monitoring and therapy during the case but to avoid placing the catheter after anticoagulants or antiplatelet agents have been administered. General anesthesia is preferred, allowing for BP manipulation (hypotension before aneurysm embolization versus hypertension with thrombo-occlusive complications), better image quality with a motionless patient, ICP management (sedation), and rapid response to intraprocedural complications (eg, barbiturates, ventriculostomy, craniotomy with intraoperative rupture). Neurophysiologic monitoring has proven useful in identifying intraprocedural thromboembolic events and aneurysmal rupture before it is recognized on an angiographic study and is preferred when readily available. The neurointerventionist should be able to view the BP, pulse oximetry, and ICP values while viewing the imaging screens. The anesthesiologist should be ready to deliver protamine, decrease MAP, and administer barbiturates for cerebral protection in case of intraprocedural vessel rupture. The technicians should understand the treatment plan before beginning the procedure so that they may have all needed catheters, coils, stents, or other devices out and ready for immediate use. These individuals must also maintain a log of all devices used during the procedure. The nurses should prepare all necessary drugs, including sedatives, ICP control agents, anticoagulants, antiplatelet agents, and reversal agents (see Table 2). They must ensure that the crash cart is supplied with resuscitation drugs and supplies for emergent surgical airway control or ventriculostomy while monitoring vital signs and access line patency to maintain irrigation and prevent air embolism. After the procedure, patients often receive heparin or antiplatelet agents when high suspicion for a thromboembolic event exists. The BP cap is liberalized slightly over 24 hours before allowing it to increase as part of hypervolemic, hypertensive, and hemodilution therapy for vasospasm.

Vascular malformations (arteriovenous malformations)

In the neurointerventional suite, patients with cerebral AVMs can be classified into those with ICH as the result of rupture versus those who present electively for staged embolization before definitive surgical/radiosurgical treatment or definitive endovascular AVM obliteration. Issues regarding ICP control and use of anticoagulants in patients with ICH caused by AVM rupture are similar to those in patients with aneurysmal SAH as discussed in the previous section. General anesthesia provides a theoretic benefit for most AVM embolization procedures by minimizing patient movement during microcatheterization of multiple pedicles, allowing for tight MAP control and providing cerebral protection in the face of a complication [12]. The physician or technician must prepare embolic agents in a timely fashion so that they have been mixed to the proper consistency when the interventionist is ready to inject them. The anesthesia team is responsible for lowering the MAP to allow for better AVM nidus penetration during embolization. After the procedure, the BP must be kept strictly under control to avoid normal perfusion pressure breakthrough and subsequent hemorrhage.

Cerebral vasospasm

Patients who have failed maximal medical therapy for vasospasm arrive in the neurointerventional suite in a hypertensive state because they have been treated with vasopressors and in a state of hypervolemia because of increased intravenous fluid loads. These patients are often intubated and are receiving some form of cerebral protection with high-dose sedatives or barbiturates. The anesthesia team must maintain the hypertensive and hypervolemic state during the angioplasty procedure. The interventionist and technician prepare the balloon microcatheter

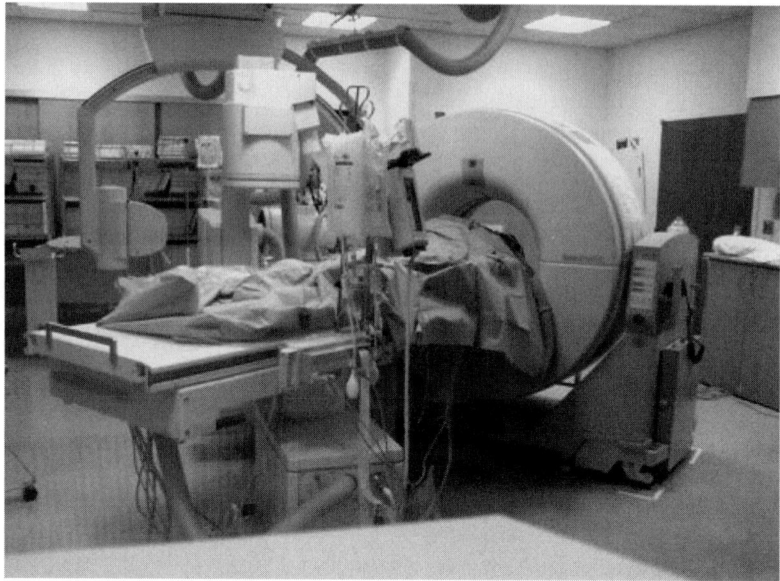

Fig. 1. Use of portable CT scanner in the neurointerventional suite.

while the nurse prepares adequate infusion volumes of intra-arterial papaverine, calcium channel antagonists, or other vasodilators [13,14].

Future directions

With the growth of endovascular technologies and techniques, a larger patient population with a greater diversity of neurovascular disorders may be treated in the neurointerventional suite. The challenge is to train an adequate number of neurointerventionists with a fundamental understanding of the neurovascular patient and the disease process. This should allow the field to grow beyond urban academic medical centers to community and rural medical centers, where time-dependent therapies like stroke intervention may become more successful. In the future, the use of mobile angiography units with telemedicine capabilities may allow the performance of neurointerventional procedures outside the classic neurointerventional suite. Portable CT and MRI scanners may allow for the performance of non-invasive cerebral physiologic studies (eg, Xenon CT blood flow, CT perfusion, MRI diffusion and perfusion) within the neurointerventional suite (Fig. 1). As the number of tools available to the interventionist expands, one must remember the captain of the ship principle. The interventionist must understand how each tool applies to its intended disease and should adequately prepare the neurointerventional team and supervise the coordinated execution of each member's tasks, always being prepared to mobilize emergency plans in the case of a complication.

References

[1] Smith AL, Wollman H. Cerebral blood flow and metabolism: effects of anesthetic drugs and techniques. Anesthesiology 1972;36:378–400.

[2] Siesjo BK. Cerebral circulation and metabolism. J Neurosurg 1984;60:883–908.

[3] Strandgaard S, Olesen J, Skinhoj E, Lassen NA. Autoregulation of brain circulation in severe arterial hypertension. BMJ 1973;1:507–10.

[4] Vishteh A, Raudzens P, Spetzler R, et al. Anesthesia in cerebrovascular disease. In: Winn H, editor. Youman's neurological surgery. 5th edition. Philadelphia: WB Saunders; 2004. p. 1503–15.

[5] Scheller MS, Tateishi A, Drummond JC, Zornow MH. The effects of sevoflurane on cerebral blood flow, cerebral metabolic rate for oxygen, intracranial pressure, and the electroencephalogram are similar to those of isoflurane in the rabbit. Anesthesiology 1988;68:548–51.

[6] Werner C, Kochs E, Hoffman W, et al. The effects of sevoflurane on neurological outcome from incomplete ischemia in rats. J Neurosurg Anesthesiol 1991;3:237.

[7] Martin ML, Lennox PH. Sedation and analgesia in the interventional radiology department. J Vasc Interv Radiol 2003;14:1119–28.

[8] Branston NM, Symon L, Crockard HA, Pasztor E. Relationship between the cortical evoked potential and local cortical blood flow following acute middle cerebral artery occlusion in the baboon. Exp Neurol 1974;45:195–208.
[9] Lesnick JE, Michele JJ, Simeone FA, DeFeo S, Welsh FA. Alteration of somatosensory evoked potentials in response to global ischemia. J Neurosurg 1984;60:490–4.
[10] Lopez JR, Chang SD, Steinberg GK. The use of electrophysiological monitoring in the intraoperative management of intracranial aneurysms. J Neurol Neurosurg Psychiatry 1999;66:189–96.
[11] Kharrazi M. Anesthesia for carotid stent procedures. J Endovasc Surg 1996;3:211–6.
[12] Armonda RA, Thomas JE, Rosenwasser RH. The interventional neuroradiology suite as an operating room. Neurosurg Clin N Am 2000;11:1–20.
[13] Badjatia N, Topcuoglu MA, Pryor JC, et al. Preliminary experience with intra-arterial nicardipine as a treatment for cerebral vasospasm. AJNR Am J Neuroradiol 2004;25:819–26.
[14] Feng L, Fitzsimmons BF, Young WL, et al. Intraarterially administered verapamil as adjunct therapy for cerebral vasospasm: safety and 2-year experience. AJNR Am J Neuroradiol 2002;23:1284–90.

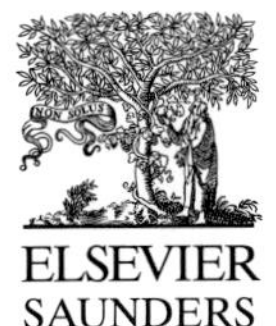
ELSEVIER
SAUNDERS

Neurosurg Clin N Am 16 (2005) 241–248

NEUROSURGERY
CLINICS
OF NORTH AMERICA

Indications for Catheter-Based Angiography of the Cerebrovasculature

Brian Jankowitz, MD[a], Elad I. Levy, MD[b,*], L. Nelson Hopkins, MD, FACS[b], Lee R. Guterman, PhD, MD[b]

[a]*Department of Neurological Surgery, University of Pittsburgh Medical Center, 200 Lothrop Street, Suite B-400, Pittsburgh, PA 15213, USA*

[b]*Department of Neurosurgery and Toshiba Stroke Research Center, School of Medicine and Biomedical Sciences, State University of New York at Buffalo, 3 Gates Circle, Buffalo, NY 14209, USA*

Cerebral angiography has long remained the "gold standard" for the evaluation and diagnosis of cerebrovascular pathologic changes. Advances in interventional techniques and noninvasive imaging modalities have resulted in a transformation of the indications for catheter-based angiography. Most angiographic procedures are now performed with an intention to treat the underlying pathologic findings. Furthermore, imaging modalities like CT angiography (CTA) and magnetic resonance angiography (MRA) have supplanted catheter-based interventions for diagnosis because of their near-equivalent sensitivity and specificity as well as the associated reduced use of resources in terms of staffing, equipment, and cost. In this article, we review the current indications for catheter-based cerebral angiography for radiographic diagnosis, intraoperative decision making, initiation of endovascular therapy, and postprocedural monitoring.

Haschek and Lindenthal [1] and Moniz pioneered the development of cerebral angiography [2–4]. Luessenhop and Velasquez [5] subsequently validated the technique by exploring intracranial vessels with balloon-tipped catheters. Today, the process involves percutaneous entry into the femoral, radial, or brachial artery by use of a modified Seldinger technique [6]. The procedure is often performed on an elective basis; in light of competition from noninvasive studies, much scrutiny has been given to complication rates, efficacy, and cost.

Using the results of a cooperative study of the American Society of Interventional and Therapeutic Neuroradiology, American Society of Neuroradiology, and Society of Interventional Radiology, Citron et al [7] reported a neuroangiography success rate of 98%, as defined by an evaluation that adequately established or excluded pathologic findings of the extracranial or intracranial circulation, with a complication rate of 2.5% for reversible neurologic deficit and 1% for permanent neurologic deficit. Several studies have assessed the risk of thromboembolic events associated with diagnostic cerebral angiography in patients with cerebrovascular disease, subarachnoid hemorrhage (SAH), cerebral aneurysm, and arteriovenous malformation (AVM) [8–12]. The overall risk of thromboembolism-related complications occurring during or within 24 hours of the angiogram ranged from 1.0% to 2.6%. Permanent neurologic deficits occurred in 0.1% to 0.7% of cases. Complication rates in nonacademic settings are reported to be as low as 0.5% for stroke and 0.4% for transient ischemic attack [13]. Factors predisposing patients to increased risk of angiography-related complications include advanced age, severe atherosclerosis, symptomatic cerebrovascular disease, acute SAH, and vascular dysplasia [7]. Other factors that increase this risk include procedure length, number of catheter exchanges, catheter size, catheter manipulation, and amount of contrast media.

* Corresponding author.
E-mail address: elevy@buffns.com (E.I. Levy).

1042-3680/05/$ - see front matter
doi:10.1016/j.nec.2004.08.002

Expense assumes greater importance with the advent of rising medical costs and limited reimbursement. Clinical studies increasingly take into account the cost of cerebrovascular imaging modalities. U-King-Im et al [14] evaluated MRA versus digital subtraction angiography (DSA) for carotid imaging, showing approximately a 2.4-fold increase in cost for DSA. Findings such as these prompt physicians to pay greater attention to preprocedural suspicion of the underlying pathologic changes as they evaluate cost-effectiveness and risk-benefit.

There are no absolute contraindications to catheter-based angiography. Relative contraindications include iodinated contrast media allergy, hypotension, severe hypertension, coagulopathy, renal insufficiency, and congestive heart failure. The possibility of contrast-induced nephropathy in patients with renal insufficiency remains the most common cause of avoiding angiography. A recent meta-analysis of seven randomized controlled trials reaffirms that hydration and *N*-acetylcysteine remain the treatment of choice to prevent contrast nephropathy in such patients, with an overall 56% reduction in the relative risk of developing nephropathy [15].

Atherosclerotic disease

Catheter-based angiography in cerebrovascular atherosclerotic disease may define occlusive morphology when CT or MRI techniques are of poor quality, equivocal, contraindicated, or inadequate. Angiography can better depict tandem lesions. The hemodynamic significance of a lesion can be determined by evidence of more than 50% reduction in luminal diameter, less than 2 mm of residual lumen, external carotid artery opacification preceding internal carotid artery (ICA) opacification, delayed ocular choroidal blush, or early opacification of the contralateral vasculature after ipsilateral dye injection [16]. Angiography is diagnostic and a means of immediate therapy. Current therapies include intra-arterial administration of thrombolytic agents, mechanical thrombolysis or thrombectomy, angioplasty, and stent placement.

Extracranial carotid stenosis has provided fertile ground for the comparison of imaging modalities. CTA, MRA, and ultrasonography (US) allow excellent visualization of the extracranial vasculature; however, many surgeons are reticent to perform surgery based on the findings of a single noninvasive study. MRA technology is notorious for overestimation of the severity of stenosis. In a study involving 91 patients with 70% to 99% stenosis by MRA evaluation, 19 patients had 50% to 69% stenosis and 5 patients had less than 50% stenosis by DSA [17]. Another study has shown a sensitivity and specificity of 95% and 90%, respectively, for identification of carotid stenosis greater than or equal to 70% with MRA as compared with DSA [18]. CTA has a reported 89% agreement with catheter-based angiography [19]. The collaborators of the North American Symptomatic Carotid Endarterectomy Trial concluded that transcranial Doppler (TCD) US was 59.3% sensitive and 80.4% specific for stenosis exceeding 70% [20]. More recently, sensitivities ranging from 81% to 93% in the anterior circulation, with a negative predictive value of 94%, have been reported [21].

DSA remains the method of choice for delineating occlusion versus trickle flow in near-occluded lesions of the ICA, although Chen et al [22] found a 100% correlation between DSA and CTA in differentiating total versus near occlusion in 57 patients. In light of a push toward noninvasive neuroimaging modalities for presurgical evaluation, a review panel sought to determine the most appropriate imaging studies to guide endarterectomy in 203 clinical settings of carotid artery disease [23]. As a result of their review, the panel recommended (1) conventional angiography or two concordant noninvasive studies (US, CTA, or MRA) in the setting of moderate symptomatic disease, (2) US plus another modality or MRA and CTA alone in the setting of severe asymptomatic disease, and (3) one noninvasive imaging study in the setting of severe symptomatic disease. When assessing patients, physicians must keep in mind that previous studies have reported a 6% to 7.9% misclassification of ICA stenosis, even when two noninvasive imaging strategies are combined [24,25]. The Warfarin-Aspirin Symptomatic Intracranial Disease (WASID) trial, which was recently funded by the National Institutes of Health, requires performance of angiography along with TCD US and MRA [26–28]. This trial provides an opportunity for critical evaluation of these noninvasive tests. The Stroke Outcomes and Neuroimaging of Intracranial Atherosclerosis trial is being conducted in collaboration with the WASID trial to define the TCD US and MRA parameters that determine severe (50%–99%) intracranial stenosis of large proximal arteries on catheter angiography [27].

DSA may help to guide intraoperative decision making. Aleksic et al [29] sought to determine whether DSA findings could predict the need for the placement of a shunt during carotid endarterectomy. A cross-flow toward the contralateral hemisphere noted during preoperative angiography had a sensitivity of 91% in obviating the need for intraoperative shunt placement during carotid surgery performed under local anesthesia. Further studies may delineate a positive predictive value for the necessity of a shunt.

Although new studies are ongoing to generate support for use of noninvasive imaging, DSA remains the modality of choice in the event of discordant noninvasive studies or when assessing patients for whom CEA would pose significant risk. A three-vessel angiogram remains the most effective method of determining the adequacy of collateral circulation.

Intracranial aneurysm

Cerebral aneurysms represent a focal dilation of an artery. The management and elimination of these lesions have gained much notoriety with the advent of approaches for endovascular repair. Spontaneous SAH demands immediate diagnostic angiography. DSA can provide a means to obtain the diagnosis and administer therapy. Questions remain with respect to the most appropriate initial study as well as the need for angiography after therapy or in the event of a nondiagnostic study, however. Another concerning topic involves the resolution of MRA and CTA in detecting aneurysms less than 5 mm in diameter. Rebleeding does not correlate with aneurysm size. Clinicians have to take this into account, because these smaller ruptured aneurysms may escape detection. Piotin et al [30] studied the volumetric assessment of intracranial aneurysms. Rotational DSA was more accurate than MRA or CTA, prompting these authors to recommend DSA for the evaluation of cerebral aneurysms.

The accuracy of MRA for detecting aneurysms larger than 3 mm approaches 90%; however, this falls to less than 40% for aneurysms smaller than 3 mm [16]. An early assessment of MRA for the screening of unruptured intracranial aneurysms in 200 patients revealed a 99.5% correlation between DSA and MRA; detection of a single 3-mm posterior communicating artery aneurysm was missed by MRA [31]. More recently, Watanabe et al [32] studied the ability of three-dimensional (3D) MRA to plan a surgical approach in 106 patients with SAH secondary to an intracranial aneurysm. Forty-six percent of patients had surgery on the basis of the MRA findings alone. The remaining patients required further imaging, consisting of CTA or DSA. Functional limitations of MRA included poor image quality (because of motion artifact), slow flow in the aneurysm, thrombosis, or subacute clot. Anatomy limited the proper surgical evaluation primarily in the following locations: basilar artery, ICA, or high-position anterior communicating artery. Blood flow is represented on MRA; therefore, turbulent flow may cause poor visualization, such as in the tortuous carotid siphon. Low perfusion, sluggish flow, or thrombus may obscure imaging, such as in giant aneurysms.

CTA has an accuracy of 90% when compared with DSA for depiction of aneurysms [33]. The advantage of CTA lies in its mechanism of distinguishing contrast flow from blood flow. CTA is even more sensitive than DSA in delineating the presence of contrast media, and it can differentiate the thrombus within a vessel. Although this makes CTA a useful adjunct for detecting the sluggish flow within giant aneurysms, bony artifact and acute blood can obscure the pathologic changes; thus, aneurysms in the cavernous sinus may be missed. In a recent report by Hoh et al [34], CTA was used as the sole imaging study for the prospective evaluation of 223 patients with intracranial aneurysms. Of these patients, 18% underwent a further pretreatment evaluation with DSA. All aneurysms responsible for the patients' presenting symptoms and 97% of multiple aneurysms were detected by CTA. Reasons for obtaining DSA after an initial evaluation with CTA included the necessity to clarify the relation of the aneurysm to the parent vessel or perforating branches or to assess further the morphology of the aneurysm and the anatomy of the aneurysm neck.

Yasui et al [35] conducted a study to delineate further the limitations of CTA as compared with DSA. CTA displayed a particular weakness in the evaluation of the posterior circulation. Perforators of the posterior cerebral artery, a small posterior communicating artery, and infundibular dilation of the posterior communicating artery could not be detected.

Infectious or mycotic aneurysms represent a subset of disease particularly suited to DSA evaluation. In a retrospective review, Venkatesh and colleagues [36] related a 90% incidence in the distal vasculature. All aneurysms were less than 10 mm, and most were 3 to 5 mm. Chun et al [37] recommend endovascular therapy in stable patients with ruptured infectious aneurysms, further supporting DSA as the imaging modality of choice.

Angiographically negative SAH remains another disease subset that is particularly suited to evaluation with DSA. Topcuoglu et al [38] conducted a retrospective review of patients with SAH without evident cause, concluding that noninvasive imaging with MRA and CTA provides little diagnostic value. Of those presenting with nonperimesencephalic SAH, only DSA elucidated a cause on follow-up evaluation.

Aneurysms are evaluated after coil embolization to assess for patency or residual neck and flow. Standard follow-up imaging often includes repeat DSA at 3, 12, and 36 months after the last embolization. Nome and colleagues [39] compared MRA and DSA in the follow-up evaluation of 51 patients treated with Guglielmi detachable coils (GDCs; Boston Scientific Target, Fremont, California). The sensitivity of MRA for detecting residual flow within the aneurysm was 97%. The patency status of parent artery and branch vessel flow was correctly identified in all but a single patient. The limitations of MRA included signal loss in the vicinity of the coil mass, reduced flow signal in adjacent vessels, and misinterpretation of high signal intensity from thrombus as circulating blood. Considering these deficiencies, DSA is recommended as the initial follow-up study, with a transition to MRA or CTA when these issues have been ruled out.

Cerebral vasculitis

The diagnosis of cerebral vasculitis represents a challenge to all clinicians. Inflammatory changes in the vessel result in narrowing and obliteration of the vascular lumen that can progress to thrombotic occlusion, necrosis, and rupture. Pathologic features of vasculitis include spasm, edema, cellular infiltration, and proliferation. Diagnosis is often beyond the resolution of conventional radiography, with the reported sensitivity of DSA being 24% to 33% [40,41]. Cloft et al [42] found a relatively poor correlation between MRA and DSA in the evaluation of patients with primary angiitis of the central nervous system, with MRA showing no pathologic features in 34% of abnormal territories. Although DSA is limited, it remains the standard of radiographic diagnosis.

Arteriovenous malformations and arteriovenous fistulas

AVMs are congenital anomalies of blood vessels that usually cause symptoms in the third or fourth decade of life. These lesions consist of dilated feeding arteries and a core or nidus of tangled vascular loops and terminate in draining veins. CT and MRI are excellent diagnostic adjuncts, although DSA is still considered the gold standard. Mori et al [43] reported rates of sensitivity and specificity of 87% and 100%, respectively, for MRA in diagnosing hemodynamic features of AVMs. Farb et al [44] found MRA to be equivalent to DSA for depiction of AVM components in 70% to 90% of cases. Aside from diagnosis, DSA may be useful in predicting hemorrhage. Using time-density curves obtained by DSA to elucidate hemodynamic risk factors for AVM hemorrhage, Todaka et al [45] showed a significant difference in the mean number of draining veins, the median transit time of the feeding artery, and the ratio of the mean transit time of the draining to the feeding vessels. DSA is also necessary for radiosurgical assessment. St. George et al [46] found that MRI localization of the AVM nidus before treatment was not predictable and that discrepancies with DSA findings were occasionally significant, thus precluding safe radiosurgical planning that relies on MRI as the sole imaging modality [46]. Concerning evaluation after treatment, empiric evidence supports initial DSA for immediate and initial postprocedure follow-up and MRA for long-term evaluation.

Arteriovenous fistulas represent an abnormal communication between high-pressure (arterial structures) and low-pressure (venous structures) systems. The vessels collateralize into a prominent network and are usually dural based. Although DSA remains the study of choice, with recent advances in endovascular treatment supporting this opinion, the diagnostic use of noninvasive imaging must be evaluated. Noguchi et al [47] attempted to define the diagnostic criteria on MRA by evaluating patients with angiographically proven moderate- to high-flow intracranial dural arteriovenous fistulas. Two blinded neuroradiologists evaluated the images. Sensitivity and specificity for the identification of multiple high-intensity structures adjacent to the sinus wall, high-intensity areas in the venous sinus, and early filling of the venous sinus were 100% and 100%, 76% and 86%, and 87% and 100%, respectively.

Intraoperative utility

As neurosurgeons gained familiarity with and appreciated the usefulness of DSA, a natural progression moved toward the application of this imaging modality for intraoperative evaluation. Early use of intraoperative angiography focused on the evaluation of surgically treated aneurysms. Studies show that angiography prompted a change in surgical treatment 7% to 14% of the time, resulting in a complication rate of 0% to 0.5% [48–50]. Tang et al [49] found that residual aneurysm and vessel compromise were the most common cause for a change in surgical strategy. In multivariate logistic regression analysis, location in the proximal ICA and size were the factors relating to the increased revision rates. Surgical procedures for the clipping of aneurysms in the superior hypophyseal artery and clinoidal region were fraught with the highest revision rates. Surgery for giant (>24 mm) and large (15–24 mm) aneurysms was revised in 29% and 22% of cases, respectively. Moreover, in a prospective assessment of intraoperative angiography during aneurysm surgery, Klopfenstein et al [48] found that experienced cerebrovascular surgeons could not predict the need for angiography. The group of patients labeled "intraoperative angiography unnecessary" before surgery had a surgical alteration rate equal to that for the "intraoperative angiography necessary" group. The most common causes for surgical revision in the group for whom intraoperative angiography was considered necessary were residual aneurysms and parent vessel occlusion, in addition to previously undiagnosed aneurysms. These findings prompted Klopfenstein et al [48] to recommend consideration of intraoperative angiography for most aneurysm cases.

Catheter-based angiography has been used to assess graft patency during extracranial-intracranial bypass procedures and has displayed branch occlusion in 7% to 16% of cases [50,51]. Using this approach to monitor graft patency, Yanaka et al [50] were able to open the occluded graft in all cases, resulting in a graft patency rate of 100% after surgery.

Concerning vascular malformations, a 10% to 36% incidence of residual AVM after surgery is reported in the literature [52–54]. Intraoperative adjuncts to improve resection rates would be of great benefit in reducing future hemorrhagic incidence or repeat surgery. When using intraoperative DSA during AVM resection, Lui et al [55] discovered abnormalities in 20% of patients. In one patient, angiographic imaging displayed residual AVM in the temporal lobe near a cortical draining vein and allowed for safe completion of the resection. In another patient, angiography documented abnormal displacement of the left posterior cerebral artery. A follow-up CT scan indicated an epidural hematoma effacing the left parietal area that required urgent surgical evacuation. In this case, the angiogram had provided a warning of an acute hemorrhagic event. For smaller AVMs, intraoperative DSA may be necessary simply to locate the nidus. These instances support the use of intraoperative angiography as a means to avoid further anesthesia or repeat craniotomy. Further study must decipher which procedures would best benefit from this adjunct.

Newer methods of arterial access are being developed to facilitate intraoperative angiography. Recently, Lee and Macdonald [51] described their experience with access via the superficial temporal artery. Fourteen percent of patients had unexpected findings, including arterial occlusion and residual aneurysm.

Assessing brain death

Those whose medical specialty involves the central nervous system are often called on to perform brain death examinations. Often, a bedside examination involving a detailed assessment of brain stem function, the interpretation of which is corroborated by at least two clinicians, suffices for the diagnosis of brain death. Confounding factors that may alter an examination include severe electrolyte, acid-base, or endocrine disturbances; the presence of severe hypothermia (defined as a core temperature of ≤32°C); hypotension; and the absence of evidence of drug intoxication, poisoning, or neuromuscular blocking agents. In some European, South American, or Asian countries, routine confirmatory testing is required for the diagnosis of brain death. In the United States, such confirmation is optional in adults but recommended in children less than 1 year old [56]. Infants may not have fully developed cranial nerves, the findings of the examination may be difficult to interpret accurately, and the pediatric population has a tendency to become hypothermic when ill. On a neurosurgical service, a barbiturate-induced coma most often obviates an expedient diagnosis of brain death. When time becomes a factor (if organ donation is contemplated or examination findings are spurious), DSA can quickly provide a radiographic diagnosis of brain death. One should note absence of flow at the foramen magnum in the posterior circulation and at the petrosal portion of the carotid artery in the anterior circulation [57]. DSA may soon be supplanted by CTA in declaring brain death. Qureshi et al [58] reported CTA documentation of the absence of cerebral blood flow in patients receiving intravenous pentobarbital for burst suppression, thus allowing organ harvest or timely withdrawal of care. Further studies are necessary to evaluate the sensitivity and specificity of CTA versus DSA in brain death assessment.

Trauma

Blunt carotid injury is an uncommon but potentially devastating injury, with an incidence approaching 1% for all cases of blunt trauma injury [59]. Delayed symptoms complicate early diagnosis; thus, efforts have been made to devise a screening algorithm. Diagnostic studies are indicated in the face of hemorrhage of presumed carotid origin, cervical bruits, history of external cervical trauma with altered mental status, suspicious mechanism of injury, or lateralizing neurologic deficits unexplained by parenchymal damage [60]. Subtle vessel dissections and skull base anatomy present limitations for duplex scanning [61]. Regardless of its efficacy, MRA is often a logistic impossibility with trauma patients. Although CTA is becoming the favored diagnostic study, DSA remains the study of choice for the radiographic diagnosis of blunt carotid injury. When a liberalized screening method based on neurologic examination and mechanism of injury was used by Kerwin et al [62], 21 (44%) of 48 patients exhibited abnormal angiographic findings. Fracture through the foramen transversarium, unexplained hemiparesis, basilar skull fracture, unexplained neurologic examination results, and anisocoria revealed angiographic abnormalities in 60%, 44%, 42%, 38%, and 33% of patients, respectively, justifying the use of DSA in this patient population.

To evaluate noninvasive imaging in establishing a diagnosis of blunt cerebrovascular injury, Biffl et al [63] evaluated 62 trauma patients with a suspicious injury or examination by CTA or MRA. DSA was then used for comparison. Among patients with normal CTA results, 30% were found to have occult vascular injury by DSA, providing a sensitivity and specificity of 68% and 67%, respectively. Anatomic limitations secondary to bony artifact include the ICA in its petrous and cavernous segments and the vertebral artery within the vertebral foramina. Of those patients with normal MRA findings, 11% had a false-negative study, with a sensitivity and specificity of 75% and 67%, respectively. Aside from the logistic concerns, pseudoaneurysms presented difficulties for MRA assessment because of their turbulent flow. The findings led the authors to conclude that noninvasive imaging is not ready to replace DSA for the evaluation of trauma patients with suspected blunt cerebrovascular injury.

Summary

Catheter-based cerebral angiography remains an important method of garnering information about the cerebrovasculature. Although noninvasive imaging continues to supplant this gold standard, evidence-based medicine regarding the equivalence of these imaging modalities to DSA is lacking and studies need to be completed. When clinicians rely on a study to make surgical decisions, they must concede to the existing evidence when choosing the optimal method of diagnostic evaluation.

References

[1] Haschek E, Lindenthal OT. Ein Beitrag zur praktischen verwerthung der photographie nach rontgen. Wien Klin Wochenschr 1896;9:63–4.

[2] Antunes JL. Egas Moniz and cerebral angiography. J Neurosurg 1974;40:427–32.

[3] Moniz E. L'encephalographic artérielle, son importance dans la localisation des tumeurs cérébrales. Rev Neurol (Paris) 1927;2:72–90.

[4] Wolpert SM. Neuroradiology classics. AJNR Am J Neuroradiol 1999;20:1752–3.

[5] Luessenhop AJ, Velasquez AC. Observations on the tolerance of the intracranial arteries to catheterization. J Neurosurg 1964;21:85–91.

[6] Seldinger SI. Catheter replacement of the needle in percutaneous arteriography; a new technique. Acta Radiol 1953;39:368–76.

[7] Citron SJ, Wallace RC, Lewis CA, et al. Quality improvement guidelines for adult diagnostic neuroangiography: cooperative study between ASITN, ASNR, and SIR. J Vasc Interv Radiol 2003;14 (Suppl):S257–62.

[8] Cloft HJ, Joseph GJ, Dion JE. Risk of cerebral angiography in patients with subarachnoid hemorrhage, cerebral aneurysm, and arteriovenous malformation: a meta-analysis. Stroke 1999;30:317–20.

[9] Dion JE, Gates PC, Fox AJ, Barnett HJ, Blom RJ. Clinical events following neuroangiography: a prospective study. Stroke 1987;18:997–1004.

[10] Earnest FT, Forbes G, Sandok BA, et al. Complications of cerebral angiography: prospective assessment of risk. AJR Am J Roentgenol 1984;142: 247–53.

[11] Heiserman JE, Dean BL, Hodak JA, et al. Neurologic complications of cerebral angiography. AJNR Am J Neuroradiol 1994;15:1401–11.

[12] Theodotou BC, Whaley R, Mahaley MS. Complications following transfemoral cerebral angiography for cerebral ischemia. Report of 159 angiograms and correlation with surgical risk. Surg Neurol 1987;28:90–2.

[13] Johnston DC, Chapman KM, Goldstein LB. Low rate of complications of cerebral angiography in routine clinical practice. Neurology 2001;57:2012–4.

[14] U-King-Im JM, Hollingworth W, Trivedi RA, et al. Contrast-enhanced MR angiography vs. intra-arterial digital subtraction angiography for carotid imaging: activity-based cost analysis. Eur Radiol 2004;14:730–5.

[15] Birck R, Krzossok S, Markowetz F, Schnulle P, van der Woude FJ, Braun C. Acetylcysteine for prevention of contrast nephropathy: meta-analysis. Lancet 2003;362:598–603.

[16] Grossman R, Yousem D. Neuroradiology. 2nd edition. New York: Mosby; 2003.

[17] U-King-Im JM, Trivedi RA, Graves MJ, et al. Contrast-enhanced MR angiography for carotid disease: diagnostic and potential clinical impact. Neurology 2004;62:1282–90.

[18] Butz B, Dorenbeck U, Borisch I, et al. High-resolution contrast-enhanced magnetic resonance angiography of the carotid arteries using fluoroscopic monitoring of contrast arrival: diagnostic accuracy and interobserver variability. Acta Radiol 2004;45: 164–70.

[19] Verhoek G, Costello P, Khoo EW, Wu R, Kat E, Fitridge RA. Carotid bifurcation CT angiography: assessment of interactive volume rendering. J Comput Assist Tomogr 1999;23:590–6.

[20] North American Symptomatic Carotid Endarterectomy Trial Collaborators. Beneficial effect of carotid endarterectomy in symptomatic patients with high-grade carotid stenosis. N Engl J Med 1991;325: 445–53.

[21] Demchuk AM, Christou I, Wein TH, et al. Accuracy and criteria for localizing arterial occlusion with transcranial Doppler. J Neuroimaging 2000;10: 1–12.

[22] Chen CJ, Lee TH, Hsu HL, et al. Multi-slice CT angiography in diagnosing total versus near occlusions of the internal carotid artery: comparison with catheter angiography. Stroke 2004;35:83–5.

[23] Kennedy J, Quan H, Ghali WA, Feasby TE. Importance of the imaging modality in decision making about carotid endarterectomy. Neurology 2004;62: 901–4.

[24] Johnston DC, Goldstein LB. Clinical carotid endarterectomy decision making: noninvasive vascular imaging versus angiography. Neurology 2001;56: 1009–15.

[25] Patel SG, Collie DA, Wardlaw JM, et al. Outcome, observer reliability, and patient preferences if CTA, MRA, or Doppler ultrasound were used, individually or together, instead of digital subtraction angiography before carotid endarterectomy. J Neurol Neurosurg Psychiatry 2002;73:21–8.

[26] Chimowitz MI, Kokkinos J, Strong J, et al. Design. Progress and challenges of a double-blind trial of warfarin versus aspirin for symptomatic intracranial arterial stenosis. Neuroepidemiology 2003;22:106–17.

[27] Stroke outcome and neuroimaging of intracranial atherosclerosis (SONIA): design of a prospective, multicenter trial of diagnostic tests. Neuroepidemiology 2004;23:23–32.

[28] Hart RG. Why is WASID an important clinical trial? Neuroepidemiology 2003;22:101–2.

[29] Aleksic M, Gawenda M, Heckenkamp J, Matoussevitch V, Coburger S, Brunkwall J. Prediction of cerebral ischemic tolerance during carotid cross-clamping by angiographic criteria. Eur J Vasc Endovasc Surg 2004;27:640–5.

[30] Piotin M, Gailloud P, Bidaut L, et al. CT angiography, MR angiography and rotational digital subtraction angiography for volumetric assessment of intracranial aneurysms. An experimental study. Neuroradiology 2003;45:404–9.

[31] Nakagawa T, Hashi K, Tanabe S. Efficacy of MRA for detection of unruptured cerebral aneurysms in the "brain dock". Nosotchu No Geka 1994;22: 187–90.

[32] Watanabe Z, Kikuchi Y, Izaki K, et al. The usefulness of 3D MR angiography in surgery for ruptured cerebral aneurysms. Surg Neurol 2001;55: 359–64.

[33] Korogi Y, Takahashi M, Katada K, et al. Intracranial aneurysms: detection with three-dimensional CT angiography with volume rendering—comparison with conventional angiographic and surgical findings. Radiology 1999;211:497–506.

[34] Hoh BL, Cheung AC, Rabinov JD, Pryor JC, Carter BS, Ogilvy CS. Results of a prospective protocol of computed tomographic angiography in place of catheter angiography as the only diagnostic and pretreatment planning study for cerebral aneurysms by a combined neurovascular team. Neurosurgery 2004; 54:1329–42.

[35] Yasui T, Kishi H, Komiyama M, et al. The limitations of three-dimensional CT angiography (3D-CTA) in the diagnosis of cerebral aneurysms. No Shinkei Geka 2000;28:975–81.

[36] Venkatesh SK, Phadke RV, Kalode RR, Kumar S, Jain VK. Intracranial infective aneurysms presenting with haemorrhage: an analysis of angiographic findings, management and outcome. Clin Radiol 2000;55:946–53.

[37] Chun JY, Smith W, Halbach VV, Higashida RT, Wilson CB, Lawton MT. Current multimodality

management of infectious intracranial aneurysms. Neurosurgery 2001;48:1203–14.

[38] Topcuoglu MA, Ogilvy CS, Carter BS, Buonanno FS, Koroshetz WJ, Singhal AB. Subarachnoid hemorrhage without evident cause on initial angiography studies: diagnostic yield of subsequent angiography and other neuroimaging tests. J Neurosurg 2003;98:1235–40.

[39] Nome T, Bakke SJ, Nakstad PH. MR angiography in the follow-up of coiled cerebral aneurysms after treatment with Guglielmi detachable coils. Acta Radiol 2002;43:10–4.

[40] Alrawi A, Trobe JD, Blaivas M, Musch DC. Brain biopsy in primary angiitis of the central nervous system. Neurology 1999;53:858–60.

[41] Hankey G. Isolated angiitis/angiopathy of the CNS. Prospective diagnosis and therapeutic experience. Cerebrovasc Dis 1991;1:2–15.

[42] Cloft HJ, Phillips CD, Dix JE, McNulty BC, Zagardo MT, Kallmes DF. Correlation of angiography and MR imaging in cerebral vasculitis. Acta Radiol 1999;40:83–7.

[43] Mori H, Aoki S, Okubo T, et al. Two-dimensional thick-slice MR digital subtraction angiography in the assessment of small to medium-size intracranial arteriovenous malformations. Neuroradiology 2003; 45:27–33.

[44] Farb RI, McGregor C, Kim JK, et al. Intracranial arteriovenous malformations: real-time auto-triggered elliptic centric-ordered 3D gadolinium-enhanced MR angiography—initial assessment. Radiology 2001;220:244–51.

[45] Todaka T, Hamada J, Kai Y, Morioka M, Ushio Y. Analysis of mean transit time of contrast medium in ruptured and unruptured arteriovenous malformations: a digital subtraction angiographic study. Stroke 2003;34:2410–4.

[46] St. George EJ, Butler P, Plowman PN. Can magnetic resonance imaging alone accurately define the arteriovenous nidus for gamma knife radiosurgery? J Neurosurg 2002;97:464–70.

[47] Noguchi K, Melhem ER, Kanazawa T, Kubo M, Kuwayama N, Seto H. Intracranial dural arteriovenous fistulas: evaluation with combined 3D time-of-flight MR angiography and MR digital subtraction angiography. AJR Am J Roentgenol 2004;182: 183–90.

[48] Klopfenstein JD, Spetzler RF, Kim LJ, et al. Comparison of routine and selective use of intraoperative angiography during aneurysm surgery: a prospective assessment. J Neurosurg 2004;100:230–5.

[49] Tang G, Cawley CM, Dion JE, Barrow DL. Intraoperative angiography during aneurysm surgery: a prospective evaluation of efficacy. J Neurosurg 2002;96:993–9.

[50] Yanaka K, Fujita K, Noguchi S, et al. Intraoperative angiographic assessment of graft patency during extracranial-intracranial bypass procedures. Neurol Med Chir (Tokyo) 2003;43:509–13.

[51] Lee MC, Macdonald RL. Intraoperative cerebral angiography: superficial temporal artery method and results. Neurosurgery 2003;53:1067–75.

[52] Anegawa S, Hayashi T, Torigoe R, Harada K, Kihara S. Intraoperative angiography in the resection of arteriovenous malformations. J Neurosurg 1994;80:73–80.

[53] Martin NA, Bentson J, Vinuela F, et al. Intraoperative digital subtraction angiography and the surgical treatment of intracranial aneurysms and vascular malformations. J Neurosurg 1990;73:526–33.

[54] Pietila TA, Stendel R, Jansons J, Schilling A, Koch HC, Brock M. The value of intraoperative angiography for surgical treatment of cerebral arteriovenous malformations in eloquent brain areas. Acta Neurochir (Wien) 1998;140:1161–5.

[55] Lui W, Fan Y, Cheng P, Wong W. The use of intraoperative angiography in the management of neurovascular disorders. Annals of the College of Surgeons of Hong King 2002;6:36–41.

[56] American Academy of Pediatrics Task Force on Brain Death in Children. Report of special task force. Guidelines for the determination of brain death in children. Pediatrics 1987;80:298–300.

[57] Bradac GB, Simon RS. Angiography in brain death. Neuroradiology 1974;7:25–8.

[58] Qureshi AI, Kirmani JF, Xavier AR, Siddiqui AM. Computed tomographic angiography for diagnosis of brain death. Neurology 2004;62:652–3.

[59] Biffl WL, Moore EE. Identifying the asymptomatic patient with blunt carotid arterial injury. J Trauma 1999;47:1163–4.

[60] Biffl WL, Moore EE, Ryu RK, et al. The unrecognized epidemic of blunt carotid arterial injuries: early diagnosis improves neurologic outcome. Ann Surg 1998;228:462–70.

[61] Fry WR, Dort JA, Smith RS, Sayers DV, Morabito DJ. Duplex scanning replaces arteriography and operative exploration in the diagnosis of potential cervical vascular injury. Am J Surg 1994;168:693–6.

[62] Kerwin AJ, Bynoe RP, Murray J, et al. Liberalized screening for blunt carotid and vertebral artery injuries is justified. J Trauma 2001;51:308–14.

[63] Biffl WL, Ray CE Jr, Moore EE, Mestek M, Johnson JL, Burch JM. Noninvasive diagnosis of blunt cerebrovascular injuries: a preliminary report. J Trauma 2002;53:850–6.

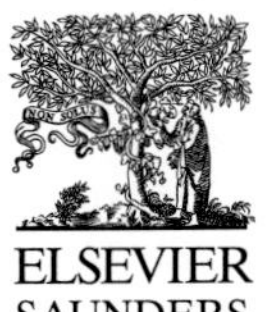
ELSEVIER
SAUNDERS

Neurosurg Clin N Am 16 (2005) 249–256

NEUROSURGERY
CLINICS
OF NORTH AMERICA

Temporary and Permanent Occlusion of Cervical and Cerebral Arteries

Richard J. Parkinson, MD[a,*], Bernard R. Bendok, MD[a,b], Brian A. O'Shaughnessy, MD[a], Ali Shaibani, MD[b], Eric J. Russell, MD[b], Christopher C. Getch, MD[a], Issam A. Awad, MD[a], H. Hunt Batjer, MD[a]

[a]*Department of Neurological Surgery, Feinberg School of Medicine, Northwestern University, 233 East Erie Street, Suite 614, Chicago, IL 60611, USA*

[b]*Department of Radiology, Feinberg School of Medicine, Northwestern University, 676 North Clair Street, Suite 800, Chicago, IL 60611, USA*

Permanent occlusion of cervical vessels is a solution to many vascular diseases and has been practiced for almost 200 years. John Hunter pioneered ligation as a therapeutic technique by ligating the popliteal artery to treat an aneurysm. Carotid occlusion was initially used to treat penetrating injuries of the carotid artery. In 1804, Abernethy ligated the common carotid artery after trauma; unfortunately, the patient died from a subsequent stroke [1]. Astley Cooper (1768–1841) described his experience with carotid ligation for aneurysms in 1836, with the first successful procedure being performed in 1808. Victor Horsley made the diagnosis of a giant carotid aneurysm at surgical exploration and successfully ligated the carotid artery a few days later [2]. The later developments of cerebral angiography by Egas Moniz in the 1920s, surgical clipping of aneurysms by Dandy in the 1930s, and gradual vascular occlusion of the carotid and other vessels by the use of adjustable clamps [1,3] as well as by endovascular techniques in the 1970s stimulated interest in the use of endovascular balloon occlusion as a minimally invasive alternative to open ligation of a parent vessel and using endovascular techniques to test cerebral reserve [3]. The development of Hunterian strategies to treat unclippable aneurysms of posterior and anterior cerebral circulations was pioneered by Drake et al [4].

Approximately 80% of patients tolerate carotid occlusion or the loss of a nondominant or codominant vertebral artery [5,6]. The issue of determining which patients can safely tolerate a permanent occlusion led to the evolution of balloon test occlusion (BTO) as a pretreatment test [7–9]. Temporary endovascular balloon occlusion to test cerebrovascular reserve before cervical or cerebral artery sacrifice is a relatively recent diagnostic test [5], the sensitivity and specificity of which are still under review [10]. The primary indications for this procedure are surgically untreatable aneurysms [7,11,12,26,27]; control of hemorrhage associated with trauma, aneurysm rupture, or tumor invasion [3,8]; skull base or cervical tumors intimately associated with arteries [1,8,13–15]; traumatic or nontraumatic arterial fistulae (not otherwise manageable); and dissection (Box 1). In addition, BTO, combined with other adjunctive tests, such as CT angiography (CTA), magnetic resonance angiography (MRA), digital subtraction angiography (DSA), CT or magnetic resonance perfusion [16] studies, clinical examination, induced hypotension [14], acetazolamide challenge test [9,14], transcranial Doppler ultrasonography and electroencephalogram (EEG) monitoring, carotid stump pressure

* Corresponding author.
E-mail address: Rparky34@aol.com (R.J. Parkinson).

1042-3680/05/$ - see front matter
doi:10.1016/j.nec.2004.08.003

Box 1. Indications for temporary or permanent balloon occlusion

1. Surgically untreatable aneurysms
   - Giant
   - Fusiform
   - Cavernous
   - Petrous
   - Cervical carotid aneurysms
2. Head and neck cancer: carotid or vertebral artery sacrifice required for en bloc resection or devascularization
3. Control of hemorrhage
4. Arteriovenous fistulae (not otherwise manageable)
5. Assessment presacrifice of injured vessel (eg, dissection)

measurement, and xenon-cerebral blood flow (CBF) or single photon emission computed tomography (SPECT) quantitative CBF measurement, can provide useful information about the cerebral arterial anatomy and physiology of a particular patient [4,5,7,8,17,18]. These tests, when properly performed and interpreted, can provide a high degree of certainty that permanent occlusion of a given vessel will or will not result in a deficit related to hypoperfusion or ischemic infarction [7,8,19,20]. If the occlusion is not tolerated, consideration must be given to the abandonment of permanent arterial sacrifice or preocclusion revascularization via a surgical bypass procedure.

There is no doubt, however, that despite the satisfactory outcome of provocative tests, a few patients treated with a Hunterian strategy are at risk of stroke or neurologic deficit because of hypoperfusion or postocclusion thromboembolism [8]. Our institution therefore uses a selective revascularization protocol (Table 1) unlike some other institutions, which advocate a universal revascularization approach [21]. Briefly, a selective approach involves using provocative testing and performing revascularization based on the results of the provocative testing, and the universal approach involves distal revascularization for all vessels requiring sacrifice. The assessment of cerebrovascular reserve before a contemplated parent artery sacrifice or an extended temporary occlusion (eg, as may be necessary in the reconstruction of a giant aneurysm) at our institution has been previously described [7]. Essentially, cerebrovascular reserve is assessed using four modalities: neuroclinical, hemodynamic, neurophysiologic, and provocative. These modalities are assessed together in an effort to predict tolerance to parent artery sacrifice. Neuroclinical assessment involves examination of the awake patient for any corresponding deficits during BTO. Hemodynamic assessment during temporary occlusion involves observation of cross-flow on DSA from the contralateral to ipsilateral hemisphere and radionuclide CBF studies (^{99m}Tc-hexamethylpropyleneamine oxime–SPECT) with maintenance of normotension. Neurophysiologic testing involves EEG assessment for any changes during occlusion. Provocative testing involves pharmacologically reducing the patient's mean arterial pressure to approximately two thirds of baseline during temporary occlusion and a neuroclinical reassessment [7,14,22]. This testing has been associated with a high correlation to tolerance of permanent sacrifice of the carotid artery in 18 of 19 patients [22].

Van Rooij et al [23], in a study of 17 patients who underwent successful BTO of the cervical internal carotid artery with neurologic and neurophysiologic monitoring (no complications noted) followed by permanent occlusion of the carotid artery, demonstrated that not a single patient had suffered an ischemic event at the 21-month follow-up. Mathis and colleagues [8], in their extensive experience of 500 temporary internal and common carotid artery balloon occlusions, found a 0.4% permanent neurologic complication rate. Overall, in the literature, the

Table 1
Indications for bypass from temporary balloon occlusion: institutional protocol

Clinical	EEG	SPECT	Hypotension	Intervention
Pass	Pass	Pass	Pass	PO
Pass	Fail	Fail	Fail	PO + low-flow bypass (STA-MCA)
Fail	Fail	Fail	Fail	PO + high-flow bypass (venous/radial artery bypass)
Pass	Pass	Fail	Fail	PO + low-flow bypass (STA-MCA)

Abbreviations: PO, permanent occlusion; STA-MCA, superficial temporal artery to middle cerebral artery.

complication rate associated with BTO is approximately 1.5% [7]. The generally good outcome in patients who have permanent occlusion is evident when considering the Cooperative Study of Intracranial Aneurysms and Subarachnoid Hemorrhage [24], in which 100 of 129 patients with unruptured aneurysms had a good outcome with a Hunterian strategy with no provocative testing. Echoing these results are those of Drake et al [4], who reported ischemic complications in 3 of 114 patients who underwent parent artery occlusion (all complications were thought to result from thromboembolism rather than hypoperfusion—this may represent a technical failure), again, with no provocative testing. Graves et al [25] found a permanent neurologic complication rate of 1 of 19 patients in their endovascular internal carotid occlusion series.

The techniques of parent vessel test occlusion have also been refined to place the balloon immediately proximal to the lesion to be occluded, even quite distally in the cerebral circulation, so as to minimize the column of thrombus that develops beyond the balloon; reduce the risk of recanalization related to collaterals to the arterial segment just proximal to the lesion; and minimize trauma and ischemia to proximal collaterals, perforators, and end arteries [7]. This more selective approach may also result in a better occlusion rate and improved resolution of giant aneurysms because of greater relative flow reduction within them [7]. In addition, the technique can be used to assess collaterals during occlusion of posterior circulation vessels, such as the posterior cerebral artery P1 segment, the distal vertebral artery, the posterior inferior cerebellar artery, and even the proximal basilar artery [7,21,25]. The issues of collateral flow, perforator occlusion, and ischemia are particularly relevant in these regions.

Technique and devices for balloon test occlusion

The following is a description of the protocol used at our institution. Before the procedure, the patient is assessed medically, particularly from a cardiovascular reserve point of view (in terms of evaluation of fitness for induction of hypotension). An anesthesiologist is in attendance for hemodynamic monitoring and supervision of induced hypotension. The patient is examined for femoral and leg pulses. A baseline neurologic examination is performed. An arterial line, intravenous line, electrocardiogram (EKG) monitor, EEG monitor, and Foley catheter are placed. The patient is given antibiotics (cephalothin or oxacillin). Femoral line sheaths (6.5-French right and 5.5-French left) of appropriate lengths are then placed via micropuncture access and a modified Seldinger technique. Once the sheaths are in position, a loading dose of heparin (60 U/kg) is intravenously administered to achieve an activated coagulation time (ACT) of 300 seconds. At our institution, it is also routine practice for a diagnostic cerebral angiogram to be performed before BTO is attempted. Bilateral external carotid angiography is also performed to assess the anatomy of the superficial temporal arteries, should these vessels be required for bypass surgery. If angiography has been performed, we start with an arch run to image the cervical and intracranial vessels. This serves as a baseline anatomic reference, which is repeated after trial balloon occlusion. After diagnostic angiography, the vessel to be occluded is selected with a 6-French guide catheter using over-the-wire and roadmap techniques. If access is particularly difficult (eg, because of an anomalous origin of the left common carotid artery [ie, the so-called "bovine arch"]), an exchange length wire can be left in the vessel of interest along with the diagnostic catheter. The guide catheter is then navigated to the vessel of interest over the exchange length wire. It is our practice to keep all catheters that might be exchanged during the procedure connected to a heparinized saline drip via rotating hemostatic adapters so as to avoid thromboembolic complications. Once the guide catheter is in an appropriate position proximal to the target occlusion site, contrast is gently injected to ensure that placement of the guide catheter did not cause a dissection. The diameter of the target vessel is then measured using standard calibration techniques. With modern three-dimensional (3D) noninvasive imaging (MRA and CTA), a measurement can also be obtained before BTO. It is our practice to confirm the measurements of any previous angiographic study with those obtained during this study. The appropriate balloon is then prepared in standard fashion as outlined by the particular manufacturer. It is critical to avoid air pockets in any balloon system and to study diameter and volume curves of the balloon carefully. Balloons used for extracranial BTO are compliant balloons (Figs. 1 and 2). One example of a compliant balloon is the HyperForm nondetachable balloon

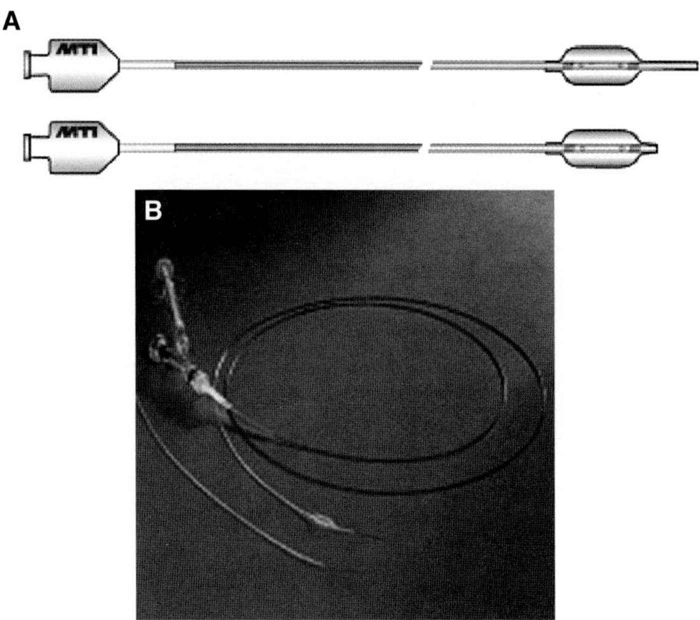

Fig. 1. HyperForm temporary occlusion balloon catheters (Micro Therapeutics, Irvine, California).

(Micro Therapeutics, Irvine, California). We have also used coronary balloons for intracranial BTO because of the greater diameter precision achieved with these balloons. When the internal carotid artery is targeted for occlusion, we place the guide catheter below the petrous (C2) segment of the internal carotid artery and carefully avoid the more distal petrous segment of the carotid artery, because a greater risk of vessel dissection is associated with catheter placement in this region. Baseline blood pressure and SPECT perfusion values are obtained before the procedure. Before the balloon is inflated, a baseline neurologic examination is performed

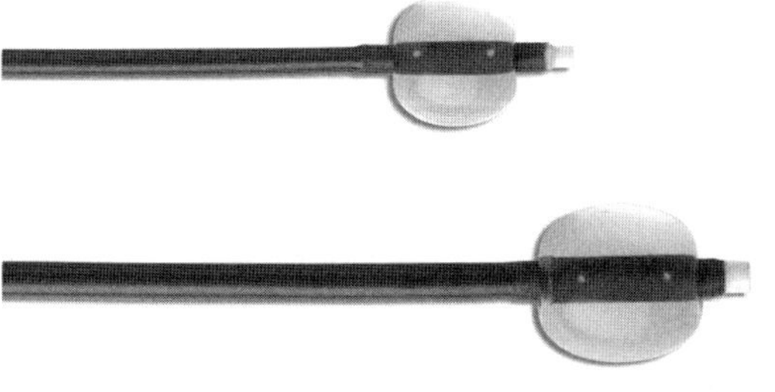

Fig. 2. The Concentric Balloon Guide Catheter (Concentric Medical, Mountain View, California), a commonly used balloon test occlusion catheter.

and an EEG tracing is obtained in the angiography suite. Sedation is given (fentanyl, no benzodiazepines). Once the guide catheter is in position and the balloon is ready for use, we navigate the balloon to the area of chosen temporary occlusion. After the balloon has been positioned, it is carefully inflated to the previously determined vessel diameter (Fig. 3). Contrast is gently injected through the guide catheter to confirm occlusion. Most compliant balloons can slowly deflate, so it is our practice to check for occlusion every 5 minutes. A contrast column below the balloon, which can be seen fluoroscopically, gives some assurance that the vessel is indeed occluded and can be followed to confirm continuous occlusion. Once occlusion has been achieved, a neurologic examination is performed every 5 minutes. At approximately 15 minutes, if the results of the neurologic examination are unchanged, the anesthesiologist is asked to reduce the mean arterial pressure to 30% below baseline. Ideally, the patient is monitored for 15 minutes at normotension and for 15 minutes with hypotension (30% below baseline mean arterial pressure). An arch angiogram of the intracranial circulation is performed to assess collateral flow while the target vessel is temporarily occluded (see Fig. 3). Alternatively, a selective angiogram of

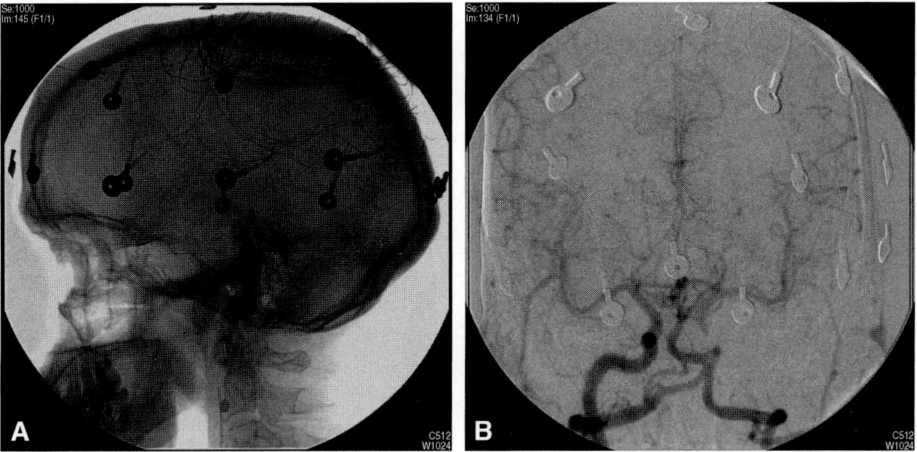

Fig. 3. A case of a patient with head and neck cancer who underwent temporary balloon occlusion of the left internal carotid artery before carotid artery sacrifice during radical resection. (*A*) MediTech (Watertown, Massachusetts) balloon in situ in the left internal carotid artery. (*B*) Arch angiogram showing good collateral flow to the left hemisphere from the right internal carotid artery via the anterior communicating artery.

the other relevant cervical vessels can be performed to assess collateral flow (Fig. 4). A ^{99m}Tc (Pertechnetate) tracer is intravenously administered at this stage. If the patient develops a deficit or EEG changes during BTO, the balloon is immediately deflated and an angiogram is performed. Embolic occlusion of distal vessels should be ruled out by observing capillary phase runs to assess the perfusion of the entire parenchyma. If no EEG or clinical change occurs during BTO, the balloon is deflated after 30 minutes; final angiography is performed of the target vessel to rule out a dissection and thromboembolic complications. As with any angiographic run to assess parenchymal perfusion, imaging is extended to the capillary and venous phases. The balloon and diagnostic catheters are then removed, followed by the sheath. The puncture site is closed with a Perclose device (Abbott, Redwood City, California), or when the ACT is less than 150 seconds, bleeding at the site can be controlled with manual compression. It is our practice not to give protamine unless a hemorrhagic complication occurs. The patient is then transferred to the nuclear medicine unit, and a repeat SPECT scan is performed. The patient is admitted to the neurointensive care unit for 24 hours after the procedure, where routine postangiography checks (eg, groin site observations, leg pulses, leg movement) and hourly neurologic examinations are performed. A postprocedure EKG is obtained.

Technique of permanent occlusion of the vertebral or carotid artery

If the BTO does not show evidence of neurologic compromise, permanent occlusion is planned via an endovascular or surgical approach. If an endovascular option is chosen, the patient is given heparin to achieve an ACT of 300 seconds after sheath placement. Patients usually receive a loading dose of clopidogrel (75 mg daily for 3 days before the procedure) and aspirin (325 mg daily beginning 10 days before occlusion).

The endovascular procedure is performed with an anesthesiologist in attendance for hemodynamic monitoring and to maintain normotension. An arterial line, intravenous lines, EKG and EEG monitors, and a Foley catheter are placed. Midazolam and fentanyl are administered for sedation. Baseline neurologic and leg pulse examinations are performed. Bilateral 6.5-French femoral sheaths are placed, and intravenous heparin (to an ACT of 300 seconds) and antibiotics (usually cefazolin) are given. The vessel to be occluded is approached using a 6-French Envoy catheter. A single-vessel cervical and intracranial injection is then performed. Because of the current limited availability of detachable vascular balloons, platinum microcoils are packed into the parent vessel until angiographic occlusion is achieved. It has been our practice to use a guide catheter capable of temporarily occluding the parent vessel, such as the Concentric Balloon

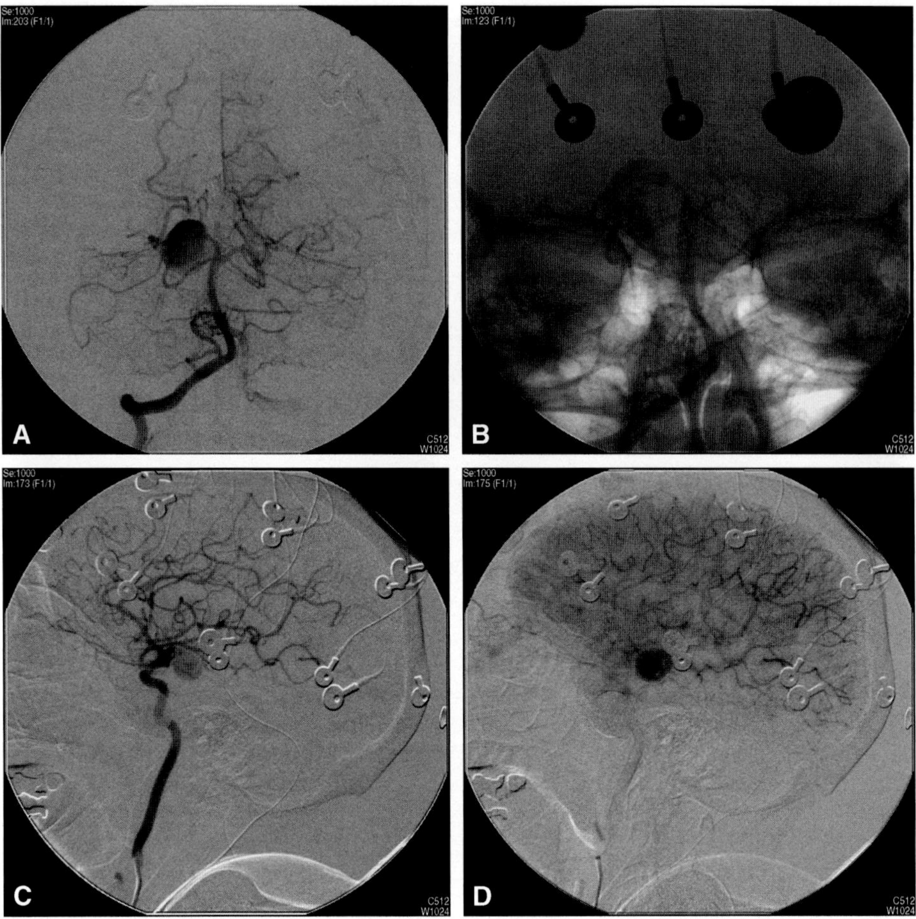

Fig. 4. A case of a patient with a large right P1 segment aneurysm incorporating the right posterior communicating artery origin. Potential P1 sacrifice with or without P1 distal bypass was planned. (*A*) Anteroposterior vertebral artery angiogram, demonstrating the P1 aneurysm. (*B*) HyperForm balloon (Micro Therapeutics, Irvine, California) in situ in the right P1. (*C, D*) Late arterial phase and capillary phase lateral right internal carotid artery angiograms with the balloon inflated showing filling of the aneurysm from the posterior communicating artery. The patient therefore required P1 sacrifice with distal bypass.

Guide Catheter (Concentric Medical, Mountain View, California). This guide catheter allows for flow arrest until a stable coil mass has been deployed and can be exchanged with the Envoy catheter. One or two oversized (relative to the parent vessel) "basket coils" are initially placed proximal to the aneurysm. The basket coil mass is then filled with helical detachable coils or pushable coils until vessel occlusion has been achieved (Fig. 5). A three-vessel cerebral angiogram can then be performed with an aortic pigtail catheter to assess collateral flow, or a selective study can be performed (see Fig. 5C). The sheaths are then removed, and bleeding at the puncture site is controlled with manual compression when the ACT has normalized, or the site is closed with the Perclose device. Protamine is not given. The patient is then re-examined neurologically; leg pulse and groin checks are performed, and a CT scan is obtained. The patient is admitted to the neurointensive care unit for 48 hours, where strict normotension is maintained and hourly neurologic checks are done. The patient is gradually mobilized on postprocedure day 2 and kept in the hospital for a total of approximately 5 days. A repeat CT/MRI perfusion study is performed while the patient is still in the hospital, and the results are compared with the baseline study. The

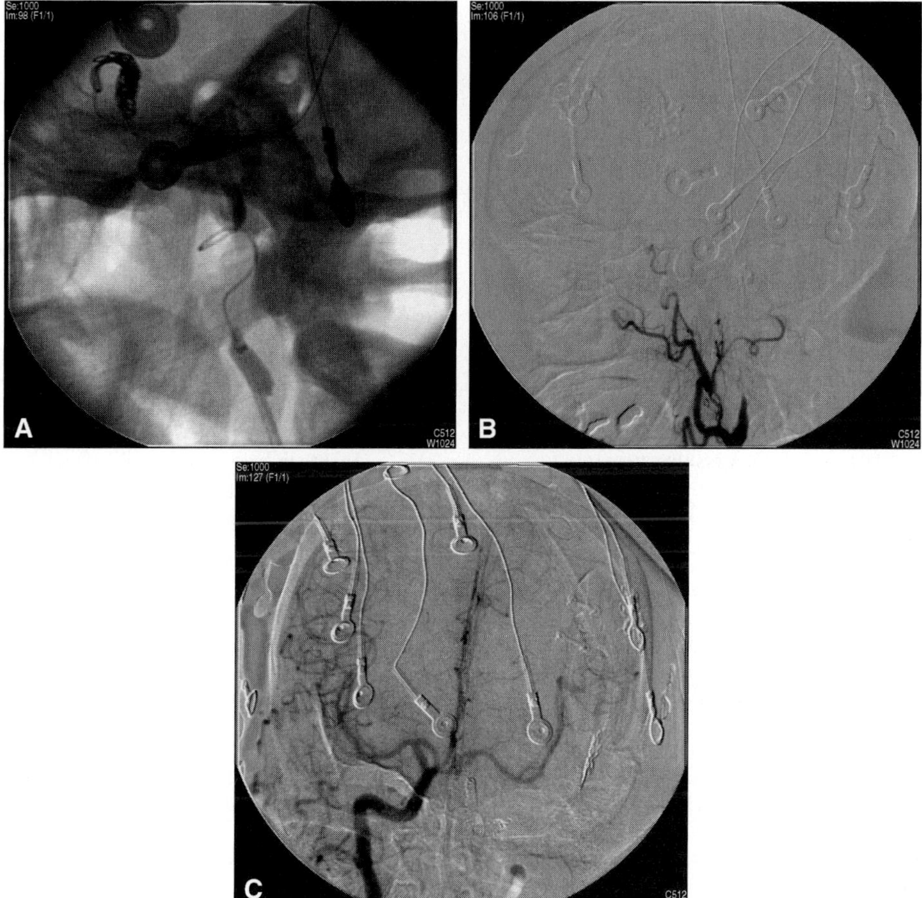

Fig. 5. Permanent sacrifice of the left internal carotid artery in a patient who previously tolerated temporary balloon occlusion. (*A*) Proximal carotid balloon occlusion with a Concentric balloon (Concentric Medical, Mountain View, California) and definitive distal coil placement. (*B*) After occlusion, stasis of contrast is seen in the left internal carotid artery with flow diversion into the external carotid artery. (*C*) Right internal carotid artery study showing effective occlusion of the left internal carotid artery and good collateral flow into the left anterior circulation via the anterior communicating artery.

clopidogrel and aspirin is continued for 1 month; thereafter, the patient is maintained on aspirin only.

Summary

We believe that temporary and permanent endovascular balloon occlusions are safe and effective procedures for the assessment and treatment of conditions for which parent vessel sacrifice is contemplated. In selected patients, BTO can predict the outcome of parent vessel sacrifice with a high degree of accuracy. This avoids the potential morbidities of a universal revascularization strategy (ie, the risks of revascularization when it may not be required) or ischemic stroke after parent vessel sacrifice when inadequate collaterals exist. In addition, in experienced hands, permanent occlusion of intracranial arteries using endovascular techniques can be done with a high degree of safety [25]. Endovascular occlusion may permit vessel sacrifice closer to the lesion than is typically possible with open surgical techniques.

References

[1] Lee S, Huddle D, Awad IA. Indications and management strategies in therapeutic carotid occlusion. Neurosurg Q 2000;10:211–23.

[2] Greenblatt SH, editor. A history of neurosurgery. AANS Press; 1997. p. 264–26.

[3] Lee S, Awad IA. Therapeutic carotid occlusion: current management paradigms. Clin Neurosurg 2000; 46:363–91.

[4] Drake CG, Peerless SJ, Ferguson GG. Hunterian proximal arterial occlusion for giant aneurysms of the carotid circulation. J Neurosurg 1994;81:656–65.

[5] Eckard DA, Purdy PD, Bonte FJ. Temporary balloon occlusion of the carotid artery combined with brain blood flow imaging as a test to predict tolerance prior to permanent carotid sacrifice. AJNR Am J Neuroradiol 1992;13:1565–9.

[6] Dare AO, Chaloupka JC, Putman CM, Fayad PB, Awad IA. Failure of the hypotensive provocative test during temporary balloon test occlusion of the internal carotid artery to predict delayed hemodynamic ischemia after therapeutic carotid occlusion. Surg Neurol 1998;50:147–56.

[7] O'Shaughnessy BA, Salehi SA, Mindea SA, Batjer HH. Selective cerebral revascularization as an adjunct in the treatment of giant anterior circulation aneurysms. Neurosurg Focus 2003;14(3).

[8] Mathis JM, Barr JD, Jungreis CA, Yonas H, Sekhar LN, Vincent D, et al. Temporary balloon test occlusion of the internal carotid artery: experience in 500 cases. AJNR Am J Neuroradiol 1995;16:749–54.

[9] Marshall RS, Lazar RM, Young WL, Solomon RA, Joshi S, Duong DH, et al. Clinical utility of quantitative cerebral blood flow measurements during internal carotid artery test occlusion. Neurosurgery 2002;50:996–1005.

[10] Sorteberg A, Sorteberg W, Bakke S, Lindegaard K, Boysen M, Nornes H. Varying impact of common carotid artery digital compression and internal carotid artery balloon test occlusion on cerebral hemodynamics. Head Neck 1998;20:687–94.

[11] Gupta DK, Young WL, Hashimoto T, Halim AX, Marshall RS, Lazar RM, et al. Characterization of the cerebral blood flow response to balloon deflation after temporary internal carotid artery test occlusion. J Neurosurg Anasthesiol 2002;14:123–9.

[12] Sluzewski M, Brilstra EH, van Rooij WJ, Wijnalda D, Tulleken CAF, Rinkel GJE. Bilateral vertebral artery balloon occlusion for giant vertebrobasilar aneurysms. Neuroradiology 2001;43:336–41.

[13] George B, Ferrario C, Blanquet A, Kolb F. Cavernous sinus exenteration for invasive cranial base tumors. Neurosurgery 2003;52:772–82.

[14] Dare AO, Gibbons KJ, Gillihan MD, Guterman LR, Loree TR, Hicks WL Jr. Hypotensive endovascular test occlusion of the carotid artery in head and neck cancer. Neurosurg Focus 2003;14(3).

[15] Feiz-Erfan I, Han PP, Spetzler RF, Lanzino G, Ferriera MAT, Gonzalez LF, et al. Salvage of advanced squamous cell carcinomas of the head and neck: internal carotid artery sacrifice and extracranial-intracranial revascularization. Neurosurg Focus 2003; 14(3).

[16] Michel E, Liu H, Remley KB, Martin AJ, Madison MT, Kucharczyk J, et al. Perfusion MR neuroimaging in patients undergoing balloon test occlusion of the internal carotid artery. AJNR Am J Neuroradiol 2001;22:1590–6.

[17] Okudaira Y, Arai H, Sato K. Cerebral blood flow alteration by acetazolamide during carotid balloon occlusion. Stroke 1996;27:617–21.

[18] Eckert B, Thie A, Carvajal M, Groden C, Zeumer H. Predicting hemodynamic ischemia by transcranial Doppler monitoring during therapeutic balloon occlusion of the internal carotid artery. AJNR Am J Neuroradiol 1998;19:577–82.

[19] Sudhakar KV, Sawlani V, Phadke RV, Kumar S, Ahmed S, Gujral RB. Temporary balloon occlusion of internal carotid artery: a simple and reliable clinical test. Neurol India 2000;48:140–3.

[20] McIvor NP, Willinsky RA, TerBrugge KG, Rutka JA, Freeman JL. Validity of test occlusion studies prior to internal carotid artery sacrifice. Head Neck 1994;16(1):11–6.

[21] Spetzler RF, Carter LP. Revascularization and aneurysm surgery: current status. Neurosurgery 1985; 16:111–6.

[22] Standard SC, Ahuja A, Guterman LR, et al. Balloon test occlusion of the internal carotid artery with hypotensive challenge. AJNR Am J Neuroradiol 1995; 16:1453–8.

[23] van Rooij WJ, Sluzewski M, Metz NH, et al. Carotid balloon occlusion for large and giant aneurysms: evaluation of a new test occlusion protocol. Neurosurgery 2000;47:116–22.

[24] Nishioka H. Report on the cooperative study of intracranial aneurysms and subarachnoid hemorrhage. Section VIII, part I: results of the treatment of intracranial aneurysms by occlusion of the carotid artery in the neck. J Neurosurg 1966;25:660–82.

[25] Graves VB, Perl J II, Strother CM, Wallace RC, Kesava PP, Masaryk TJ. Endovascular occlusion of the carotid or vertebral artery with temporary proximal flow arrest and microcoils: clinical results. AJNR Am J Neuroradiol 1997;18:1201–6.

[26] Field M, Jungreis CA, Chengelis N, Kromer H, Kirby L, Yonas H. Symptomatic cavernous sinus aneurysms: management and outcome after carotid occlusion and selective cerebral revascularization. AJNR Am J Neuroradiol 2003;24:1200–7.

[27] Sorteberg A, Sorteberg W, Bakke SJ, Lindegaard KF, Boysen M, Nornes H. Cerebral hemodynamics in internal carotid artery trial occlusion. Acta Neurochir (Wien) 1997;139:1066–73.

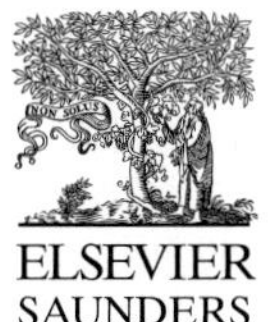

ELSEVIER
SAUNDERS

Neurosurg Clin N Am 16 (2005) 257–258

NEUROSURGERY
CLINICS
OF NORTH AMERICA

Cervical Carotid Revascularization: Indications from a Surgical Perspective

Brian E. Snell, MD[a,*], Christopher M. Loftus, MD[b]

[a]*Department of Neurological Surgery, Medical College of Wisconsin, 9200 W. Wisconsin Avenue, Milwaukee, WI 53226, USA*

[b]*Department of Neurosurgery, Temple University School of Medicine, 3401 North Broad Street, Parkinson Pavilion, Suit 580, Philadelphia, PA 19140, USA*

Atherosclerotic narrowing and ulceration at the carotid bifurcation is a major cause of thromboembolic stroke. The results of several prospective randomized trials for symptomatic and asymptomatic carotid occlusive disease have provided evidence-based data for treatment of the same. By 1990, seven trials were planned or in progress. Four of these trials addressed asymptomatic carotid occlusive disease (Carotid Artery Stenosis Asymptomatic Narrowing Operation Versus Aspirin study, Mayo Asymptomatic Carotid Endarterectomy study, Veterans Administration Asymptomatic Stenosis Trial [VAAST], and the Asymptomatic Carotid Atherosclerosis Study [ACAS]) [1–4]. Patients could not have symptoms from ipsilateral cerebral ischemia secondary to carotid occlusive disease, although contralateral symptoms were permitted in the VAAST and ACAS. The four trials used similar exclusion criteria. Patients with neurologic (eg, seizures, dementia), cardiac (eg, atrial fibrillation, severe valvular disease), or general medical conditions (eg, diabetes, renal failure) that might affect stroke outcome were also excluded [5]. There is one ongoing asymptomatic carotid surgery randomized trial in the United Kingdom and Europe, the Asymptomatic Carotid Surgery Trial [6]. No results are available from this trial at the present time.

The ACAS randomized 1662 patients with greater than 60% stenosis (by angiography or Doppler ultrasound) to surgery versus best medical management. All patients received daily aspirin (325 mg). Nonwhite populations comprised only 5% of the study group. The projected risk of ipsilateral stroke at 5 years (mean follow-up of 2.7 years) was 5.1% for the surgical group and 11% for medical management. This represented an overall relative risk reduction of 53%. This risk reduction was more apparent for men and independent of degree of stenosis or contralateral disease. The calculated stroke risk for the medical management arm was 2.2% per year. The perioperative risk of stroke and death was 2.3% plus an additional risk of 1.2% for arteriography. Surgical benefit was noted at 10 months after randomization and remained statistically significant at 3 years [4].

Three trials focused on symptomatic carotid occlusive disease (North American Symptomatic Carotid Endarterectomy Trial [NASCET], Veterans Administration Symptomatic Stenosis Trial [VASST], and European Carotid Surgery Trial [ECST]) [7–10]. All three of these trials were terminated early. The NASCET and VASST maintained that participating centers must have surgical morbidity rates of less than 6%. Inclusion criteria were relatively similar among the trials and included transient retinal ischemia, transient cerebral ischemia, or minor completed stroke within 120 days of randomization in the distribution of the carotid artery lesion [11].

The NASCET was terminated early secondary to significant risk reduction in patients with greater than 70% stenosis in the surgical arm. Six hundred fifty-nine patients with symptomatic carotid stenosis between 70% and 99% were randomized to surgical (328 patients) and nonsurgical (331 patients) treatment arms. Ipsilateral stroke

* Corresponding author.
E-mail address: bsnell@neuroscience.mcw.edu

doi:10.1016/j.nec.2004.08.019

risk at 2-year follow-up was 9% for the surgical group versus 26% for the nonsurgical group. This represented a 71% relative risk reduction ($P < 0.001$). According to these findings, one stroke could be prevented for every 6 to 7 endarterectomies performed. A significant correlation was noted between severity of stenosis and surgical benefit. The protective effect of endarterectomy was durable over time and independent of age, gender, and stroke risk factors [7]. At 5-year follow-up for 2226 patients with 50% to 69% stenosis randomized to nonsurgical and surgical arms, the ipsilateral stroke rate was 22.2% versus 15.7% (nonsurgical versus surgical; $P = 0.045$). Author estimates were that 15 endarterectomies would have to be performed to prevent one stroke in a 5-year period. Those individuals with less than 50% stenosis did not benefit from endarterectomy. Contralateral occlusion was a strong risk factor for stroke, though contralateral stenosis was not [8]. Timing of surgery did not affect surgical risk.

The ECST stenosis criterion was 0% to 99%. The trial randomized 3018 patients, 1807 to surgery and 1211 to best medical management. The trial was terminated early at an interim analysis of 2200 patients. Follow-up was 5 years, with a mean of 2.7 years for those with less than 30% stenosis and 3.0 years for those with greater than 70% stenosis. Sample size was 374 for the less than 30% stenosis group and 395 for the greater than 70% stenosis group. The primary end point was ipsilateral stroke. The mild stenosis group (<30%) revealed no statistically significant difference between surgical and nonsurgical arms with respect to stroke incidence. The severe stenosis group (>70%) revealed a benefit to the endarterectomy arm, with a 10.3% total risk of stroke (ie, 7.5% risk of stroke or death within 30 days plus an additional 2.8% risk of stroke) versus a 16.8% risk in the nonsurgical arm. The total 3-year risk of disabling or fatal stroke was 6.0% versus 11.0% in the surgical versus nonsurgical arms, respectively. Surgical benefit outweighed best medical management risk in patients with 70% to 80% stenosis. This benefit was realized 2 to 3 years after randomization [10]. ECST data reanalysis using NASCET criteria revealed a significant surgical benefit for patients with 70% stenosis.

A critical analysis of these studies provides convincing evidence for the surgical treatment of carotid occlusive disease in asymptomatic patients with greater than 60% stenosis and symptomatic patients with greater than 50% stenosis [12,13]. Note, however, that surgical benefit for women in the ACAS was not apparent and that nonwhite patients comprised only 5% of the study population. Also, ACAS and VAAST surgeons and patients were specifically selected for low surgical risk (perioperative morbidity and mortality <3%). In the symptomatic carotid stenosis trials, benefit of endarterectomy was observed in the setting of low surgical risk. Surgical benefit in nonselected populations may be less predictable.

References

[1] CASANOVA Study Group. Carotid surgery versus medical therapy in asymptomatic carotid stenosis. Stroke 1991;22:1229–35.

[2] Mayo Asymptomatic Carotid Endarterectomy Study Group. Results of a randomized controlled trial of carotid endarterectomy for asymptomatic carotid stenosis. Mayo Clin Proc 1992;67:513–8.

[3] Hobson RW, Weiss DG, Fields WS, et al. Efficacy of carotid endarterectomy for asymptomatic carotid stenosis. N Engl J Med 1993;328:221–7.

[4] Executive Committee for the Asymptomatic Carotid Atherosclerosis Study. Endarterectomy for asymptomatic carotid artery stenosis. JAMA 1995;273: 1421–8.

[5] Harrison GS, Mayberg MR. Prospective randomized studies for carotid endarterectomy. Neurosurg Clin N Am 2000;11:225–34.

[6] Halliday AW. The Asymptomatic Carotid Surgery Trial (ACST) rationale and design. Eur J Vasc Surg 1994;8:703–10.

[7] North American Symptomatic Carotid Endarterectomy Trial Collaborators. Beneficial effect of carotid endarterectomy in symptomatic patients with high-grade carotid stenosis. N Engl J Med 1991;325: 445–53.

[8] Barnett HJ. Status report on the North American Symptomatic Carotid Surgery Trial. J Mal Vasc 1993;18:202–8.

[9] Mayberg MR, Wilson SE, Yatsu F, et al. Carotid endarterectomy and prevention of cerebral ischemia in symptomatic carotid stenosis. JAMA 1991;266: 3289–94.

[10] European Carotid Surgery Trialists' Collaborative Group. Randomised trial of endarterectomy for recently symptomatic carotid stenosis: final results of the MRC European Carotid Surgery Trial (ECST). Lancet 1998;351:1379–87.

[11] Harrison GS, Mayberg MR. Prospective randomized studies for carotid endarterectomy. Neurosurg Clin N Am 2000;11:221–34.

[12] Loftus CM. Current indications for carotid endarterectomy. Neurol Med Chir (Tokyo) 1998;38: 268–74.

[13] Brennan JJ, Loftus CM. Carotid endarterectomy: current indications for surgery. Neurosurg Focus 5(6):Article 1, 1998.

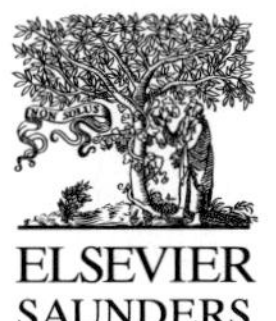
ELSEVIER
SAUNDERS

Neurosurg Clin N Am 16 (2005) 259–261

NEUROSURGERY
CLINICS
OF NORTH AMERICA

Cervical Carotid Revascularization: Indications From an Endovascular Perspective

William A. Gray, MD

Swedish Medical Center, Swedish Cardiovascular Research, Suite 1020, 1221 Madison, Seattle, WA 98104, USA

The benefit of prophylactic treatment of extracranial carotid bifurcation disease with surgical endarterectomy was established for symptomatic and asymptomatic stenosis in the 1990s in several landmark trials. More recently, the results of the Asymptomatic Carotid Atherosclerosis Study (ACAS) have been confirmed by a much larger trial demonstrating the effectiveness of endarterectomy in asymptomatic patients versus maximum modern medical therapy [1]. In an understandable effort to eliminate confounding variables, however, these trials excluded patients with significant medical and surgical comorbidities; in the North American Symptomatic Carotid Endarterectomy Trial (NASCET), two of three patients screened were ineligible for the study on the basis of one or more high-risk qualities [2]. In fact, these patients comprise between 20% and 50% of the population in whom endarterectomy would otherwise be considered appropriate therapy in clinical practice [3,4]. Moreover, in surveys performed after the NASCET and ACAS, the 30-day mortality rate at high-volume nontrial hospitals was greater than twice that at NASCET centers and almost three times that at low-volume nontrial hospitals [2], suggesting a patient selection issue or operator and/or facility issue.

In several subsequent nonrandomized analyses, the high-risk features excluded in the NASCET and ACAS have been associated with a significant increase in adverse outcomes. Specifically, death, stroke, and myocardial infarction (MI) at 30 days ranged between 7.8% and 9.9% for patients older than 75 years of age [5,6]. The risk of stroke and death alone is typically more than twice that seen in the ACAS and NASCET in patients with congestive heart failure (8.6%) [5], the presence of angina pectoris or coexistent coronary disease necessitating bypass surgery (9.9%–18.7%) [5,6], prior carotid endarterectomy (CEA) with recurrent stenosis (7.6%–10.9%) [7,8], contralateral occlusion (14.3%) [9], and renal insufficiency (8.2%–13%) [10,11]. In a retrospective study performed by the Cleveland Clinic on more than 3000 patients undergoing CEA in a 10-year period, patients with coronary artery disease, chronic obstructive pulmonary disease, and chronic renal insufficiency (creatinine level >3.0 mg/dL) were found to have three times the in-hospital stroke and death rate compared with patients in a normal risk category [3]. Although there are also data relating outcomes to operator and/or center volumes, most observers believe that the extrapolation of the NASCET and ACAS results to these high-risk patients has resulted in these less than favorable outcomes, which are significantly worse than those reported in the original trials.

At about the same time that the role of endarterectomy was being clarified in the United States, an evolution in device technology with the advent of self-expanding stents allowed the consideration of an endovascular alternative to surgery to address its apparent deficiencies in the high-risk patient. Although early work with carotid angioplasty in Europe dates back to the 1980s, the results were suboptimal, and carotid stenting did not start in earnest in the United States until the early to mid-1990s. Those early reports demonstrated the potential of this new technology in high-risk patients, even if the stroke and death rates ranged between 7% and 11% [12,13]. After these single-center reports, the first

E-mail address: william.gray@swedish.org

1042-3680/05/$ - see front matter
doi:10.1016/j.nec.2004.11.001

attempt at a randomized trial versus endarterectomy was the Wallstent Carotid Trial (1997–1999), which enrolled largely standard-risk patients [14]. The trial was halted prematurely after approximately 200 patients were enrolled, because it seemed as though the noninferiority end points would not be satisfied. Although there were no significant differences between the treatment groups, there was a trend favoring endarterectomy. Critique of this early trial focused on several key issues: the lack of a dedicated stent (the original Wallstent [Boston Scientific, Natick, Massachusetts] was a tracheobronchial device; it has since been modified for carotid application), the lack of cerebral embolic protection, the inexperienced nature of most operators, the absence of a phase I feasibility trial, and trial design (eg, end point definitions, statistical underpinnings).

Armed with the lessons of this trial and with a better understanding of device, operator, and trial requirements, technology evolved to include dedicated, low-profile, and nitinol stents as well as embolic protection devices and an expanded pool of experienced operators, and the concept of initiating trials in high-risk surgical patients evolved. Although not entirely exclusive, the overlap between a surgical high-risk feature and an endovascular approach to carotid treatment is generally quite limited. Accordingly, the next phase of study involved the high-risk patients in whom endarterectomy was proving difficult. Importantly, those investigating carotid stenting also recognized the importance of independent neurologic auditing of results [15], and it was incorporated into those trials going forward.

The first multicenter randomized control trial ever to examine outcomes of surgery in patients with high-risk features, the Stenting and Angioplasty with Protection in Patients at High Risk for Endarterectomy (SAPPHIRE) study, was conducted as a pivotal trial for device approval (Precise nitinol stent [Cordis Endovascular; Johnson & Johnson, New Brunswick, New Jersey] and Angioguard filter embolic protection device [Johnson & Johnson]) for Cordis Endovascular/Johnson & Johnson [16]. Patients with severe carotid stenosis (>50% in symptomatic patients and >80% in asymptomatic patients) and high-risk features were randomized to endarterectomy or carotid stenting after agreement as to their appropriateness among a team consisting of an experienced surgeon, an experienced interventionist, and a neurologist at each site. High-risk comorbidities were defined in two broad categories: anatomic and medical. The anatomic inclusions were contralateral carotid occlusion or laryngeal nerve palsy, prior neck irradiation, prior endarterectomy with recurrent stenosis, difficult surgical access, and tandem lesions. Medical inclusion criteria were severe left ventricular dysfunction (ejection fraction <30%) or New York Heart Association class III/IV heart failure, open heart surgery within 6 weeks, easily provoked angina or an acute coronary syndrome, severe pulmonary disease, and age greater than 80 years. In addition to the 334 patients randomized (310 treated), 407 patients considered to be at excessive surgical risk were entered into a stent registry and 7 patients in whom stenting was considered prohibitive were entered into an endarterectomy registry. The randomized phase of the trial was halted before completion because of lack of enrollment once other nonrandomized registries were in place as preferred alternatives for patients and treating physicians. The 360-day primary end point of all death, all stroke (to 30 days) and ipsilateral stroke (to 360 days), and MI (to 30 days) was 12.2% for the stent arm and 20.1% for endarterectomy ($P = 0.053$), fulfilling the prespecified end point of noninferiority. The risk of stroke out to 2 years was not different for the two treatments, 5.9% for stenting and 5.8% for surgery, and the low 1-year clinically driven target lesion revascularization rates, 0.6% and 3.6%, respectively, demonstrated durability of the initial results in both arms. Subsequent analysis revealed that the ipsilateral stroke rate in both treatment arms was comparable to those in the NASCET and ACAS trials. Based on the results of this randomized control trial, on April 21, 2004, the device advisory panel to the US Food and Drug Administration (FDA) recommended approval of the Precise stent and Angioguard embolic protection system for patients in whom carotid revascularization was indicated and who had high-risk surgical features as defined in the trial.

Several other pivotal device trials followed the SAPPHIRE study but in registry rather than randomized formats according to agreements with the FDA. In these studies, a weighted historical control is used as the comparator to the stent results and is constructed based on a continuously updated review of the literature for outcomes specific to the proportion of each high-risk inclusion group in the trial. The inclusion criteria in these later studies were similar to those of the SAPPHIRE trial, as were the end points, with the notable exception that the SAPPHIRE study included all death to 1 year, whereas these studies only included death to 30 days as one of the primary measures of procedural safety along with stroke and MI. The ACCULINK for the Revascularization of Carotids in High Risk Patients (ARCHeR), Registry to Evaluate the NeuroShield Bare Wire Cerebral Protection System and Xact Stent in Patients at High Risk for Carotid Endarterectomy (SECuRITY), and Boston Scientific EPI: A Carotid Stenting Trial for High-Risk Surgical Patients (BEACH) studies have all reported 30-day data [17–19], and the ARCHeR trial has reported 1-year primary end point results [20]. The 30-day stroke, death, and MI rates in those trials ranged between 5.4% and 7.8%, and the 1-year freedom from death, ipsilateral stroke, and MI in the ARCHeR study was 90%, statistically better than the historical surgical control. These trial results are remarkable for their low rates of major complications (especially when compared with surgery), their consistency across devices and operators, and their durability in stroke prevention, and they solidify the indication for carotid stenting with embolic protection in the high surgical risk patient.

Carotid stenting with embolic protection is now moving into the standard-risk patient cohorts with the Carotid Revascularization Endarterectomy versus Stent Trial (CREST), sponsored by the National Institute of Neurological Disorders and Stroke (NINDS) of the National Institutes of Health (NIH), in which symptomatic patients are being randomized to receive surgery or stenting. An enrollment of approximately 2500 patients at 70 sites is anticipated over the next several years. In addition, randomized trials in standard-risk asymptomatic patients are being contemplated and should address the role of stenting in the most common cohort currently undergoing CEA in this country.

References

[1] Asymptomatic Carotid Surgery Trial. Lancet 2004.

[2] Wennberg DE, Lucas FL, Birkmeyer JD, et al. Variation in carotid endarterectomy mortality in the Medicare population: trial hospitals, volume, and patient characteristics. JAMA 1998;279:1278–81.

[3] Ouriel K, Hertzer NR, Beven EG, et al. Preprocedural risk stratification: identifying an appropriate population for carotid stenting. J Vasc Surg 2001; 33:728–32.

[4] Lepore MR Jr, Sternbergh WC III, Salartash K, et al. Influence of NASCET/ACAS trial eligibility on outcome after carotid endarterectomy. J Vasc Surg 2001;34:581–6.

[5] Goldstein LB, Samsa GP, Matchar DB, et al. Multicenter review of preoperative risk factors for endarterectomy for asymptomatic carotid artery stenosis. Stroke 1998;29:750–3.

[6] McCrory DC, Goldstein LB, Samsa GP, et al. Predicting complications of carotid endarterectomy. Stroke 1993;24:1285–91.

[7] Das MB, Hertzer NR, Ratliff NB, et al. Recurrent carotid stenosis. A five-year series of 65 reoperations. Ann Surg 1985;202:28–35.

[8] Meyer FB, et al. Recurrent carotid stenosis. In: Sundt's occlusive cerebrovascular disease. 2nd edition. Philadelphia: WB Saunders; 1994. p. 310–21.

[9] Gasecki AP, Eliasziw M, Ferguson GG, et al. Long-term prognosis and effect of endarterectomy in patients with symptomatic severe carotid stenosis and contralateral carotid stenosis or occlusion: results from NASCET. North American Symptomatic Carotid Endarterectomy Trial (NASCET) Group. J Neurosurg 1995;83:778–82.

[10] Wong JH, Findlay JM, Suarez-Almazor ME. Regional performance of carotid endarterectomy. Appropriateness, outcomes, and risk factors for complications. Stroke 1997;28(5):891–8.

[11] Hamdan AD, Pomposelli FB Jr, Gibbons GW, et al. Renal insufficiency and altered postoperative risk in carotid endarterectomy. J Vasc Surg 1999;29: 1006–11.

[12] Diethrich E, Ndiaye M, Reid DB. Stenting in the carotid artery: initial experience in 110 patients. J Endovasc Surg 1996;3:42–62.

[13] Yadav JS, Roubin GS, Iyer S, et al. Elective stenting of the extracranial carotid arteries. Circulation 1997; 95:376–81.

[14] Gray WA, et al. Presented at the American Stroke Association National Meeting. February 2001.

[15] Rothwell, Slattery J, Warlow CP. A systematic review of the risks of stroke and death due to endarterectomy for symptomatic carotid stenosis. Stroke 1996;27:260–5.

[16] Yadav J. Presented at the American Heart Association Meeting. 2002.

[17] Wholey M. Presented at the American College of Cardiology Annual Sessions. 2003.

[18] Whitlow P. Presented at the American Heart Association National Meeting. 2003.

[19] White C. Presented at All That Jazz Meeting. April 2004.

[20] Gray W. Presented at the American College of Cardiology National Meeting. March 2004.

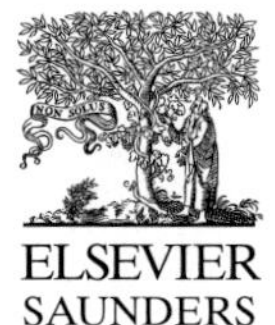
ELSEVIER
SAUNDERS

Neurosurg Clin N Am 16 (2005) 263–278

NEUROSURGERY
CLINICS
OF NORTH AMERICA

Cervical Carotid Revascularization: The Role of Angioplasty with Stenting

Ricardo A. Hanel, MD, Elad I. Levy, MD, Lee R. Guterman, PhD, MD, L. Nelson Hopkins, MD, FACS*

Department of Neurosurgery, Radiology, and Toshiba Stroke Research Center, School of Medicine and Biomedical Sciences, State University of New York at Buffalo, 3 Gates Circle, Buffalo, NY 14209–1194, USA

Stroke is the third largest cause of death after heart diseases and cancer and is the leading cause of permanent disability and disability-adjusted loss of independent life-years in Western countries [1–3]. Approximately 700,000 people in the United States experience a stroke annually, which results in an estimated $53.6 billion in direct and indirect costs [1]. By the year 2050, an estimated 1 million persons will suffer from stroke every year because of aging in the population and changes in the ethnic distribution [4].

Approximately 25% of the strokes occurring annually are attributable to ischemic events related to occlusive disease of the cervical internal carotid artery (ICA) [5]. Carotid stenosis caused by atherosclerotic disease increases the risk of ischemic stroke by acting as an embolic source or by causing hypoperfusion of the ipsilateral cerebral hemisphere. Introduced in the early 1950s [6], carotid endarterectomy (CEA) involves the performance of an arteriotomy of the cervical carotid artery with subsequent removal of the atherosclerotic plaque. Historically, CEA gained widespread acceptance [7] and was validated by the performance of several randomized trials, including the North American Symptomatic Carotid Endarterectomy Trial (NASCET) [8] and the Asymptomatic Carotid Atherosclerosis Study (ACAS) [9]. With some limitations, these studies have shown that CEA substantially reduces the stroke risk and increases the survival rate for patients with symptomatic carotid stenosis greater than 50% and asymptomatic stenosis greater than 60% [8–10]. During the past few years, carotid angioplasty with stenting (CAS) has evolved as an alternative to CEA, particularly for those patients in whom CEA is associated with a higher risk of complications [11–13]. The aim of this article is to review the relative indications and limitations for CEA and CAS and to describe the technique and results for CAS.

Carotid endarterectomy

Several randomized, multicenter, prospective trials have demonstrated evidence of the safety and efficacy of CEA in patients with symptomatic and asymptomatic carotid stenosis. Since the publication of the NASCET results in 1991 [8], CEA has been the standard of care for the revascularization of extracranial carotid stenosis [11]. In the preamble to this article, Snell and Loftus have reviewed the indications for cervical carotid revascularization from a surgical perspective. It is being increasingly recognized that certain patients who undergo CEA have a high risk of perioperative complications with increased mortality and morbidity, however [11].

Major carotid endarterectomy trials

One should keep in mind that selection criteria in the major CEA trials were restrictively defined. Exclusion criteria in the NASCET included a previous ipsilateral endarterectomy; an intracranial lesion that was more severe than the surgically accessible lesion; no angiographic depiction of the

* Corresponding author.

1042-3680/05/$ - see front matter
doi:10.1016/j.nec.2004.08.005

carotid arteries and their intracranial branches; and organ failure of the lung, liver, or kidney. Temporary exclusion criteria included uncontrolled hypertension, diabetes mellitus, or unstable angina pectoris; myocardial infarction (MI) within the previous 6 months; contralateral CEA within the previous 4 months; signs of progressive neurologic dysfunction; and a major surgical procedure within the previous 30 days. These patients could be included in the trial if the disorder responsible for their ineligibility resolved within 120 days of their qualifying cerebrovascular event. Similar restrictive inclusion and exclusion criteria were used in the European Carotid Surgery Trial (ECST) [10], ACAS [10], and Asymptomatic Carotid Surgery Trial [14]. In effect, the stringent criteria used to select patients in the major CEA trials excluded those with the highest risk of complications (ie, the group in whom the benefits of CEA might not have been evident).

Moreover, the benefits of carotid revascularization surgery demonstrated by the NASCET [8,15], ACAS [9], and ECST [16] are lost if the 30-day rate of perioperative stroke or death exceeds 6% for patients with symptomatic carotid stenosis or 3% for those with asymptomatic carotid stenosis.

Clinical practice versus clinical trials

Substantial evidence in the literature shows that the complication rates in clinical practice often exceed those in clinical trials. Wennberg et al [17], when comparing the perioperative mortality among 113,300 Medicare patients undergoing CEA during 1992 and 1993 at NASCET and ACAS hospitals and at nontrial hospitals, found that the mortality rate was almost two times greater at nontrial hospitals (2.5% at nontrial hospitals versus 1.4% at trial hospitals). In a similar study, Hsia et al [18] reported that the 30-day mortality rate among Medicare beneficiaries undergoing CEA was 2.5%, a rate much higher than the 1.0% mortality rate described in the clinical trials. Chaturvedi et al [19] reported 30-day combined rates of major stroke and death of 11.1% for symptomatic patients and 5.6% for asymptomatic patients in a prospective small series of patients undergoing operations and routine neurological examinations at an academic center, suggesting an underestimation of complication rates on the basis of those obtained in clinical trials.

Operator experience is probably an important factor contributing to this significant difference in complication rates. Careful patient selection has been found to be the key determinant in maintaining a low perioperative complication rate, however. Certain patient groups have been found to have a higher risk for perioperative complications with CEA [11,20–22]. CAS is an alternative modality for carotid revascularization that could benefit these high-risk patients.

High-risk surgical candidates

The risk of CEA associated with medical comorbidities has been well documented in the literature with respect to neurologic complications, such as stroke, as well as nonneurologic complications, such as MI [23]. In an analysis of the NASCET results, CEA was approximately 1.5 times more likely to be associated with medical complications in patients with a previous history of MI, angina, or hypertension [22]. Because patients with other significant coexistent diseases were excluded from the major CEA trials, the indications for and the results of surgery in this subgroup of patients have not been established. Factors that increase the risk of perioperative morbidity and mortality are reviewed here.

Age

Older patients seem to have a higher rate of perioperative complications with CEA. When assessing perioperative mortality of 113,300 Medicare patients, Wennberg et al [17] found that patients 85 years of age or older were three times more likely to die than those younger than 70 years of age. In a multicenter review of 1160 CEA procedures, Goldstein et al [20,21] reported a postoperative stroke or death rate of 7.5% in asymptomatic patients 75 years of age or older versus a rate of 1.8% in patients younger than 75 years. Similarly, the risk of postoperative MI associated with CEA was 6.6% in symptomatic patients 75 years of age or older versus 2.3% in patients younger than 75 years [20,21]. A NASCET subgroup analysis performed by Alamowitch et al [24] found that patients aged 75 years or older actually derived a greater benefit from CEA than those in younger age groups, however. The absolute risk reduction was 28.9% for patients aged 75 years or older (n = 71), 15.1% for those between 65 and 74 years (n = 285), and 9.7% for patients younger than 65 years of age (n = 303). Hence, although CEA definitely seems to benefit older individuals, it is reasonable to ask the question whether CAS could achieve similar benefits with a lower perioperative complication rate in older patients [20,25].

Congestive heart failure

Patients with congestive heart failure have a higher rate of perioperative stroke or death with CEA. In a multicenter review of patients undergoing CEA, Goldstein et al [20,21] found a perioperative stroke or death rate of 8.6% in patients with congestive heart failure as opposed to 2.3% in patients without this condition. CAS might be considered an alternative to CEA for this patient population.

Severe coronary artery disease

Coronary artery disease is one of the most important factors to consider when evaluating the perioperative risk of CEA. The coexistence of severe carotid artery stenosis and symptomatic coronary artery disease presents the physician with a management dilemma [22,26]. The surgical repair of one condition cannot be accomplished without a substantial risk of complication from the other. In an analysis of the NASCET results, a history of treatment of coronary artery disease was associated with a lower CEA complication rate when compared with previously undiagnosed coronary artery disease [27]. This incongruity may be the result of improved cardiac and general medical care in patients undergoing treatment for coronary artery disease, many of whom may not have previously received regular long-term medical care.

Adjunct to coronary bypass surgery

Significant carotid artery disease places patients who are undergoing coronary artery bypass grafting (CABG) at an increased risk for stroke, embolization (air or atheromatous), or both. Faggioli et al [28] reported on a series of 539 patients who underwent noninvasive evaluation (with carotid Doppler ultrasonography and ocular pneumoplethysmography) for the detection of carotid artery occlusive disease before undergoing CABG. They found that greater than 75% carotid artery stenosis was an independent predictor of stroke risk (odds ratio = 9.9) during CABG.

For patients with significant coexistent disease of the carotid and coronary arteries, there is little debate that revascularization is appropriate for both conditions; however, controversy exists regarding the timing of the procedures. Surgical options include the performance of a simultaneous procedure or a staged approach in which one procedure is performed several days after the other. Reports of combined CEA and CABG suggest that the risk of stroke or death ranges from 7.4% to 9.4%, which is roughly 1.5 to 2.0 times the independent risk of each operation [22]. In a multicenter review, the composite risk of stroke and death was higher in patients who had CEA performed in conjunction with CABG (18.7%) than in those who had CEA alone (2.1%) [21].

Conversely, patients who undergo CEA before CABG also have a higher risk of perioperative complications [26,29]. In this high-risk subgroup, avoiding a major operation or general anesthesia by performing angioplasty with stenting may represent a valid alternative to CEA [30]. The CEA guidelines published by the American Heart Association report a composite incidence of stroke, MI, and death of 16.4% for combined carotid and coronary operations, 26.2% for CEA proceeded by CABG, and 16.4% for CABG proceeded by CEA [31]. These high rates of complications would clearly offset the long-term benefit from secondary stroke prevention. At our center, revascularization with CAS was performed before planned CABG in 49 patients with concomitant coronary artery and carotid artery diseases (carotid artery stenosis >70%) [30]. The 30-day mortality rate for the combined procedure was 8%, and the stroke rate for the same period was 2%. These complication rates seem to be substantially lower than those associated with combined CABG and CEA or with CABG followed by CEA. In addition, no clinically significant recurrent stenosis was noted during a mean follow-up interval of 27 months. Although the numbers in this report are small, the data support the consideration of CAS as a valid alternative to CEA in patients with coexistent clinically significant coronary artery disease when CABG is needed (Fig. 1).

Anatomic features and tandem lesions

Anatomic variations may increase the technical difficulty of CEA and adversely affect the results. A high carotid bifurcation near the skull base, especially in a patient with a short or thick neck, or a long carotid artery stenosis that extends to the skull base can be difficult to expose surgically. Surgical dissection of the carotid artery in these cases can be difficult and, at times, extremely traumatic. These patients could be candidates for CAS (Fig. 2).

The presence of tandem lesions, where the distal lesion is more severe than the proximal lesion, was an exclusion criterion for the NASCET [8]. Among symptomatic patients with ipsilateral carotid siphon stenosis, the risk of postoperative stroke or death associated with CEA in a multicenter review of 1160 procedures was 13.9% versus

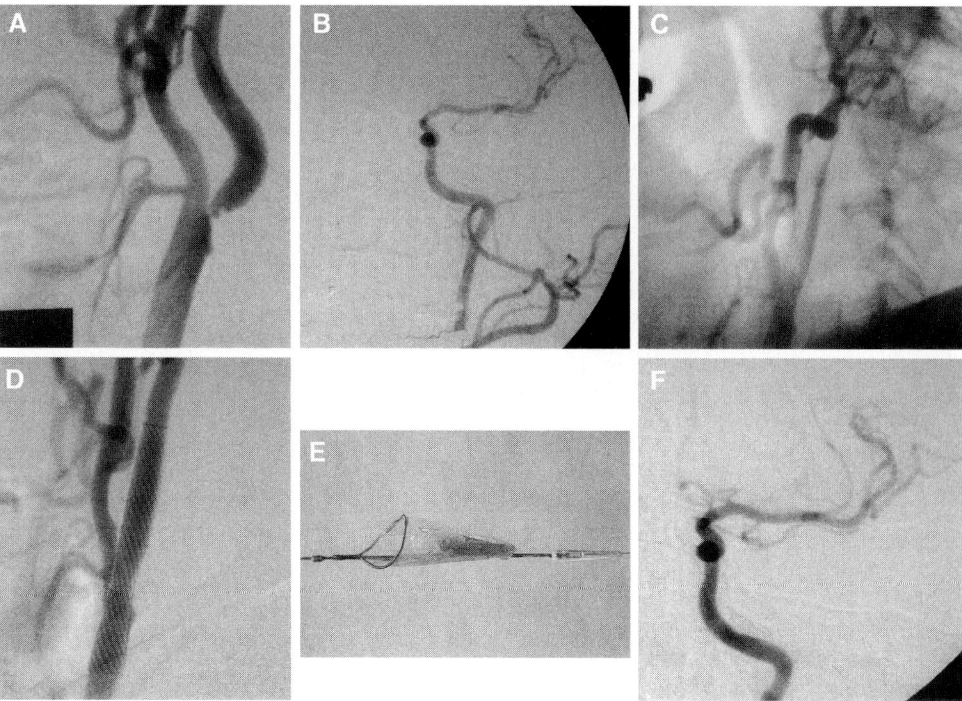

Fig. 1. This 58-year-old man presented with stable angina. Preoperative carotid Doppler ultrasound imaging demonstrated increased systolic velocities in the right carotid artery (419 cm/s). (*A*) Cerebral angiogram demonstrating the presence of severe stenosis involving the origin of the right internal carotid artery (ICA). (*B*) Intracranial image, frontal view, revealing lack of filling of the anterior cerebral artery, which suggests a flow-limiting effect of the cervical lesion or hypoplastic A1 segment of the anterior cerebral artery. Right carotid angioplasty with stenting was performed using a combination of an EPI FilterWire (Boston Scientific, Natick, Massachusetts) and a Wallstent (Boston Scientific). (*C*) After the poststent deployment angioplasty was performed, slowing of filling of the right ICA was noticed. This finding was attributed to the presence of debris in the filter. (*D*) After filter retrieval, normal flow was re-established in the right ICA. (*E*) Inspection of the filter demonstrated the presence of a large piece of plaque. (*F*) Intracranial image after cervical revascularization demonstrated flow augmentation with filling of the anterior cerebral artery territory in spite of the presence of a hypoplastic A1 segment.

7.9% in patients without distal stenosis [20]. Angioplasty was performed with and without stent placement in 11 patients with tandem lesions at our center [32]. The proximal lesion was considered to be the flow-limiting lesion and was the only lesion treated in 10 of these patients. In the remaining patient, both lesions were treated. No perioperative stroke or cardiac event or deaths occurred in this series. Hence, angioplasty with or without stenting could be considered a safe and viable alternative to CEA for patients with surgically inaccessible tandem carotid artery lesions.

Ipsilateral intraluminal thrombus

In a multicenter review of 1160 procedures, the risk of postoperative stroke or death with CEA was found to be 17.9% in symptomatic patients with ipsilateral intraluminal thrombus versus 8.1% in those without thrombus [20]. In a subgroup analysis of 53 patients enrolled in the NASCET who had intraluminal clot superimposed on atherosclerotic plaque identified by angiographic procedures, the 30-day risk of stroke was 10.7% in those randomly assigned to receive medical treatment and 12% in those who underwent CEA [33]. The high morbidity rate in this subgroup is related to the presence of fresh clot and the substantial risk of emboli dislodgment during surgical dissection of the carotid artery. Theoretically, CAS is an attractive alternative for these patients.

Contralateral occlusion

Patients with recent symptoms referable to severe carotid artery stenosis and coexistent contralateral carotid artery occlusion have a

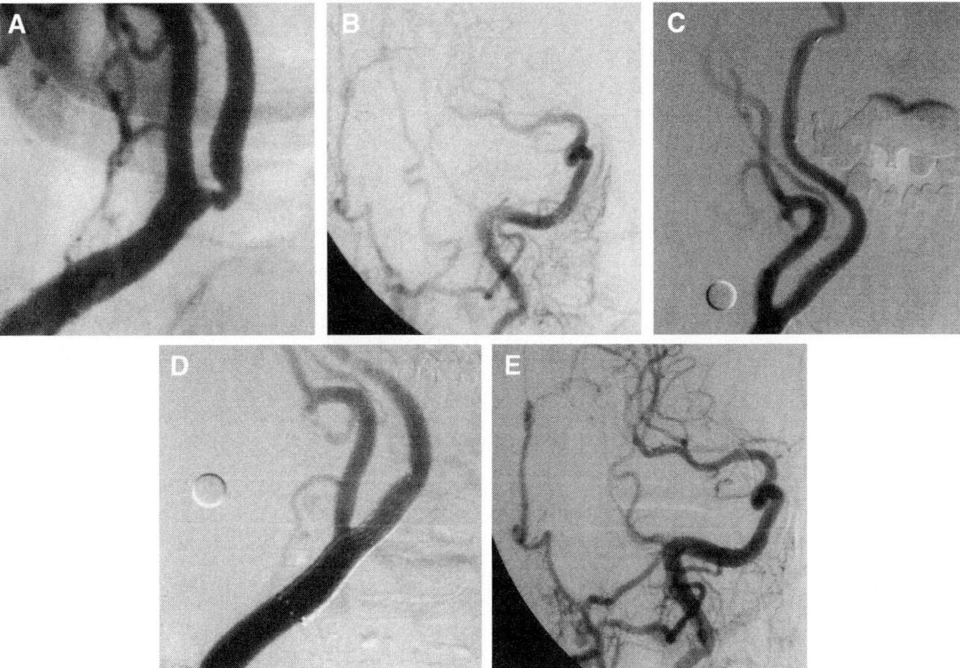

Fig. 2. This 86-year-old woman presented with progressively increasing Doppler ultrasound velocities in the right carotid artery. (*A*) Cerebral angiogram demonstrating the presence of a severe stenosis involving the origin of the right internal carotid artery (ICA). Because of her age (>80 years) and the fact that the lesion extended up to the body of C2, she was enrolled in the Carotid Revascularization with ev3 Arterial Technology Evolution (CREATE), a high-risk population carotid revascularization registry. (*B*) Intracranial image, frontal view, revealing delayed filling of ICA branches (when compared with the external carotid artery) as well as lack of filling of the anterior cerebral artery territory. (*C*) Right carotid artery stenting was performed using a combination of a Spider distal embolic protection device (ev3; Plymouth, Minnesota) and a Protégé Stent (ev3). Angiographic image after stenting demonstrates excellent revascularization of the vessel (*D*), with improvement of flow to the intracranial circulation (distal ICA branches filling before distal external carotid artery branches; anterior cerebral artery filling) (*E*).

high risk of ipsilateral ischemic stroke [34]. In the NASCET, the risk of ipsilateral stroke in medically treated patients with severe stenosis of the symptomatic carotid artery and occlusion of the contralateral carotid artery was 69.4% at 2 years [34]. Although CEA led to a significant reduction in stroke risk in this group, the perioperative risk of stroke or death in the presence of contralateral carotid artery occlusion was a high 14.3%. This increased risk may be related to the use of carotid artery shunting during CEA for patients with contralateral occlusions in up to 83% of cases [34]. In this subgroup, CAS represents a valid alternative to CEA, obviating the need for temporary occlusion in the presence of an already reduced cerebrovascular reserve. The preliminary combined results for phases 1 and 2 of the three-phase Acculink for Revascularization of Carotids in High Risk Patients (ARCHeR) trial showed a 30-day composite rate of stroke, MI, and death of 4.5% for the 66 patients with contralateral carotid occlusion included in this study [35].

Restenosis after carotid endarterectomy

Recurrent carotid artery stenosis is a potential problem after CEA (Fig. 3) [36]. Technically, a repeat operation is far more challenging than the initial procedure because of scarring around the arteries, friability of the recurrent plaque, and the necessity for more complex anastomosis techniques. Among 82 patients undergoing operations for recurrent carotid stenosis at the Mayo Clinic, the composite rate of major morbidity and mortality was 10.8%, a rate that was five times the risk associated with primary CEA at the same institution [36]. AbuRahma et al [37] found an increased risk of cerebral ischemic events associated with CEA for recurrent stenosis. The 30-day rates of

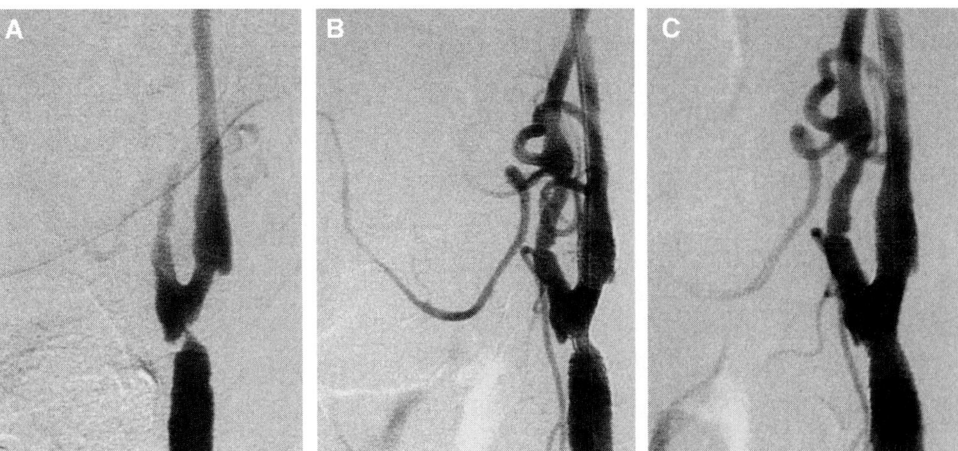

Fig. 3. This 57-year-old man presented with symptomatic recurrent stenosis of the left cervical carotid artery 2 years after endarterectomy. (*A*) Diagnostic cerebral angiogram demonstrating the presence of severe stenosis involving the distal segment of the left common carotid artery just proximal to the bifurcation. Left carotid artery stent placement with adjunctive distal embolic protection (EPI FilterWire; Boston Scientific Embolic Protection, San Carlos, California) was successfully performed. (*B*) Position of the filter after deployment of the stent (Precise Rx; Cordis, Miami Lakes, Florida). (*C*) Improvement in vessel diameter after poststent deployment angioplasty.

perioperative stroke and transient ischemic attacks (TIAs) were 4.8% and 4%, respectively, in the reoperation group, as compared with 0.8% and 1%, respectively, in the primary endarterectomy group. They also found a high rate (17%) of cranial nerve palsy with reoperation. In a review of the results of CAS performed at our center in a similar group of 18 patients with postendarterectomy recurrent carotid stenosis, only a single case of TIA and no perioperative stroke were identified [38]. The preliminary combined results of the ARCHeR 1 and 2 trials suggest that CAS is a technically feasible alternative to surgical re-exploration for patients with recurrent carotid artery stenosis [35]. The 30-day composite rate of stroke, MI, and death for the 141 patients receiving treatment with CAS for postendarterectomy recurrent stenosis in this study was 0.7%.

Radiation-induced carotid stenosis

Accelerated radiation-induced carotid stenosis is another factor that increases the risk of perioperative complications, primarily because of the technical pitfalls associated with a surgical approach. The presence of a long lesion, lack of well-defined dissection planes, and scarring around the vessels make the surgery more difficult [39,40], exposing these patients to a higher risk of wound infections and cranial nerve palsies. Carotid angioplasty and stent placement could provide a more effective method for treatment of carotid stenosis associated with radiation.

Carotid angioplasty and stenting

Background and preliminary results

Two major issues compelled the development of CAS: the need for a better therapeutic option for high-risk patients (as described previously) and the wave of minimally invasive surgery. After its introduction approximately 20 years ago by such pioneers as Kerber et al [41], Mathias et al [42], and Mullan et al [43], the field of endovascular treatment of carotid occlusive disease remained stationary, whereas the field of coronary and peripheral percutaneous transluminal angioplasty was developing at a rapid pace. In a review of the literature published up to 1996, Kachel [44] found only 523 carotid angioplasty procedures performed from 1980 to 1995.

Publication of the results obtained with stent-assisted balloon angioplasty in the coronary literature undoubtedly provided a new impetus for endovascular treatment of carotid artery occlusive disease [45] and prompted the performance of studies in which carotid angioplasty with or without stenting and CEA were compared. The purported advantages of stent placement over simple angioplasty included avoidance of plaque dislodgment, intimal dissection, and late recurrent stenosis as well as diminution of vessel recoil.

The Carotid and Vertebral Artery Transluminal Angioplasty Study (CAVATAS), the results of which were published in 2001, was the first randomized comparison of endovascular versus surgical treatment in patients with carotid artery stenosis [46]. Between March 1992 and July 1997, patients from 22 centers in Europe, Australia, and Canada were randomly assigned to endovascular treatment (n = 251) or CEA (n = 253). Stents suitable for use in the carotid arteries were developed during the course of the study. Despite the fact that the use of a stent in this trial was approved from 1994 onward, only 55 (26%) of the patients in the endovascular treatment group received a stent (the remainder received balloon angioplasty alone). Similar rates of stroke and death were reported for endovascular and surgical treatment. The number of recurrent strokes, with a mean follow-up period of approximately 2 years, was also similar in both groups. The 8-year follow-up report, which was presented in 2002, showed equivalent efficacy in stroke prevention for both therapeutic options [47].

Several other groups have reported on the effectiveness, safety, and durability of CAS. Roubin et al [12], in a review of their 5-year experience with a series of 528 consecutive patients undergoing CAS, described a 30-day major stroke or death rate of 2.6%. In 1996, Gil-Peralta et al [48] reported a series of 85 patients who underwent percutaneous angioplasty for symptomatic carotid artery stenosis over the course of a 4-year period. No deaths occurred within 30 days after the procedure, and the major morbidity rate at 30 days was 4.9%. Our group [49] has reported a 30-day major stroke or death rate of 5% in 80 high-risk patients who were considered ineligible for the NASCET according to the exclusion criteria of that study.

Distal embolic protection (DEP), initially introduced by Theron et al [50], is considered to be an important advance in the endovascular treatment of carotid occlusive disease. The rationale for using this technique is based on the concept that an embolic shower released from carotid plaque during CAS causes neurologic deficits in the periprocedural period [50]. Preliminary studies have demonstrated the potential benefit of DEP. Jaeger et al [51] reported the occurrence of cerebral ischemia (detected by diffusion-weighted MRI) in 29% (20 of 70) of patients undergoing CAS without cerebral embolic protection. This rate decreased to 7.1% with the use of embolic protection devices [52]. Whitlow et al [53] reported a multicenter experience in which a balloon device (PercuSurge GuardWire; PercuSurge, Sunnyvale, California) was used during CAS. Among the 75 patients treated with this device, no single case of periprocedural death or major stroke was noted.

The Carotid Revascularization Using Endarterectomy or Stent Systems (CARESS) Trial is a multicenter, prospective, nonrandomized clinical trial sponsored by the International Society for Endovascular Specialists (ISES) in collaboration with industry, the US Food and Drug Administration (FDA), and the Centers for Medicare and Medical Services [54]. This trial was designed as an equivalence cohort study to determine whether the rate of stroke or death after CAS with DEP is comparable with that for CEA. Patients with 50% or greater symptomatic carotid stenosis or 75% or greater asymptomatic carotid stenosis were enrolled in this trial. The population represented a broad-risk population typical of those treated in a general vascular practice. The CEA/CAS enrollment ratio at each clinical site was designed to be 2:1. The primary end point for comparison was the 30-day death and stroke rate. In phase 1 of this trial, 439 patients were enrolled from 14 clinical sites (254 CEA patients and 143 CAS patients; ratio of 1.8:1). Overall, 68% of the patients treated were asymptomatic, with a similar distribution in each group. The medical history before treatment was similar in both groups, with the exception of a more frequent history of previous CEA in the CAS group (30% versus 11% in the CEA group). The MI, stroke, and death rates were 0.8%, 2.4%, and 0.4%, respectively, in the CEA group and 0%, 2.1%, and 0%, respectively, in the CAS group. Statistically, the results of this study represented equivalence between the two revascularization modalities.

The Stent and Angioplasty with Protection for Patients at High Risk for Endarterectomy (SAPPHIRE) trial also demonstrated the benefit of DEP [55]. Patients from 29 centers in the United States were enrolled in this trial. Eligible study patients were those who were asymptomatic with greater than 80% stenosis (by Doppler ultrasound) or symptomatic with greater than 50% stenosis plus at least one feature that would place them at high risk for CEA (older than 80 years of age, congestive heart failure, severe chronic obstructive pulmonary disease, postendarterectomy recurrent carotid stenosis, previous radiation therapy, or previous radical neck surgery). Eligible patients were then screened by a team that included a vascular surgeon, an interventionist, and a neurologist. Consensus that patients were good candidates for either procedure was required before randomization; those rejected as candidates for surgery underwent stenting and were included in a stent registry, whereas those rejected for stenting had surgery and were included in a surgical registry. At the end of the enrollment period in June 2002, 409 patients had been included in the stenting registry (CEA risk considered excessively high) and 7 patients in the surgical registry (CAS risk deemed excessive). A total of 307 patients were randomized: 156 to CAS and 151 to CEA. The devices used for CAS in this trial were the PRECISE nitinol stent (Johnson & Johnson, Warren, New Jersey) and the AngioGuard (Johnson & Johnson) distal protection device. The preliminary results have been presented but not published [56,57]. The 30-day composite stroke and death rate was similar for both groups (4.5% for CAS group versus 6.6% for CEA group). When the rate of MI was taken into consideration, the CAS group did better, with a major adverse cardiovascular event (MACE) rate of 5.8%, compared with a 12.6% MACE rate in the CEA group. The 1-year follow-up data for this study demonstrated overall MACE rates of 11.9% for the CAS group and 19.9% for the CEA group. At 1 year of follow-up, the incidence of major ipsilateral stroke was significantly higher in the CEA group (3.3%) versus the CAS group (0%). Regarding ipsilateral minor stroke, there was a trend toward more minor strokes in the CAS group (3.8% in the CAS group versus 2% in the CEA group; $P = 0.5$) [57].

The 30-day results of all three phases of the ARCHeR trial were presented as well as the 1-year follow-up data for phases 1 and 2 of the ARCHeR trial [35]. This trial included a total enrollment of 581 patients at 48 sites in the Unite States, Europe, and South America. Eligibility criteria included carotid artery stenosis that was asymptomatic and greater than 80% (by angiography) or symptomatic and greater than 50%. High-risk factors established for inclusion in this trial were the presence of two or more of the following criteria: (1) two or more coronary vessels with 70% or greater stenosis, (2) MI within 30 days, (3) CABG or valve surgery within 30 days, (4) unstable angina, and (5) contralateral carotid occlusion as well as one or more of the following criteria: (1) ejection fraction less than 30% or New York Heart Association functional class III or greater, (2) forced expiratory volume in the first second (FEV_1) less than 30% (predicted), (3) dialysis-dependent renal failure, (4) uncontrolled diabetes, (5) postendarterectomy recurrent stenosis, (6) history of radical neck surgery or radiation therapy, (7) surgically inaccessible lesion, (8) spinal immobility, (9) tracheostomy stoma, and (10) contralateral laryngeal nerve paralysis. Eligible patients were assessed by an independent neurologist before enrollment and throughout the CAS follow-up period. Enrollment in the trial included 158, 278, and 145 patients in phases 1, 2, and 3 of the trial, respectively. In phase 1 of the ARCHeR trial, patients were treated with use of the Acculink Stent (Guidant/Advanced Cardiovascular Systems, Menlo Park, California) alone. In phase 2 of the ARCHeR trial, patients were treated with a combination of the stent and the AccunetFilter (Guidant) for DEP. In phase 3 of the ARCHeR trial, next-generation rapid-exchange versions of the filter and stent were used. The ARCHeR trial results are summarized in Table 1 [58]. Further data analysis will be possible after the results of the study have been published.

The 30-day results of the Boston Scientific EPI: A Carotid Stenting Trial for High-Risk Surgical Patients (BEACH) were also recently presented and are provided in Table 1. In this trial, devices used were the EPI FilterWire EZ (Boston Scientific, Fremont, California) as DEP and the monorail Wallstent (Boston Scientific). The BEACH is a single-arm, prospective, nonrandomized trial in which 747 patients from 47 sites across the United States were enrolled. The high-risk inclusion criteria for the study population were similar to those described previously for the SAPPHIRE and ARCHeR studies.

Several other carotid stent registries are being maintained in the United States (Table 2). One randomized controlled trial currently under way is the Carotid Revascularization Endarterectomy versus Stent Trial (CREST), which is jointly sponsored by the National Institutes of Health and Guidant Corporation (Indianapolis, Indiana). The results of CREST and other carotid stent studies are expected to provide the level I evidence necessary for FDA approval for CAS as an optimal technique for carotid revascularization.

Endovascular management protocol and procedural technique

The technique of CAS varies slightly for each case depending on the clinical situation. The following is a description of the management

Table 1
Summary of single-arm registry results already presented

	ARCHeR 1 (n = 158)	ARCHeR 2 (n = 278)	ARCHeR 3 (n = 145)	BEACH
Major stroke at 30 days	1.9%	1.4%	1.4%	1%
Minor stroke at 30 days	2.5%	4.3%	4.8%	2.5% (1.9% ipsilateral)
MI at 30 days	2.5%	2.9%	0.7%	0.8%
Stroke-related death at 30 days	0.6%	0.7%	0	1.5% (all deaths)
Non–stroke-related death at 30 days	1.9%	1.4%	1.4%	
Major stroke from day 31 to 1 year	0	0.3%	N/A	Spring 2005
Minor ipsilateral stroke from day 31 to 1 year	0.6%	1%	N/A	Spring 2005
Stroke-related death from day 31 to 1 year	0	0	N/A	Spring 2005

Abbreviations: ARCHeR, Acculink for Revascularization of Carotids in High Risk Patients; ARCHeR 1, stent alone; ARCHeR 2, stent plus distal embolic protection; ARCHeR 3, rapid exchange version of stent and filter; BEACH, Boston Scientific EPI: A Carotid Stenting Trial for High Risk Surgical Patients; MI myocardial infarction; N/A, not available.

protocol and procedural technique used for most patients at our center.

Medical management

Endovascular procedures carry an inherent risk of intimal injury and subsequent thrombosis and vessel occlusion. Moreover, all stents are thrombogenic [59]. Therefore, patient preparation for stenting hinges on adequate administration of antiplatelet and anticoagulation therapies. Consideration must be given not only to the selection and dosing of antithrombotic medications but to minimizing the potential for associated hemorrhagic complications. Most information about treatment with these medications must be obtained from the cardiac literature, because clinical data in the neurosurgical literature are limited. Aspirin is a cyclooxygenase-1 inhibitor that irreversibly inhibits platelet aggregation but does not impede platelet adhesion or platelet-activated mitogenic activity. Clopidogrel is a thienopyridine derivative with potent antiplatelet action that inhibits adenosine phosphate–induced platelet aggregation. This drug works synergistically with aspirin, and evidence from the cardiac literature supports the use of combination antiplatelet regimens [60]. Clopidogrel, in combination with aspirin, has become the standard treatment for patients undergoing coronary angioplasty and stenting. When possible, patients are pretreated with aspirin (325 mg daily) and clopidogrel (75 mg daily) for at least 3 days before CAS or are given a loading dose of clopidogrel (300–600 mg) early on the day of the procedure.

For most stenting procedures, an intravenous bolus dose of heparin (50–75 U/kg) is administered after catheterization of the common carotid artery (CCA). Saline solutions used for irrigation of the catheters are prepared with heparin (1 U/mL), and catheter systems are flushed continuously with this solution. The activated coagulation time (ACT) is maintained in the range of 250 to 300 seconds for the duration of the procedure.

The use of platelet glycoprotein (GP) IIb-IIIa inhibitors (eg, abciximab, eptifibatide) in conjunction with CAS is controversial. These agents block the final common pathway of platelet aggregation by preventing the binding of fibrinogen to platelets and are the most potent of the antiplatelet drugs [61]. Our preliminary experience suggests that the administration of GP IIb-IIIa inhibitors places patients with chronic cerebral ischemia at an elevated risk of intracranial hemorrhage; therefore, such agents should be reserved for patients who experience thromboembolic complications during or soon after the procedure [61]. Abciximab can be given as an initial loading dose at 0.25 mg/kg immediately before the procedure is performed, followed by a 12-hour intravenous infusion at a rate of 10 μg/min. Eptifibatide may be administered as a loading dose at 180 μg/kg, followed by a 20- to 24-hour infusion at 0.5 to 2 mcg/kg. When the use of GP IIb-IIIa inhibition is recommended after the procedure, we suggest obtaining a CT scan before beginning the infusion to check for intracerebral hemorrhage, which would contraindicate the administration of these agents. In our daily practice, the use of such agents is reserved for the treatment of thromboembolic complications; we do not recommend the routine periprocedural administration of these agents.

Bradycardia occurs occasionally during angioplasty, particularly when the plaque involves the

Table 2
Carotid angioplasty and stenting trials

Study (manufacturer or sponsor)	Design	Clinical characteristics and percentage of stenosis	Stent	Distal protection device
ARCHeR 3 (Guidant)	Prospective single-arm registry (1-year follow-up results to be presented)	High risk Asymptomatic >80% Symptomatic >50%	Acculink RX	Accunet RX
BEACH (Boston Scientific)	Prospective single-arm registry (1-year follow-up results to be presented)	High risk Asymptomatic >80% Symptomatic >50%	Monorail Wallstent	EPI FilterWire EZ
CABERNET (Boston Scientific and EndoTex)	Prospective single-arm registry	High risk Asymptomatic >60% Symptomatic >50%	NexStent	EPI FilterWire
CARESS (NIH) (excludes CREST patients)	Prospective double-arm registry, physician chooses treatment, 2:1 CEA to CAS ratio	Asymptomatic >75% Symptomatic >50%	Physician's choice	Physician's choice
CREST (NIH, Guidant)	Randomized trial	Symptomatic >50%	Acculink	Accunet
MAVErIC 2 (Medtronic AVE)	Prospective single-arm registry	High risk Asymptomatic >80% Symptomatic >50%	Medtronic AVE Self-Expanding Stent System	PercuSurge
SECURITY (Perclose)	Prospective single-arm registry	High risk Asymptomatic >80% Symptomatic >50%	X-Act	NeuroShield
CREATE (ev3)	Prospective single-arm registry	High risk Asymptomatic >70% Symptomatic >50%	Protégé	Spider

Abbreviations: ARCHeR 3, Acculink for Revascularization of Carotids in High Risk Patients; BEACH, Boston Scientific EPI: A Carotid Stent for High Risk Surgical Patients; CAS, carotid artery angioplasty with stenting; CABERNET, Carotid Artery Revascularization Using Boston Scientific EPI FilterWire and EndoTex Stent; CARESS, Carotid Revascularization with Endarterectomy or Stenting Systems; CEA, carotid endarterectomy; CREATE, Carotid Revascularization with ev3 Arterial Technology Evolution; CREST, Carotid Revascularization Endarterectomy versus. Stent Trial; MAVErIC 2, Evaluation of the Medtronic AVE Self-Expanding Carotid Stent System with Distal Protection in the Treatment of Carotid Stenosis; NIH, National Institutes of Health; SECURITY, Study to Evaluate the Neuroshield Bare Wire Cerebral Protection System and X-Act Stent in Patients at High Risk for Carotid Endarterectomy.

Adapted from Levy EI, Kim SH, Bendok BR, Boulos AS, Xavier AR, Yahia AM, et al. Interventional neuroradiologic therapy. In: Mohr JP, Choi DW, Grotta JC, Weir B, Wolf PA, editors. Stroke: pathophysiology, diagnosis, and management. 4th edition. New York: Churchill Livingston; 2004. p. 1497; with permission.

carotid sinus. Atropine and a prepared dopamine solution are kept available should significant bradycardia and hypotension occur. Medical management of bradycardia during angioplasty is usually sufficient.

After stent placement, heparin therapy is generally discontinued but not reversed with protamine. In some situations, such as when an angiographically documented dissection or thrombosis is present, continued infusion of heparin is appropriate to maintain the activated prothrombin time 1.5 to 2.3 times the baseline value. Aspirin (325 mg daily) and clopidogrel (75 mg daily) are administered for at least 4 weeks after the procedure to allow for complete endothelialization of the stent [62]. Aspirin is continued indefinitely.

Preparation for the procedure

The procedure is performed in an angiography suite with biplane digital subtraction and fluoroscopic imaging capabilities. The patient is kept awake, with local anesthesia and sedatives administered to permit continuous neurologic assessment. Dorsalis pedis and posterior tibialis pulses are assessed and marked for later reference, a practice that is particularly important in patients with coexistent peripheral vascular disease. A Foley catheter and two peripheral intravenous lines are placed. Oxygen saturation, cardiac rhythm, and blood pressure are monitored throughout the procedure.

Diagnostic angiogram

A 5-French sheath is placed in the right femoral artery, and a three-vessel diagnostic angiogram is obtained (if not previously performed) using a 5-French Simmons-2 or angled glide catheter. An intracranial angiogram with the injection of contrast material into the ipsilateral CCA is necessary for later comparison should intracranial thromboembolism be suspected after angioplasty. After a working projection image of the target vessel has been obtained, measurements are made of the vessel diameter proximal and distal to the lesion, the length of the lesion, and the severity of the stenosis (using the NASCET method [8]).

Vascular access

As previously mentioned, the loading dose of heparin is administered before the guide catheter is placed within the CCA. When the ACT reaches at least 250 seconds, the diagnostic catheter is positioned in the CCA and is used to advance a 0.035 in, 300 cm long stiff glide wire into the distal external carotid artery (ECA). In the setting of stenosis or occlusion of the ECA, an Amplatz exchange "J" wire (Cook, Bloomington, Indiana) is placed in the distal CCA and used to provide support for the guide sheath. With the stiff wire in position, the diagnostic catheter is removed as well as the femoral artery sheath. A 6-French, 90 cm guide sheath (Cook) is then advanced over the wire and placed just proximal to the carotid bifurcation. For those patients who have undergone complete diagnostic cerebral angiography, a combination of a 6-French, 90 cm shuttle select catheter (Cook) and a 6.5-French, head-hunter, 125 cm shuttle slip-catheter (Cook) is used. In these cases, the shuttle is introduced primarily in the femoral artery over a 0.035 in wire (this wire can be regular, stiff, or superstiff) and parked in the descending aorta. The inner obturator and wire are removed. The head-hunter shuttle slip-catheter is then advanced into the system, and the target vessel is catheterized. At this point, the wire (a 035 in, 300 cm long stiff glide or an Amplatz exchange "J" wire, depending on the status of the ECA) is advanced, followed by the slip-catheter and shuttle. The position and integrity of the target vessel as well as those of the distal ECA territory after manipulation with the exchange wire are assessed by angiography.

Carotid angioplasty with stenting procedure

Once the guide catheter is in place, we proceed with the following steps of the CAS procedure. First, the DEP device is positioned. If necessary, prestent deployment angioplasty is performed to enlarge the stenotic region sufficiently to permit passage of the stent. The stent is then deployed, after which time, poststent deployment angioplasty is done to remodel and expand the stent fully. Finally, the DEP is retrieved. After each step, high-resolution biplanar angiograms are obtained and neurologic examinations are performed to allow for prompt recognition of any changes from the patient's baseline status.

Distal embolic protection device placement. There are three classes of devices used for DEP: filtration, balloon occlusion, and flow reversal. Retrievable filters designed to collect debris during CAS are placed distal to the stenotic region without interrupting flow within the ICA. Examples of filtration devices include the EPI FilterWire (Boston Scientific Embolic Protection, San Carlos, California), Accunet (Guidant Corp.), AngioGuard (Cordis, Miami Lakes, Florida), Mednova (Abbott Laboratories, Abbott Park, Illinois), and Spider (ev3, Plymouth, Minnesota). Balloon occlusion techniques involve inflation of a balloon and interruption of flow in the ICA distal to the stenosis for the duration of the stenting procedure. An example of a balloon occlusion DEP device is the PercuSurge balloon. The flow-reversal technique involves the placement of balloons in the ECA and CCA to interrupt flow in these vessels and to cause retrograde flow in the ICA to prevent embolization into the intracranial circulation [63].

After the guide catheter is positioned, a DEP device (the authors' preference is to use a retrievable filter) mounted on a 0.014 in microguidewire is carefully guided across the stenotic region using a biplanar road-mapping technique. When crossing the lesion, the combination of turning and slightly pushing the device is preferred rather than simply pushing it. Ideally, the device should be placed in a relatively straight segment of the distal ICA and then deployed. Once the DEP device is deployed, the operator should assess the apposition of the device to the vessel wall to obtain more effective embolic containment.

Predilation angioplasty. With lower grade lesions, predilation angioplasty may not be necessary. The selection of a predilation angioplasty balloon is based on the dimensions of the lesion. The balloon must be long enough to cover the entire length of the lesion. The inflation diameter should be undersized to avoid overinflation and to open the artery just enough to allow passage of the stent. After an angiogram of the cervical carotid artery is obtained with the DEP device in place, the angioplasty balloon is advanced and centered on the lesion. The balloon is inflated to the manufacturer's recommended nominal pressure for several seconds and then deflated. The blood pressure cuff is set at a continuous mode during angioplasty to allow rapid sequential measurement of blood pressure should bradycardia and hypotension occur.

Stent placement. Most stents currently in use for CAS are self-expanding stents, such as the Wallstent, Acculink stent, and Precise stent (Cordis). The Wallstent is composed of stainless steel, and the Acculink and Precise stents are made of nitinol, a nickel and titanium alloy. Selection of the stent is determined by the length of the lesion and the normal diameter of the CCA. The stent should be oversized 1 to 2 mm more than the normal arterial caliber and should cover the lesion completely. At diameters less than full expansion, nitinol stents exert a chronic outward radial force that serves to maintain apposition of the stent to the vessel wall after deployment. Often, the stent extends from the CCA into the ICA, crossing the bifurcation and origin of the ECA; in these cases, the stent should be sized according to the larger caliber of the CCA. Although rare, when dealing with cases of contralateral ECA occlusion, one should be prepared for the potential need for revascularization of the ipsilateral ECA if occlusion occurs after stent deployment and poststent angioplasty.

When using a retrievable filter for distal protection, the position of the stent should be angiographically verified before the stent is deployed. The use of distal balloon occlusion precludes vessel assessment. In each case, anatomic landmarks should be carefully analyzed before the stent is deployed to ensure precise positioning of the stent.

Postdilation angioplasty. After the stent is in place, poststent deployment angioplasty is performed. Balloon selection is based on the diameter of the ICA. The balloon should be kept within the segment of stented artery during the angioplasty to avoid the risk of vessel dissection, especially at the distal ICA. Slow balloon inflation can be used on those patients with known overresponsive carotid baroreceptors.

Distal embolic protection device retrieval. After completing the poststent deployment angioplasty, cervical and intracranial images are obtained to assess target vessel patency and to exclude evidence of any major intracranial vessel occlusion. Once this is done, the DEP device is withdrawn, and a final series of cervical carotid and intracranial circulation angiograms are obtained.

The course of the DEP retrieval sheath through the segment of stented vessel should be carefully observed. The retrieval catheter can get caught on the stent struts protruding into the vessel lumen. This is especially important when using stents with an open-cell design. If this occurs, several options are available. Bringing the guide sheath closer to the stent may provide enough support to allow the stent to be crossed with the retrieval sheath. An angled, 4-French, 100 cm long diagnostic catheter can be used. Substituting the retrieval sheath for this catheter may allow the operator to navigate its tip around the difficult stent segment. Another option is the use of an angioplasty balloon with a 0.035 in compatible inner lumen, which would allow capture of the DEP device. Advancing the balloon into the difficult segment with partial inflation pushes the stent struts against the vessel wall, permitting further advancement of the balloon and subsequent retrieval of the device.

When distal balloon occlusion is used for DEP, 60 mL of blood is aspirated before the balloon is deflated. The aspiration is accomplished by use of an export catheter placed just proximal to the balloon.

Access site closure

After obtaining an angiogram of the femoral entry vessel, the decision to proceed with percutaneous closure is made. If the entry point of the sheath is above the bifurcation of the common femoral artery and the vessel is free of major atherosclerotic disease, the catheter systems and femoral sheath are removed, and a percutaneous closure device, such as the Perclose (Redwood City, California) or AngioSeal (St. Jude Medical, Minnetonka, Minnesota), is used. Otherwise, the guide sheath is exchanged for a 7-French, 15 cm sheath, which is left in place and removed when the ACT has normalized.

Periprocedural management and discharge plan

After the procedure, the patient is admitted to the intensive care unit for monitoring overnight. Hourly neurologic assessments and close surveillance of hemodynamic parameters are important. A systolic blood pressure of 110 to 160 mm Hg is maintained. A baseline carotid Doppler ultrasound study is obtained within 24 hours of the procedure to assess vessel patency and to provide a reference for further Doppler ultrasound evaluations. Most patients are discharged to home on the day after the procedure. As previously mentioned, aspirin and clopidogrel are prescribed.

Limitations of carotid angioplasty with stenting

Several anatomic features can make CAS difficult to undertake. Endovascular access to the carotid system can be problematic in patients with severe peripheral vascular disease that affects the iliac or femoral arteries and in those with a bovine configuration to the aortic arch, a tortuous aortic arch, or an ectatic CCA. Near-complete occlusion of the carotid artery (string sign) can impair safe passage of a DEP device, and a tortuous distal cervical ICA can make deployment of the device difficult. Also, because antiplatelet therapy is strongly recommended, an inability to tolerate these agents might be considered a relative contraindication to carotid stent placement.

Two major concerns exist regarding the durability of carotid revascularization with CAS: the efficacy of CAS in preventing long-term recurrence of ischemic events and the occurrence of in-stent stenosis after CAS. As previously mentioned, the 8-year follow-up results of the CAVATAS trial showed 90.8% of patients with no clinical ipsilateral ischemic events [47]. Few accounts exist of the restenosis rates after stenting. In the CAVATAS trial, severe (70%–90%) restenosis was found in 14% of patients treated with angioplasty with or without stenting (only 26% of patients in the endovascular group in that study received stents versus 4% of those receiving surgery) [46]. In a recent retrospective report of 183 patients, Doppler ultrasound results of greater than 80% recurrent stenosis (confirmed by angiographic evidence) after stent placement were found in 5.2% of the lesions stented, with restenosis after CEA representing the main risk factor for in-stent stenosis [64]. Similarly, we found a 5% rate of significant (symptomatic or >80%) in-stent stenosis (by digital subtraction angiography) in our series of 141 patients [65]. To determine the rate of hemodynamically significant recurrent carotid stenosis after stent-assisted angioplasty (in-stent stenosis) for carotid occlusive disease, we analyzed Doppler ultrasound data that had been prospectively collected from October 1998 to September 2002 for patients enrolled in carotid stent trials at our center. Patients included in this analysis were those with at least 6 months of follow-up with serial Doppler studies or elevated in-stent velocities (> 300 cm/s) demonstrated on postprocedural Doppler imaging. Hemodynamically significant recurrent stenosis (≥80%) was determined using the following Doppler ultrasound criteria: peak in-stent systolic velocity greater than or equal to 330 cm/s, peak in-stent diastolic velocity greater than or equal to 130 cm/s, and peak ICA-to-CCA velocity ratio greater than or equal to 3.8. Follow-up studies were obtained at approximate fixed intervals of 1 day, 1 month, 6 months, and yearly. Angiography was performed for patients with recurrent symptoms, Doppler ultrasound evidence of hemodynamically significant stenosis, or both. Retreatment was performed in patients who were symptomatic, had angiographic evidence of severe (≥80%) recurrent stenosis, or both. In our study, stents were implanted in 142 vessels in 138 patients (all but 5 were considered to be high-risk surgical candidates); 25 patients were subsequently lost to follow-up. For the remaining 112 patients (117 vessels), the mean Doppler follow-up duration was 16.42 ± 10.58 months (range: 4–49 months). Using one or more of the Doppler ultrasound criteria, greater than or equal to 80% in-stent stenosis was detected in 6 (5%) patients. Eight patients underwent repeat angiography. Six patients (3 of whom were symptomatic) required repeat intervention (4 required angioplasty alone, 1 required conventional angioplasty plus Cutting-Balloon [Boston Scientific Internventional Technologies, San Diego, California] angioplasty, and 1 required stent-assisted angioplasty). Thus, we showed that in a subset of primarily high-risk surgical candidates treated with stent-assisted angioplasty, hemodynamically significant restenosis rates are comparable with published rates of restenosis after surgery and that the treatment of recurrent stenosis in this limited number of patients incurred no periprocedural neurologic morbidity.

In reports evaluating recurrent carotid stenosis after angioplasty alone, Kachel [44,66] found no restenosis in his series of 57 patients, whereas Higashida et al [67] found a 5.5% incidence of restenosis in a series of 100 carotid angioplasties (follow-up period: 3 months to 7 years). In a report by Yadav et al [13] describing patients treated with stent-assisted angioplasty for postoperative restenosis, no stenosis recurred in 8 of 22 patients who returned for follow-up angiography at 6 months. Perhaps the largest collection of patients from whom restenosis rates are available includes the global carotid stent registry of 12,392 procedures [68]. In this registry, the restenosis rates after carotid stenting were 2.7%, 2.6%, and 2.4% at 1, 2, and 3 years, respectively.

Summary

Carotid angioplasty with stent placement seems to be safer than CEA for some patients in the high-risk population. Studies are underway to assess the efficacy and long-term durability of this procedure (with distal protection) in NASCET- and ACAS-eligible populations.

Acknowledgment

We thank Paul H. Dressel for preparation of the illustrations.

References

[1] American Heart Association. Heart disease and stroke statistics—2004 update. Dallas: American Heart Association; 2003.

[2] Bonita R. Epidemiology of stroke. Lancet 1992;339: 342–4.

[3] Matchar DB. Cost of stroke. Stroke Clinical Update 2002;5:9–12.

[4] Taylor TN, Davis PH, Torner JC. Projected number of strokes by subtype in the year 2050 in the United States [abstract]. Stroke 1998;29:322.

[5] Dyken ML. Stroke risk factors. In: Norris JW, Hachinski VC, editors. Prevention of stroke. New York: Springer-Verlag; 1991. p. 83–102.

[6] DeBakey ME. Carotid endarterectomy revisited. J Endovasc Surg 1996;3:4.

[7] Pokras R, Dyken ML. Dramatic changes in the performance of endarterectomy for diseases of the extracranial arteries of the head. Stroke 1988;19: 1289–90.

[8] North American Symptomatic Carotid Endarterectomy Trial Collaborators. Beneficial effect of carotid endarterectomy in symptomatic patients with high-grade carotid stenosis. N Engl J Med 1991;325: 445–53.

[9] Executive Committee for the Asymptomatic Carotid Atherosclerosis Study. Endarterectomy for asymptomatic carotid artery stenosis. JAMA 1995;273: 1421–8.

[10] European Carotid Surgery Trialists' Collaborative Group. MRC European Carotid Surgery Trial: interim results for symptomatic patients with severe (70–99%) or with mild (0–29%) carotid stenosis. Lancet 1991;337:1235–43.

[11] Ouriel K, Hertzer NR, Beven EG, et al. Preprocedural risk stratification: identifying an appropriate population for carotid stenting. J Vasc Surg 2001; 33:728–32.

[12] Roubin GS, New G, Iyer SS, et al. Immediate and late clinical outcomes of carotid artery stenting in patients with symptomatic and asymptomatic carotid artery stenosis: a 5-year prospective analysis. Circulation 2001;103:532–7.

[13] Yadav JS, Roubin GS, Iyer S, et al. Elective stenting of the extracranial carotid arteries. Circulation 1997; 95:376–81.

[14] Halliday A, Mansfield A, Marro J, et al. Prevention of disabling and fatal strokes by successful carotid endarterectomy in patients without recent neurological symptoms: randomised controlled trial. Lancet 2004;363:1491–502.

[15] Barnett HJ, Taylor DW, Eliasziw M, et al. Benefit of carotid endarterectomy in patients with symptomatic moderate or severe stenosis. North American Symptomatic Carotid Endarterectomy Trial Collaborators. N Engl J Med 1998;339:1415–25.

[16] Randomised trial of endarterectomy for recently symptomatic carotid stenosis: final results of the MRC European Carotid Surgery Trial (ECST). Lancet 1998;351:1379–87.

[17] Wennberg DE, Lucas FL, Birkmeyer JD, Bredenberg CE, Fisher ES. Variation in carotid endarterectomy mortality in the Medicare population: trial hospitals, volume, and patient characteristics. JAMA 1998;279:1278–81.

[18] Hsia DC, Krushat WM, Moscoe LM. Epidemiology of carotid endarterectomies among Medicare beneficiaries. J Vasc Surg 1992;16:201–8.

[19] Chaturvedi S, Aggarwal R, Murugappan A. Results of carotid endarterectomy with prospective neurologist follow-up. Neurology 2000;55:769–72.

[20] Goldstein LB, McCrory DC, Landsman PB, et al. Multicenter review of preoperative risk factors for carotid endarterectomy in patients with ipsilateral symptoms. Stroke 1994;25:1116–21.

[21] Goldstein LB, Samsa GP, Matchar DB, Oddone EZ. Multicenter review of preoperative risk factors for endarterectomy for asymptomatic carotid artery stenosis. Stroke 1998;29:750–3.

[22] Paciaroni M, Eliasziw M, Kappelle LJ, Finan JW, Ferguson GG, Barnett HJ. Medical complications associated with carotid endarterectomy. North American Symptomatic Carotid Endarterectomy Trial (NASCET). Stroke 1999;30:1759–63.

[23] Sundt TM, Sandok BA, Whisnant JP. Carotid endarterectomy. Complications and preoperative assessment of risk. Mayo Clin Proc 1975;50:301–6.

[24] Alamowitch S, Eliasziw M, Algra A, Meldrum H, Barnett HJ. Risk, causes, and prevention of ischaemic stroke in elderly patients with symptomatic

internal-carotid-artery stenosis. North American Symptomatic Carotid Endarterectomy Trial Group. Lancet 2001;357:1154–60.

[25] Rothwell PM, Eliasziw M, Gutnikov SA, Warlow CP, Barnett HJ. Endarterectomy for symptomatic carotid stenosis in relation to clinical subgroups and timing of surgery. Lancet 2004;363:915–24.

[26] Harbaugh RE, Stieg PE, Moayeri N, Hsu L. Carotid-coronary artery bypass graft conundrum. Neurosurgery 1998;43:926–31.

[27] Ferguson GG, Eliasziw M, Barr HW, et al. The North American Symptomatic Carotid Endarterectomy Trial: surgical results in 1415 patients. Stroke 1999;30:1751–8.

[28] Faggioli GL, Curl GR, Ricotta JJ. The role of carotid screening before coronary artery bypass. J Vasc Surg 1990;12:724–31.

[29] Del Sette M, Eliasziw M, Streifler JY, Hachinski VC, Fox AJ, Barnett HJ. Internal border zone infarction: a marker for severe stenosis in patients with symptomatic internal carotid artery disease. For the North American Symptomatic Carotid Endarterectomy (NASCET) Group. Stroke 2000;31: 631–6.

[30] Lopes DK, Mericle RA, Lanzino G, Wakhloo AK, Guterman LR, Hopkins LN. Stent placement for the treatment of occlusive atherosclerotic carotid artery disease in patients with concomitant coronary artery disease. J Neurosurg 2002;96:490–6.

[31] Moore WS, Barnett HJ, Beebe HG, et al. Guidelines for carotid endarterectomy. A multidisciplinary consensus statement from the Ad Hoc Committee, American Heart Association. Stroke 1995;26: 188–201.

[32] Kim SH, Mericle RA, Lanzino G, Qureshi AI, Guterman LR, Hopkins LN. Carotid angioplasty and stent placement in patients with tandem stenosis [abstract]. Neurosurgery 1998;43:708A.

[33] Villarreal J, Silva J, Eliasziw M, et al. Prognosis of patients with intraluminal thrombus in the internal carotid artery. For the North American Symptomatic Carotid Endarterectomy Trial [abstract 18]. Stroke 1998;29:276.

[34] Gasecki AP, Eliasziw M, Ferguson GG, Hachinski V, Barnett HJ. Long-term prognosis and effect of endarterectomy in patients with symptomatic severe carotid stenosis and contralateral carotid stenosis or occlusion: results from NASCET. North American Symptomatic Carotid Endarterectomy Trial (NASCET) Group. J Neurosurg 1995;83: 778–82.

[35] Wholey M. ARCHeR (Acculink for Revascularization of Carotids in High-Risk Patients) [abstract]. Clin Cardiol 2003;26:296.

[36] Meyer FB, Piepgras DG, Fode NC. Surgical treatment of recurrent carotid artery stenosis. J Neurosurg 1994;80:781–7.

[37] AbuRahma AF, Jennings TG, Wulu JT, Tarakji L, Robinson PA. Redo carotid endarterectomy versus primary carotid endarterectomy. Stroke 2001;32: 2787–92.

[38] Lanzino G, Mericle RA, Lopes DK, Wakhloo AK, Guterman LR, Hopkins LN. Percutaneous transluminal angioplasty and stent placement for recurrent carotid artery stenosis. J Neurosurg 1999;90: 688–94.

[39] Loftus CM, Biller J, Hart MN, Cornell SH, Hiratzka LF. Management of radiation-induced accelerated carotid atherosclerosis. Arch Neurol 1987;44: 711–4.

[40] Melliere D, Becquemin JP, Berrahal D, Desgranges P, Cavillon A. Management of radiation-induced occlusive arterial disease: a reassessment. J Cardiovasc Surg (Torino) 1997;38:261–9.

[41] Kerber CW, Cromwell LD, Loehden OL. Catheter dilatation of proximal carotid stenosis during distal bifurcation endarterectomy. AJNR Am J Neuroradiol 1980;1:348–9.

[42] Mathias K. A new catheter system for percutaneous transluminal angioplasty (PTA) of carotid artery stenoses. Fortschr Med 1977;95:1007–11.

[43] Mullan S, Duda EE, Patronas NJ. Some examples of balloon technology in neurosurgery. J Neurosurg 1980;52:321–9.

[44] Kachel R. Results of balloon angioplasty in the carotid arteries. J Endovasc Surg 1996;3:22–30.

[45] Phatouros CC, Higashida RT, Malek AM, et al. Carotid artery stent placement for atherosclerotic disease: rationale, technique, and current status. Radiology 2000;217:26–41.

[46] Endovascular versus surgical treatment in patients with carotid stenosis in the Carotid and Vertebral Artery Transluminal Angioplasty Study (CAVATAS). A randomised trial. Lancet 2001; 357:1729–37.

[47] Brown MN. CAVATAS late results: does carotid balloon angioplasty fare well against endarterectomy? Transcatheter Therapeutics 2002;1(14):92.

[48] Gil-Peralta A, Mayol A, Marcos JR, et al. Percutaneous transluminal angioplasty of the symptomatic atherosclerotic carotid arteries. Results, complications, and follow-up. Stroke 1996;27:2271–3.

[49] Hanel RA, Qureshi AI, Saad M, et al. Carotid angioplasty and stent placement for the treatment of carotid stenosis in patients ineligible for the North American Carotid Endarterectomy Trial [abstract]. Neurosurgery 2002;51:580.

[50] Theron JG, Payelle GG, Coskun O, Huet HF, Guimaraens L. Carotid artery stenosis: treatment with protected balloon angioplasty and stent placement. Radiology 1996;201:627–36.

[51] Jaeger HJ, Mathias KD, Hauth E, et al. Cerebral ischemia detected with diffusion-weighted MR imaging after stent implantation in the carotid artery. AJNR Am J Neuroradiol 2002;23:200–7.

[52] Mathias K. A vast single center experience from Europe: immediate and late outcomes in >1400 patients. Transcatheter Therapeutics 2002;14:96.

[53] Whitlow PL, Lylyk P, Londero H, et al. Carotid artery stenting protected with an emboli containment system. Stroke 2002;33:1308–14.

[54] CARESS Steering Committee. Carotid revascularization using endarterectomy or stenting systems (CARESS): phase I clinical trial. J Endovasc Ther 2003;10:1021–30.

[55] Gruberg L. SAPPHIRE: stenting and angioplasty with protection in patients at high risk for endarterectomy, November 2004. Available at: http://www.medscape.com/viewarticle/445125. Accessed May 25, 2004.

[56] Gruberg L, Beyar R. Optimized combination of antiplatelet treatment and anticoagulation for percutaneous coronary intervention: the final word is not out yet!. J Invasive Cardiol 2002;14:251–3.

[57] US Food and Drug Administration. SAPPHIRE pivotal clinical study. Executive summary. Available at: http://www.fda.gov/ohrms/dockets/ac/04/briefing/4033b1_03_Executive%20Clinical%20Summary.pdf. Accessed May 25, 2004.

[58] Gray W, for the ARCHer Executive Committee. The ARCHeR trials: final one year results. Presented at the American College of Cardiology Scientific Sessions Chicago. March 7, 2004. Available at: http://www.summerinseattle.com/home/archer.pdf. Accessed May 25, 2004.

[59] Krupski WC, Bass A, Kelly AB, Marzec UM, Hanson SR, Harker LA. Heparin-resistant thrombus formation by endovascular stents in baboons. Interruption by a synthetic antithrombin. Circulation 1990;82:570–7.

[60] Yusuf S, Zhao F, Mehta SR, Chrolavicius S, Tognoni G, Fox KK. Effects of clopidogrel in addition to aspirin in patients with acute coronary syndromes without ST-segment elevation. The Clopidogrel in Unstable Angina to Prevent Recurrent Events Trial Investigators. N Engl J Med 2001;345:494–502.

[61] Qureshi AI, Suri MF, Ali Z, et al. Carotid angioplasty and stent placement: a prospective analysis of perioperative complications and impact of intravenously administered abciximab. Neurosurgery 2002;50:466–75.

[62] Qureshi AI, Luft AR, Sharma M, Guterman LR, Hopkins LN. Prevention and treatment of thromboembolic and ischemic complications associated with endovascular procedures: Part II—clinical aspects and recommendations. Neurosurgery 2000; 46:1360–76.

[63] Parodi JC, Schonholz C, Ferreira LM, Mendaro E, Ohki T. "Seat belt and air bag" technique for cerebral protection during carotid stenting. J Endovasc Ther 2002;9:20–4.

[64] Setacci C, Pula G, Baldi I, et al. Determinants of in-stent restenosis after carotid angioplasty: a case-control study. J Endovasc Ther 2003;10:1031–8.

[65] Hanel RA, Levy EI, Lau T, Bendok BR, Guterman LR, Hopkins LN. Incidence and treatment of in-stent stenosis after carotid angioplasty and stenting [abstract]. Neurosurgery 2003;53:510.

[66] Kachel R. PTA of carotid, vertebral, and subclavian artery stenoses. An alternative to vascular surgery? Int Angiol 1994;13:48–51.

[67] Higashida RT, Tsai FY, Halbach VV, Barnwell SL, Dowd CF, Hieshima GB. Interventional neurovascular techniques in the treatment of stroke—state-of-the-art therapy. J Intern Med 1995;237:105–15.

[68] Wholey MH, Al-Mubarek N. Updated review of the global carotid artery stent registry. Catheter Cardiovasc Interv 2003;60:259–66.

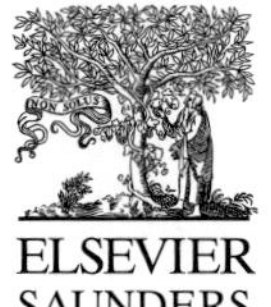
ELSEVIER
SAUNDERS

Neurosurg Clin N Am 16 (2005) 279–295

NEUROSURGERY
CLINICS
OF NORTH AMERICA

Carotid Cavernous Fistulas: Anatomy, Classification, and Treatment

Andrew J. Ringer, MD[a,b,*], Leo Salud, MD[a], Thomas A. Tomsick, MD[b]

[a]*Department of Neurosurgery, The Neuroscience Institute, Mayfield Clinic, University of Cincinnati College of Medicine, ML 0515, 231 Albert Sabin Way, Cincinnati, OH 45267, USA*

[b]*Department of Neuroradiology, The Neuroscience Institute, University of Cincinnati College of Medicine, ML 0762, 231 Albert Sabin Way, Cincinnati, OH 45267, USA*

The cavernous sinus is defined as a dural envelope through which the intracranial extradural segment of the internal carotid artery (ICA) and its branches traverse from the petrous and lacerum segments to the interdural and intradural supraclinoid segments. An abnormal communication between the ICA and external carotid artery (ECA) or any of their branches and the cavernous sinus is termed a *carotid cavernous fistula* (CCF). Patients with CCFs usually present with Dandy's triad of pulsatile exophthalmos, chemosis, and bruit.

These lesions are usually classified as direct or indirect. Direct fistulas have an abnormal communication between the ICA and the cavernous sinus. Indirect fistulas have an abnormal communication between the meningeal branches of the ICA and ECA and the cavernous sinus [1,2]. Direct CCFs are usually caused by trauma, fibromuscular dysplasia, ruptured intracavernous artery aneurysm, collagen deficiency, arterial dissection, or iatrogenic causes (eg, surgical trauma) [3–8]. The causes of indirect CCFs are unknown, but indirect CCFs have been associated with pregnancy, sinusitis, trauma, cavernous sinus thrombosis, and surgery [9–13].

Anatomy

Essential to the understanding of the causes and treatment of CCFs is a detailed knowledge of the cavernous sinus, intracavernous ICA, and meningeal branches of the ICA and ECA. Parkinson [14] first described the detailed anatomy of the cavernous sinus, which constitutes an unexpansible extradural venous plexus. The cavernous sinus communicates with adjacent regions through emissary veins in the following ways: anteriorly through the superior orbital fissure with the orbit, anteroinferiorly through the foramen rotundum with the superior portion of the pterygopalatine fossa, laterally through the foramen ovale and the foramen of Vesalius with the pterygoid region, and posteriorly through the superior petrosal sinus and inferior petrosal sinus (IPS) with the jugular vein of the upper neck (Fig. 1) [15].

The nerves in the lateral wall of the sinus (from superior to inferior) are the oculomotor, trochlear, and the first trigeminal division or ophthalmic nerves (Fig. 2). The abducens nerve courses medial to the ophthalmic nerve and lateral to the ICA. Sympathetic fibers course on the surface of the artery as it courses over the foramen lacerum. The fibers join the abducens nerve within the sinus before being distributed to the first trigeminal division, which sends sympathetic fibers that reach the pupillodilator through the long ciliary nerves by passing through the ciliary ganglion [14]. Some sympathetic fibers pass directly from the carotid plexus to the ciliary ganglion, and

* Corresponding author. c/o Editorial Office, Department of Neurosurgery, University of Cincinnati College of Medicine, ML 0515, 231 Albert Sabin Way, Cincinnati, OH, 45267–0515, USA.

E-mail address: editor@mayfieldclinic.com (A.J. Ringer).

1042-3680/05/$ - see front matter
doi:10.1016/j.nec.2004.08.004

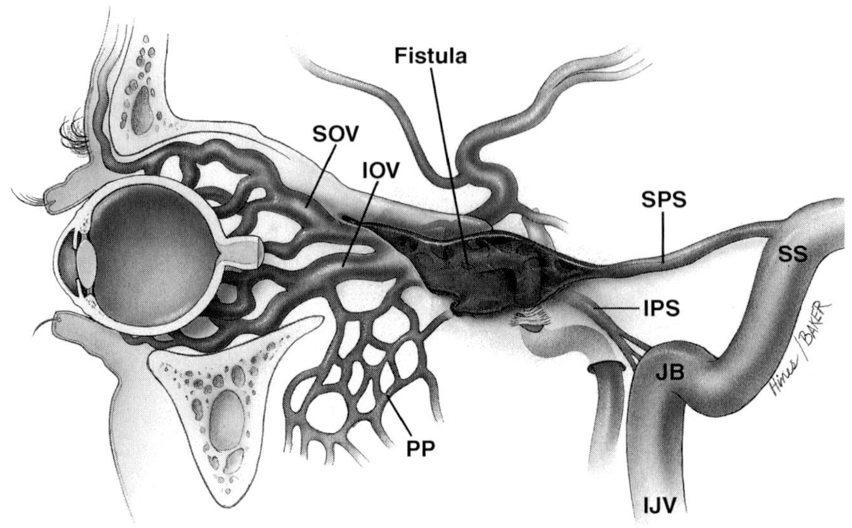

Fig. 1. Lateral view of a carotid cavernous fistula (CCF) causing enlargement of the cavernous sinus venous system and exophthalmos. IOV, inferior ophthalmic vein; IJV, internal jugular vein; IPS, inferior petrosal sinus; JB, jugular bulb; PP, pterygoid plexus; SS, sigmoid sinus; SOV, superior ophthalmic vein; SPS, superior petrosal sinus. (*Courtesy of* the Mayfield Clinic; with permission.)

other fibers may travel along the ophthalmic artery to the globe [16].

The ICA may be divided into seven anatomic segments (Fig. 3A). The cervical (C1) segment extends from the bifurcation to the skull base. The petrous (C2) segment courses through the petrous canal and terminates in the lacerum (C3) segment, where the ICA courses over the foramen lacerum. As the ICA enters the cavernous sinus, it is known as the C4 segment. The shortest segment, the clinoidal (C5) segment, extends from the distal dural ring to the ophthalmic artery. The ophthalmic (C6) segment extends to the posterior communicating artery origin, which marks the beginning of the communicating (C7) segment [17]. Debrun [4] further classified the intracavernous portion into five segments from the anterior clinoid process to the petrous canal as follows: anterior ascending segment, junction of the anterior ascending and horizontal segment, horizontal segment, and junction of the horizontal and posterior ascending segment. The clinoid or anterior ascending segment is surrounded by the anterior clinoid process laterally, the optic strut anteriorly, and the carotid sulcus medially to form a narrow space between the bone and artery. The intracavernous ICA is relatively fixed by this bony ring.

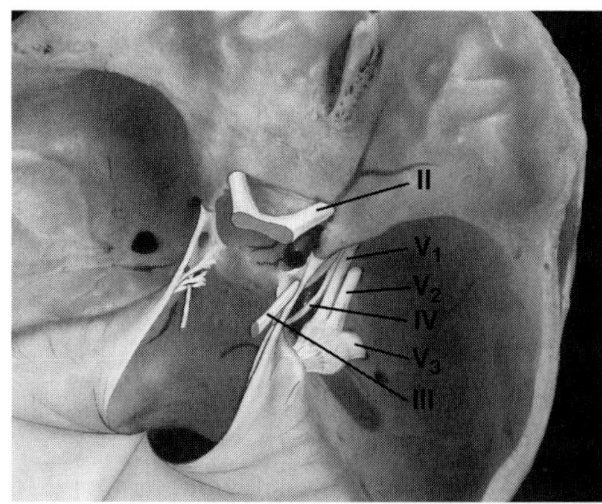

Fig. 2. The cranial nerves in and around the cavernous sinus. Optic nerve (II), oculomotor nerve (III), trochlear nerve (IV), and three divisions of the trigeminal nerve: ophthalmic (V_1), maxillary (V_2), and mandibular (V_3). (*Courtesy of* the Mayfield Clinic; with permission.)

The cavernous ICA gives off the following branches: the meningohypophyseal trunk, the inferolateral trunk or artery of the inferior cavernous sinus, McConnell's capsular artery, and, less frequently, the ophthalmic artery (Fig. 3B).

The meningohypophyseal trunk arises just before the apex of the first curve of the intracavernous ICA. This trunk is the most proximal branch of the intracavernous ICA, is fairly constant, and divides near the roof of the cavernous sinus. The meningohypophyseal trunk gives

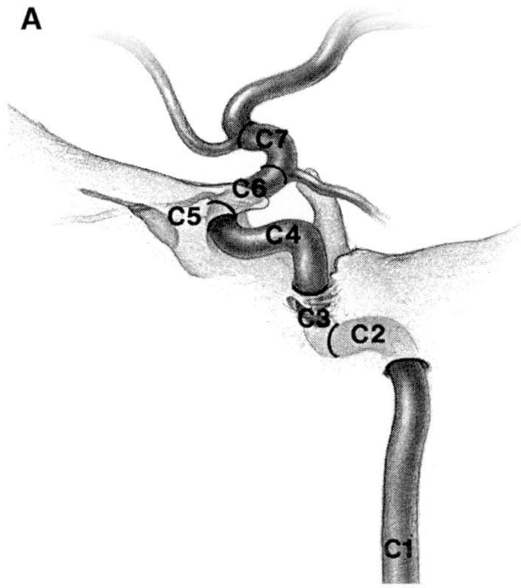

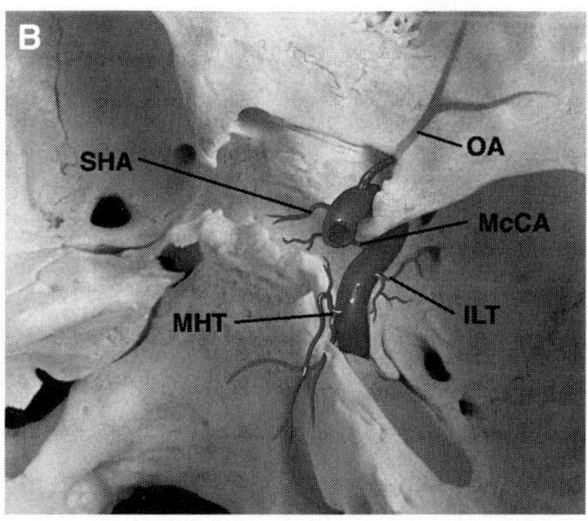

Fig. 3. (*A*) Classification of the internal carotid artery (ICA) segments includes cervical (C1), petrous (C2), lacerum (C3), cavernous (C4), clinoid (C5), ophthalmic (C6), and communicating (C7). (*From* Bouthillier A, van Loveren HR, Keller JT. Segments of the internal carotid artery: a new classification. Neurosurgery 1996;39:425–33; with permission.) (*B*) Branches of the cavernous (C4) carotid artery. ILT, inferolateral trunk; McCA, McConnell's capsular artery; MHT, meningohypophyseal trunk. The ophthalmic artery (OA) and superior hypophyseal artery (SHA) arise from the ICA just distal to the distal dural ring. (*Courtesy of* the Mayfield Clinic; with permission.)

off three branches. First, the tentorial branch or artery of Bernasconi-Cassinari, which runs along the medial edge of the tentorium, supplies the dura of the tentorium and proximal portion of cranial nerves III and IV. It is the most constant branch of the meningohypophyseal trunk and anastomoses with the meningeal branches of the ophthalmic artery. Second, the inferior hypophyseal artery courses medially to supply the posterior pituitary capsule and lobe and anastomoses with the inferior hypophyseal artery on the opposite side. Third, the dorsal meningeal artery, which passes posteriorly through the cavernous sinus to supply the dura over the clivus, sends a branch to cranial nerve VI and anastomoses with the dorsal clival artery on the opposite side.

The inferolateral trunk arises from the lateral side of the horizontal intracavernous ICA approximately 5 to 8 mm distal to the meningohypophyseal trunk [18]. The inferolateral trunk gives off four branches. First, a superior or tentorial branch supplies the roof of the cavernous sinus. Second, an anteromedial branch passes through the superior orbital fissure to supply cranial nerves V_1, III, IV, and VI, which may anastomose with the ophthalmic artery. Third, an anterolateral branch into the foramen rotundum may anastomose with the distal internal maxillary artery via the artery of the foramen rotundum. Fourth, a posterior branch passes medial and under the trigeminal ganglion. The inferolateral trunk also forms anastomoses with the proximal dural branches of the middle meningeal artery and is the branch that contributes most to cavernous sinus dural fistulas [19,20].

McConnell's capsular arteries arise from the medial side of the ICA distal to the origin of the inferolateral trunk. They supply the walls of the hypophyseal fossa and anastomose with branches of the inferior hypophyseal artery and its opposite mate [21].

The ECA contributes to the vascular network of the cavernous sinus. The accessory meningeal artery, which is a branch of the middle meningeal artery or maxillary artery, reaches the cavernous sinus through the foramen ovale or the foramen of Vesalius to form anastomoses with dural branches of the inferolateral trunk of the ICA [22]. The hypoglossal branch of the ascending pharyngeal artery gives off an ascending branch that anastomoses with the medial clival artery at the sella turcica. This anastomotic system makes it possible to see the posterior lobe of the hypophysis during injection of the ascending pharyngeal artery (Fig. 4).

The right and left cavernous sinuses communicate via a venous network localized to the clivus (Fig. 5). The cavernous sinus normally receives drainage from the superior and inferior ophthalmic veins as well as superiorly from the sphenoparietal sinus, sylvian veins, and cortical veins. The cavernous sinus drains posteriorly through the IPS and a superior petrosal sinus to the

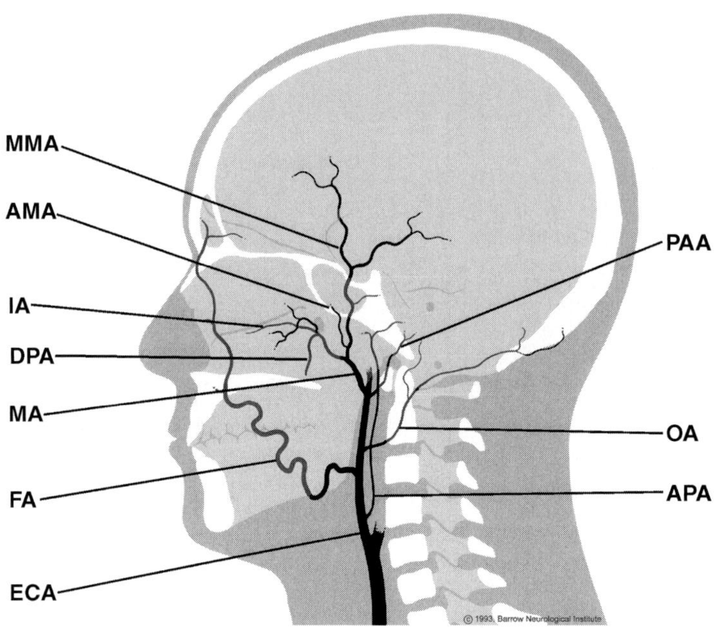

Fig. 4. Branches of the external carotid artery (ECA). AMA, accessory meningeal artery; APA, ascending pharyngeal artery; DPA, descending palatine artery; FA, facial artery; IA, infraorbital artery; MA, maxillary artery; MMA, middle meningeal artery; OA, occipital artery; PAA, posterior auricular artery. (*Courtesy of* the Barrow Neurological Institute; with permission.)

jugular bulb, inferiorly through the pterygoid plexus via emissary veins, and contralaterally through the contralateral cavernous sinus. With venous hypertension caused by an arteriovenous fistula, flow patterns may be revised.

Thus, the branches of the intracavernous ICA and ECA provide a circuit for the cavernous sinus. When one portion is occluded, this system usually provides a collateral pathway. Many of these intracavernous branches are enlarged in patients with CCFs. Thus, a detailed review of the anatomy and hemodynamics of CCFs is necessary for treatment.

Classification of carotid cavernous fistulas

CCFs have been classified by their cause (spontaneous or traumatic), hemodynamic properties (high or low flow), and anatomic variability. The etiologic classification does not consider the hemodynamic and anatomic features of the lesion in relation to prognosis and therapy. With this classification, we might not distinguish a spontaneous dural high-flow fistula from a fistula caused by a ruptured intracavernous artery aneurysm clinically. Although hemodynamic classification is important to explain symptoms and plan treatment, this classification is subjective. The determination of flow on clinical and radiologic grounds is difficult and depends significantly on the physician performing the procedure. The anatomic classification provides the clinician with the definite angioarchitecture of the lesion on which a therapeutic strategy can be based.

Barrow et al [23] distinguished four types of CCFs based on arterial supply (Fig. 6). Type A is a direct fistula between the intracavernous ICA and cavernous sinus. Type A fistulas usually present with high-flow rates. Type B fistulas have dural ICA branches to the cavernous sinus, which are relatively uncommon. Type C fistulas have dural ECA branches to the cavernous sinus. Type D fistulas have dural ICA and ECA branches to the cavernous sinus. Tomsick [24–26] subclassified type D CCFs into type D1 or D2 depending on the presence of a unilateral or bilateral supply. Peeters and Kroger [1] discussed the first three fistula types, excluding type D fistulas of Barrow's classification. Larsen et al [27] described four types of CCFs as follows: type 1 are traumatically acquired direct arteriovenous fistulas; type 2 fistulas are caused by rupture of an intracavernous aneurysm into the cavernous

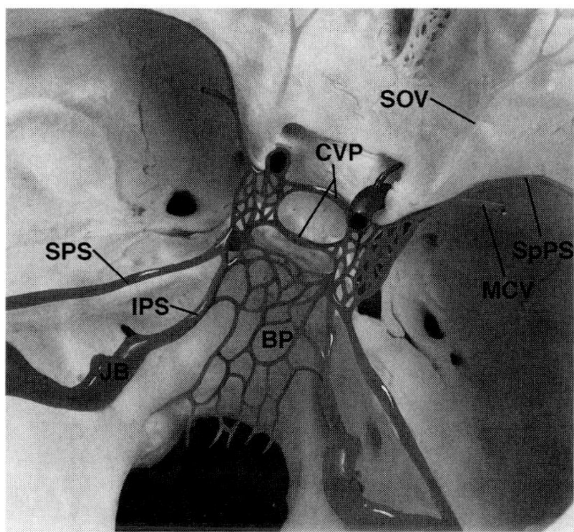

Fig. 5. Superior view of the right and left cavernous sinus communication across the sellae and clivus. BP, basilar plexus; CVP, circular venous plexus; IPS, inferior petrosal sinus; JB, jugular bulb; MCV, superficial middle cerebral vein; SOV, superior ophthalmic vein; SpPS, sphenoparietal sinus; SPS, superior petrosal sinus. (*Courtesy of* the Mayfield Clinic; with permission.)

sinus; type 3 fistulas have ECA or ICA branches to the cavernous sinus; and, finally, type 4 CCFs are a combination of direct and indirect fistula characteristics.

We discuss the classification of direct and indirect fistulas and the variations within these types.

Direct fistulas: causes and pathologic findings

Direct fistulas, type A, are acquired arteriovenous shunts between the ICA and the cavernous sinus. They are thought to be caused by a lesion in the wall of the cavernous ICA or in the wall of one of its branches, typically a result of head trauma or iatrogenic injury. Most of the lesions occur in young adults, and 20% may occur spontaneously as a result of a cavernous ICA aneurysm rupture or weakened ICA vessel walls [28]. Parkinson [28] postulated that direct CCFs are caused by tears of the ICA and meningeal vessels from the cavernous ICA. He theorized that the vessels can easily be torn by bony fractures. During trauma, movement of the artery might stretch and tear the ICA and its branches because it is fixed at the proximal petrosphenoid ligament just beyond the lacerum segment.

However, Helmke et al [29] refuted Parkinson's theories of skull fracture, tearing off, and ICA laceration. In their study of 42 cases, they found no history of skull fractures. Friedmann et al [30] showed that direct CCFs occurred in less than 1% of skull injuries and that this incidence did not parallel that of head trauma. The tearing-off hypothesis did not explain why Debrun's segment C3 is rarely involved in the genesis of direct CCFs and why most direct CCFs are localized in the C4 segment, which is always free of branches in adults. The trabeculae, which span out between the outer surface of the ICA and the outer wall of the cavernous sinus, are shown to insert tangentially into the adventitia of the ICA, not reaching the muscular layer. Thus, it seems unlikely that tugging of the trabeculae could destroy the wall of the ICA [29].

Helmke et al [29] concluded that direct CCFs develop from direct rupture of the vessel wall and that the ruptures are caused by distention of the vessel wall induced by increased intraluminal pressures. This increased tension may be caused by an intense axial acceleration of the body or by sudden compression of the carotid arteries, for example, by extreme sudden extending or bending of the neck.

Debrun et al [31] showed most direct CCFs occur in the proximal horizontal intracavernous segment. The next most common sites are the junction of the horizontal and intracavernous ascending segments, posterior ascending segment, junction of the anterior ascending and horizontal intracavernous segments, and the anterior ascending segment.

Most direct type A CCFs are high-flow shunts. Total steal, which is a complete absence of filling of the ICA above the fistula, occurs in 5% of patients at diagnosis. Type A fistulas typically range from 1 to 5 mm in size (average = 3 mm) [30]. Bilateral traumatic CCFs occur in approximately 1% to 2% of patients with traumatic CCFs [32].

Spontaneous direct CCFs usually arise from any condition that predisposes the ICA wall to weaken [33]. Predisposing factors to the development of spontaneous type A CCFs are collagen deficiency syndrome, which causes a defect in the arterial wall media, (eg, aneurysms of the cavernous ICA); Ehlers-Danlos syndrome [34]; fibromuscular dysplasia [35]; and pseudoxanthoma elasticum [36].

Clinical features of direct fistulas

Patients with direct fistulas initially may present with intracranial bruit. Most patients present

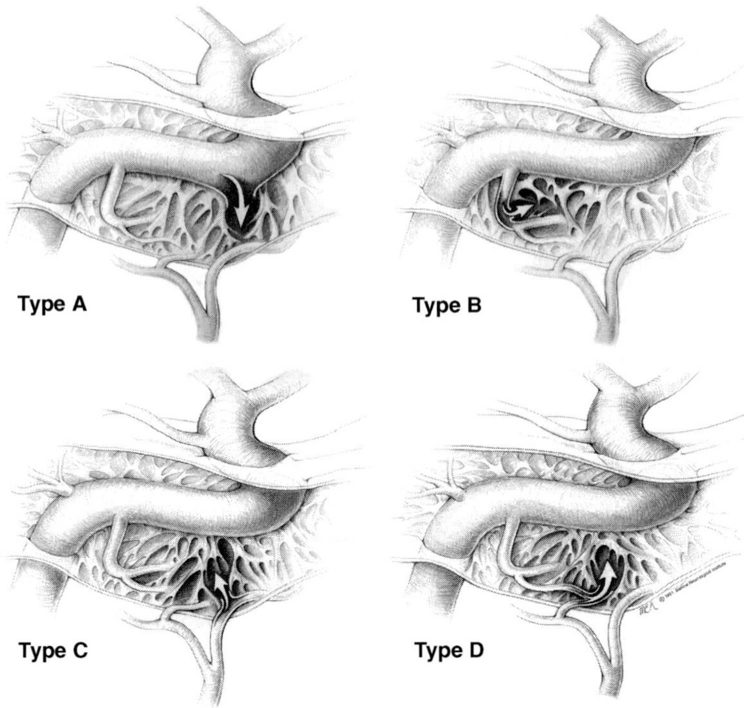

Fig. 6. Classification of carotid cavernous fistulas. (*A*) Type A fistulas involve a direct communication of the internal carotid artery (ICA) and the cavernous sinus. (*B*) Type B fistulas arise from a torn intracavernous branch of the ICA. Type C fistulas arise entirely from external carotid dural branches (*C*), whereas type D fistulas include small dural branches of the ICA and external carotid artery (*D*). Type D2 fistulas involve bilateral internal and external carotid supply. (*Courtesy of* the Barrow Neurological Institute; with permission.)

with proptosis (90%), chemosis (90%), diplopia (50%), pain (25%), trigeminal nerve dysfunction, elevated intraocular pressure, and visual loss (up to 50%) [25].

Retrograde venous drainage from the cavernous sinus into the orbit produces venous hypertension and increased orbital venous volume. This increase in orbital vascular volume also causes enlargement of the extraocular muscles, which subsequently leads to proptosis. Increased exposure of the cornea may cause corneal damage. Diplopia may also occur because of limited mobility of the extraocular muscles. Chemosis is another clinical presentation of ocular venous hypertension. The conjunctival vasculature becomes incompetent to hold fluid and then leaks into the conjunctiva, causing it to swell [19].

Normal intraocular pressure is maintained by a pressure gradient between the anterior chamber and its aqueous fluid and the episcleral vein; the former has a higher pressure than the latter. Increases in episcleral venous pressure cause a reversal of flow. Subsequently, the aqueous fluid is not reabsorbed appropriately, and intraocular pressure elevates. Visual loss may also result from decreased ocular or retinal perfusion because of orbital venous stasis. The pain in direct CCFs is presumably caused by involvement of the dural walls of the cavernous sinus [37].

Intracranial hemorrhage develops in 5% of patients, probably as venous drainage reverses into the sphenoparietal sinus with occlusion of other drainage pathways, with resultant cerebral cortical venous hypertension. One percent to 2% of these cases manifest life-threatening epistaxis caused by rupture of a pseudoaneurysmal cavernous sinus varix [25].

Radiographic evaluation

Noninvasive imaging, such as CT and MRI, is useful in the diagnostic workup of traumatic CCFs. A CT scan of the orbit usually demonstrates proptosis of the affected globe, dilatation of the cavernous sinus and superior ophthalmic vein, and enlargement of the extraocular muscles

[37]. It is also useful to identify skull fractures that may compromise the carotid artery lumen. Orbital ultrasound is another noninvasive means to image these changes. The "gold standard" for diagnosis is selective cerebral angiography, however. The initial angiographic evaluation should be tailored to obtain the following information: size and location of the fistula, presence of any associated cavernous carotid aneurysm, identification of high-risk features (eg, cortical venous drainage, pseudoaneurysm, cavernous sinus varix), venous drainage patterns, differentiation of direct from indirect lesions, and associated vascular injuries.

The angiographic workup must include the five following parts. First, assessment of the morphology of the carotid bifurcation and the origin of the ICA is performed by injection of both common carotid arteries (CCAs). Visualization of the contralateral CCA is needed to rule out a carotid dissection or stenosis, pseudoaneurysm, or contralateral CCF. Second, ipsilateral ICA and ECA angiograms can identify the location of the fistula to assess whether the CCF is of high or low flow and to determine the presence of a complete or partial steal. Complete steal is of enormous interest because it confirms that the CCF is of high flow, that the fistula tear is large, and that the patient has an excellent circle of Willis if there are no contralateral deficits [24]. In patients with high-flow fistulas, regular ICA angiography at three frames per second cannot possibly detect the morphology of the fistula. Therefore, specific maneuvers can slow down the flow through the fistula. The Mehringer-Hieshima maneuver consists of a gentle ipsilateral ICA injection and manual compression of the ipsilateral carotid artery while filming at a slower rate [2]. Use of a double-lumen balloon catheter in the ipsilateral ICA is another way to demonstrate the fistula. With the balloon in place, slow injection of contrast at 1 mL/s at one or two frames per second allows opacification of the fistula [38]. Third, assessment of the patency of the anterior communicating artery is performed by ipsilateral carotid compression of the contralateral ICA. Fourth, ipsilateral carotid compression of the vertebral artery, called the Heuber maneuver, opacifies the fistula through a patent posterior communicating artery. Fifth, assessment of venous drainage is extremely important for treatment by correlation with patient's symptoms. Patients with cranial nerve deficits usually have petrosal venous drainage. Patients with ocular symptoms usually have superior ophthalmic venous drainage. Patients with severe headaches may have cortical venous drainage and should be treated aggressively because of their predisposition to bleed. The venous route also provides excellent access for treatment.

Indirect fistulas (types B, C, and D): causes and pathologic findings

Indirect CCFs (types B, C, and D) are typically low-flow fistulas and are also called dural fistulas. They may occur spontaneously in women older than 50 years of age. The cause of these lesions is still unclear, but some evidence points to a congenital origin [39]. Congenital dural fistulas have been reported in infants as young as 5 weeks of age. Taniguchi et al [40] postulated that indirect CCFs may represent a collateral response to thrombosis of the cavernous sinus and may be a manifestation of a thrombotic tendency, which may lead to multiple dural fistulas. Barrow favors the theory of Newton and Hoyt [41], who postulated that spontaneous low-flow CCFs form after the rupture of one of the thin-walled dural arteries that normally traverse the cavernous sinus. Different factors that may predispose patients to this rupture include hypertension [42], pregnancy [11], trauma and straining [40], atherosclerotic disease [40], and collagen vascular disease.

Clinical features of indirect fistulas

The onset of symptoms of indirect CCFs is more insidious compared with direct CCFs. The symptoms and signs of the former are often fewer and less severe than those of the latter. Among 260 cases reviewed at diagnosis, signs and symptoms included red eye (90%), proptosis (89%), increased intraocular pressure (83%), double vision or cranial nerve paresis (68%), pain (40%), and bruit (39%) [37]. Diplopia is usually horizontal because of the involvement of the abducens nerve, which occurs in 50% of cases; in contrast, vertical diplopia of a trochlear nerve palsy or upward gaze occurs because of oculomotor nerve involvement. The possible causes of cranial nerve paresis are venous congestion, venous compression, or, less often, ischemia caused by arterial steal from the meningohypophyseal and inferior cavernous arterial supply to the nerves.

Spontaneous resolution of dural fistulas can occur independent of treatment. This resolution may be attributed to further thrombosis of the involved segment of the cavernous sinus. Its incidence ranges from 10% to 60% in the literature [21]. Hamby noted cases of spontaneous resolution after diagnostic angiography alone. In fact, the rate of spontaneous cure after diagnostic angiography has been reported to be as high as 43% [43]. Sasaki et al [44] reported that 18 of 19 patients with dural CCFs had complete regression of the signs and symptoms during an observation period ranging from 6 months to 8 years.

Exacerbation and remission of signs and symptoms is the hallmark of the disease, possibly because of cavernous sinus thromboses and shunting of venous flow in different directions. Redirection of blood flow to the superior ophthalmic veins may cause ocular signs and symptoms, that to the retinal vein may cause blindness, that to the spinal pial venous drainage may cause myelopathy, and that to the brain via pial veins may cause intracerebral hemorrhage. Retrograde cortical venous drainage is a well-known cause of neurologic deficits and severe headaches. In Ernst and Tomsick's study [24] of dural CCFs, 20% of patients had known pial venous cortical drainage but no hemorrhage. Halbach et al [45] noted that the risk of intracerebral hemorrhage in patients with cortical venous drainage from direct fistulas may be fatal if untreated. The incidence of hemorrhage with direct or indirect fistulas is remarkably low.

Radiographic evaluation

Angiography is the diagnostic modality of choice. Its goals are to determine the location of the fistula, define the arterial supply to the fistula and pattern of venous drainage, identify any dangerous extracranial-to-intracranial or ophthalmic collaterals, and evaluate the carotid bifurcations before initiation of carotid compression therapy. Tolerance for ICA occlusion should also be evaluated using balloon test occlusion (BTO) to aid in identification of appropriate therapeutic choices.

The angiographic workup should include selective angiography of both ICAs, including visualization of both ascending pharyngeal arteries, both internal maxillary arteries, and ipsilateral vertebral arteries. During ECA injection, the following arteries should be noted: the middle meningeal artery, accessory meningeal artery, distal internal maxillary artery (including the artery of the foramen rotundum and vidian artery), and ascending pharyngeal artery. These arteries usually supply type C and D fistulas. During ICA injections, the following arteries should be noted: the meningohypophyseal artery, inferolateral artery, and McConnell's arteries, because they supply type B and D fistulas [24].

During angiography of CCFs, dangerous anastomoses should be noted. If arterial embolization is contemplated, the following are important: the ophthalmic, meningeal, and vidian arteries and the artery of the foramen rotundum to the ICA branch; ascending pharyngeal to cavernous and petrous carotid arteries; and occipital artery communication to the ICA or vertebral artery. If transvenous embolization is contemplated, the venous phase should be studied to identify venous drainage patterns and determine the route.

Identification of the exact point of fistula in direct CCFs may be difficult because of the high-flow state. In many cases, this point may be visualized by injection of the vertebral artery during manual compression of the ipsilateral carotid artery. The source of flow in indirect CCFs can typically be identified by selective injection of the external carotid branches as mentioned previously.

Determination of the patient's ability to tolerate ICA occlusion is important before embarking on a therapeutic intervention. BTO is the currently accepted technique for evaluation. Proper evaluation requires documentation of collateral flow during ipsilateral ICA occlusion if not already demonstrated on routine angiography. Evaluation of the contralateral carotid or vertebral artery may be performed during BTO using bilateral femoral access with a diagnostic catheter or before BTO by manual compression of the ipsilateral carotid artery. Occlusion of the ICA is performed after gaining access to the CCA with a 6-French guide catheter. Although we used the Endeavor nondetachable balloon (Target Therapeutics, Fremont, California) for occlusion because of its compliant nontraumatic characteristics, this product has recently become unavailable. We now use the Hyperglide balloon (Micro Therapeutics, Irvine, California) for the same purpose. This wire-valve balloon uses a 0.010-in wire to occlude the distal exit port during inflation and has a similar compliance profile to the Endeavor. Administration of intravenous heparin (50–70 U/kg) helps the patient to achieve an activated clotting time (ACT) of greater than 300 seconds before undergoing balloon inflation. Throughout the procedure, a heparinized saline flush (2.5 U/mL at 30 mL/h) is continued via the guide catheter and the groin sheath. The ACT is checked hourly and maintained over 300 seconds. The ICA may be best occluded with the balloon positioned within the petrous (C2) segment of the ICA. The rigid carotid canal permits ICA occlusion at lower balloon volumes, thereby reducing the risk of dissection. The disadvantage of occlusion at this location is the risk of creating a steal phenomenon with retrograde filling of the fistula. This phenomenon can be recognized during evaluation of collateral flow as described previously. Passing the BTO despite a steal predicts clinical tolerance to ICA occlusion. If the patient develops neurologic signs with a steal above, it does not mean that the ICA cannot be occluded. Therefore, the occlusion test should be repeated with the ostium occluded or by trapping the ostium with two balloons.

After confirmation of ICA occlusion, the patient is evaluated clinically with detailed testing of mental status, speech, visual fields, facial animation, and motor power in all four extremities. If no deficits are noted, the patient is observed for 15 to 20 minutes and re-examined. If the patient tolerates occlusion at normal blood pressure, nitroprusside infusion is initiated and titrated to achieve a mean arterial pressure two thirds of the patient's baseline. The patient is examined again and observed for 15 to 20 minutes. Periodic visualization of the balloon ensures that it has not migrated or deflated. At our institution, standard evaluation includes single proton emission computed tomography (SPECT) to rule out significant asymmetry in perfusion during BTO. This is accomplished by intravenous injection of ^{99m}Tc-hexamethylpropyleneamine oxime during the period of ICA occlusion. A SPECT scan must be performed within 1 hour of injection because of the short half-life of the tracer. This can best be accomplished by calling for tracer injection after achieving target hypotension. The importance of SPECT evaluation, even in patients who seem to tolerate BTO during relative hypotensive challenge, was illustrated in the review by Larson et al [27], in which 2 of 58 patients apparently tolerating BTO with hypotensive challenge suffered a major stroke after permanent carotid occlusion.

Indications for emergency treatment

In a study of 155 patients with CCFs, Meyers et al [46] noted that the presence of the following angiographic features increases the risks of morbidity and mortality: pseudoaneurysm, large varix of the cavernous sinus, venous drainage to cortical veins, and thrombosis of venous outflow pathways distant from the fistula. Clinical signs and symptoms that should concern the interventionalist are increased intracranial pressure; progressive proptosis, which may signify spontaneous thrombosis of venous outflow pathways to the orbit; diminished visual acuity; hemorrhage; and transient ischemic attacks, which may signify impaired cerebral autoregulation secondary to chronic steal phenomenon. Recognition of these signs, symptoms, and radiographic findings should warrant immediate and definitive treatment to improve outcome [46].

Surgical management

Although surgical treatment of CCFs has been relegated to historical status for the last 30 years, it remains a consideration for salvage of failed endovascular attempts. The earliest technique, described in the *Lancet* in 1875, was ligation of the CCA, which was fraught with failure that resulted in symptom resolution for only one third of patients [47]. In 1935, Dandy described a conceptually more appropriate technique for trapping the fistula in which cervical ICA ligation was followed by craniotomy and ligation of the supraclinoid (C5) ICA. Although this proved more successful, a high failure rate, which was blamed on collateral supply from the ECA, remained. In 1942, Jaeger [48] addressed this problem by isolation and ligation of the supraclinoid carotid artery (C5 segment), which was followed by packing the muscle into the cervical ICA. Hamby [49] later modified this by surgically packing muscle into the entire cavernous (C4) ICA segment.

Although the aforementioned techniques are effective, sacrifice of the ICA is required. Transcavernous occlusion of a CCF may permit preservation of ICA flow as described by Parkinson [50] and Mullan [51] Parkinson exposed the C4 segment of the ICA between the trochlear nerve and the first division of the trigeminal nerve. Mullan exposed the ICA between the first and second divisions of the trigeminal nerve or packed the cavernous sinus through the superior petrosal sinus, IPS, or superior ophthalmic vein (Fig. 7). When performing surgical transvenous packing, as in transvenous endovascular repair, the surgeon must avoid occlusion of only the posterior drainage, which could result in pressurization of the superior ophthalmic vein with visual loss or

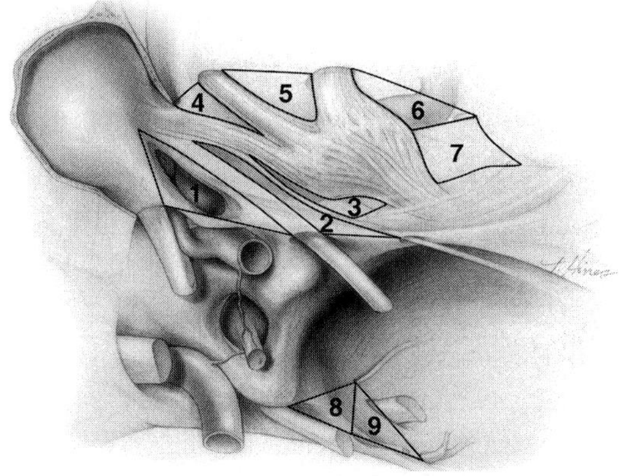

Fig. 7. Surgical view of the cavernous sinus after posterior orbitotomy and anterior clinoidectomy. Anatomic triangles of the cavernous sinus region are (1) anteromedial triangle (Dolenc), (2) paramedical triangle, (3) Parkinson's triangle, (4) anterolateral triangle (Mullan), (5) lateral triangle, (6) posterolateral triangle (Glasscock), (7) posteromedial quadrilateral (Kawase), (8) inferomedial triangle, and (9) inferolateral triangle. (*From* Tew JM, van Loveren HR, Keller JT. Atlas of operative microneurosurgery, vol. 2. Philadelphia: WB Saunders; 2001. p. 76–7; with permission.)

occlusion of the anterior drainage with cortical venous pressurization.

Indications for surgical repair include compromised proximal arterial access that prevents endovascular repair or failure of transarterial and transvenous endovascular repair. Preoperative evaluation should include complete angiographic definition of the fistula and BTO as described previously. The appearance and condition of the superficial temporal artery should also be noted when extracranial-to-intracranial bypass is needed. Although the details of surgical technique and management are beyond the scope of this article, the topic is expertly described by van Loveren et al [52].

Endovascular repair: type A carotid cavernous fistulas

Balloon occlusion

The large carotid defect commonly present in type A CCFs frequently permits transarterial balloon occlusion of the fistula with preservation of the ICA. The earliest procedures were performed with latex balloons hand-tied to the delivery catheter with latex strips. The development of the gold-valve balloon (GVB) permitted selection of a preformed detachable balloon fashioned for manual attachment to the delivery catheter. The balloon was mounted on a 2-French Teflon microcatheter that was passed through the delivery catheter, typically a 3-French catheter, and was detached by manual traction on the catheter. The Heishima detachable silicone balloon (DSB) made use of a miter valve that required a slightly higher detachment force than the GVB. When the US Food and Drug Administration (FDA) limited the use of implanted latex devices, the DSB became the preferred method for balloon occlusion of CCFs.

The technique for DSB occlusion of a CCF involves transfemoral access to the proximal CCA with a 7-French guide catheter or long 6-French sheath. If the ICA origin arises at an oblique angle from the CCA, an angled tip to the guide catheter may aid by directing the balloon during advancement. Once femoral access is gained, the patient undergoes anticoagulation with intravenous heparin (50–70 U/kg) and an ACT is confirmed over 300 seconds. The ACT is checked again hourly, and supplemental heparin is given as needed.

After the guide catheter is positioned, angiography is performed to document the anatomy of the lesion and define the site of the fistula. The specific DSB chosen depends on the size of the venous compartment that needs to be filled and the flow rate through the fistula. Selection of a balloon too small for the cavernous sinus compartment into which the fistula opens results in a persistent or recurrent fistula. For high-flow fistulas, selection of a balloon with a low detachment force may risk premature detachment, whereas a balloon with a high detachment force may not detach safely on reaching the target.

Next, the uninflated balloon is advanced to the distal end of the guide catheter; at this point, roadmap imaging is used for further balloon positioning. Partial inflation and deflation advance the balloon within the artery, permitting blood flow to carry the balloon distally. In many cases, the high flow of the fistula directs the balloon into the cavernous sinus. If the balloon is carried distal to the fistula within the ICA, a nondetachable balloon may be advanced first and inflated distal to the fistula, thus occluding distal flow. Subsequent attempts to advance the DSB should result in deflection into the cavernous sinus through the fistula. On entering the cavernous sinus, the DSB is inflated and drawn back against the fistula. Angiography is performed to document occlusion of the fistula. If flow persists through the fistula, the DSB is inflated further and the process is repeated until the fistula is occluded (Fig. 8). When occlusion is documented, the balloon is detached by withdrawal of the delivery catheter from the balloon. The force required for detachment depends on the type of balloon chosen.

The advantage of balloon occlusion of a CCF is its ability to occlude the fistula rapidly with preservation of the ICA. Potential disadvantages include fistula recurrence and ICA compromise as the inflated balloon protrudes through the fistula site to narrow the adjacent ICA lumen. Although this compromise may require prolonged anticoagulation after completion of the procedure, it rarely restricts distal flow. The fistula may recur if the balloon migrates, deflates, or ruptures. The concern raised in the past with silicone balloons was that filling with a hypotonic solution could cause osmotic loss of fluid volume and partial deflation. For this reason, many interventionalists chose to inflate the DSB with mildly hypertonic saline or metrizamide solutions or with permanent solid material, such as silicone [53] or hydroxyethyl methacrylate [54]. Laboratory research implies that deflation rarely occurs by osmotic fluid loss and that saline-diluted contrast is safe for DSB inflation, however [55]. In cases of traumatic CCFs, we have seen balloons punctured by bony spicules and migration of balloons without deflation presumably because of dilation of the venous compartment by the balloon. The DSB was most recently available from Target Therapeutics and came in three sizes, with each available in low (20–30 g), medium (30–40 g), and high (40–55 g) force of detachment ranges. Like the nondetachable Endeavor balloon, the DSB has been discontinued, making detachable balloon treatment currently unavailable in the United States.

Coil occlusion

Coil occlusion for CCFs became popular after FDA approval of the Guglielmi detachable coil (GDC) system in 1995. The advantages of coil occlusion of CCFs include ease of access and availability of a variety of sizes of the embolic device when compared with balloon embolization. Potential disadvantages include slower gradual occlusion of the fistula, which increases procedure time, and the risk of incomplete fistula occlusion with loss of transarterial access; this loss would then require a second transvenous approach. As with intracranial aneurysms, coil compaction with recurrence remains a concern. This compaction may be minimized by oversizing the first coils used for framing and by keeping the microcatheter tip well into the cavernous sinus. These steps allow for some expansion of the venous compartment during embolization and for dense coil packing distal to the fistula site, thus preventing coil compaction or early loss of microcatheter access.

Our approach to coil embolization of CCFs is similar to balloon occlusion. Transfemoral access is gained before anticoagulation using the heparin dosing outlined previously. As with balloon occlusion, an ACT of 250 to 300 seconds is acceptable as long as parent vessel occlusion is not planned. The small caliber of the microcatheters used in coiling enables access to the ICA with a 6-French guide. If distal balloon occlusion is required to access the fistula as described previously, supplemental heparin may be required to

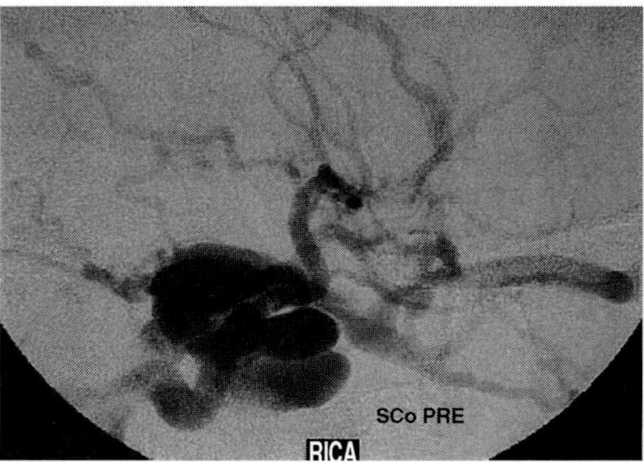

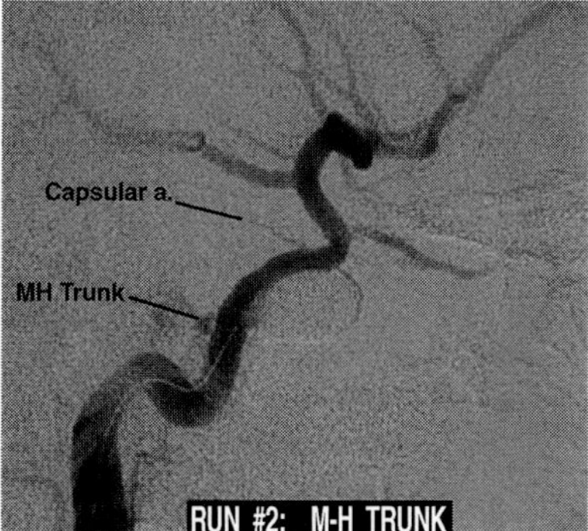

Fig. 8. Before and after angiograms of a direct (type A) carotid cavernous fistula treated with balloon occlusion. During an assault, this patient suffered fractures of the orbit, resulting in a direct fistula. Proptosis and chemosis at presentation later improved after balloon occlusion of the fistula. (*Courtesy of* the Mayfield Clinic; with permission.)

achieve an ACT greater than 300 seconds. The fistula is entered using roadmap guidance after full angiographic definition of the fistula and collateral flow. Dense coil packing is performed using the same principles of aneurysm coiling. We choose our first coil, often a three-dimensional coil, based on the size of the venous compartment opacified on angiography. As in aneurysm coiling, we begin by framing the compartment to be embolized with large coils to protect the fistula site, thus preventing coil prolapse or loss of microcatheter access before fistula occlusion. The fistula remains partially open on angiography in most cases until coil packing is quite dense. For this reason, it is usually advisable to choose coils with some resistance to stretching or unraveling as the coiling progresses.

We have used the GDC system in all our CCF coiling cases, taking advantage of the "stretch-resistant" coils in the latter stages of embolization (Fig. 9). After the fistula is closed by angiography, additional coils should only be passed if no resistance is met during advancement. If coil advancement becomes unsafe because of coil prolapse or loss of microcatheter access, the transarterial embolization may be aborted and the fistula may be occluded via a transvenous approach. Complications of transarterial coil embolization include thromboembolus, ICA compromise from protruding coil mass, and ICA dissection. When compared with balloon occlusion, coil occlusion is associated with lower rates of ICA compromise and similar rates of other complications.

Transvenous occlusion may be necessary in cases of inadequate transarterial access or incomplete occlusion after transarterial embolization (see Fig. 9D). The performance of transvenous occlusion requires arterial side angiography to allow complete visualization of the fistula. For this reason, we typically gain venous and arterial access in opposite groins to avoid confusion. The 5-French venous catheter is advanced under roadmap guidance through the

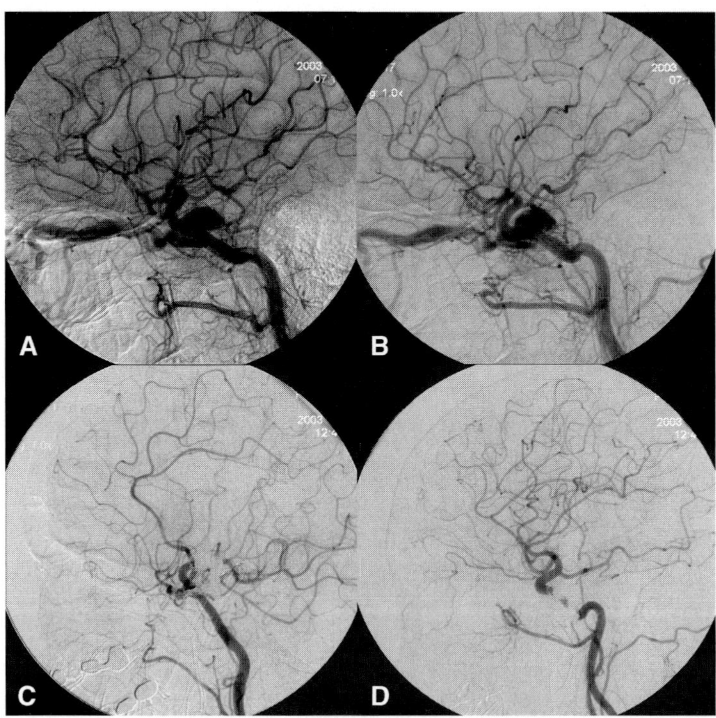

Fig. 9. Coil occlusion of direct (type A) carotid cavernous fistula. (*A*) During an automobile accident, this patient suffered multiple injuries, including a dissecting pseudoaneurysm of the right internal carotid artery. During observation with anticoagulant therapy, he acutely developed exophthalmos with an audible bruit. Angiography demonstrated the fistula (*B*), which was initially treated with transarterial coil occlusion with incomplete closure (*C*). (*D*) Subsequent transvenous coil occlusion cured the fistula. (*Courtesy of* the Mayfield Clinic; with permission.)

inferior vena cava to the superior vena cava and the internal jugular vein. On reaching the jugular bulb, we typically perform a venogram for road-map visualization of the IPS. A dual-tipped microcatheter is subsequently advanced through the IPS into the cavernous sinus to perform the coiling. The same principles of coiling or balloon occlusion apply as were described for transarterial embolization. Throughout the procedure, a 4-French diagnostic catheter is positioned in the ipsilateral CCA for control angiography. The procedure may be terminated when fistula flow is occluded. We prefer to maintain a heparinized saline flush through the 5-French venous guide catheter and the 4-French arterial diagnostic catheter. Alternatively, the arterial catheter may be withdrawn after accessing the cavernous sinus and reinserted for control angiograms. Potential complications include thromboembolus or coil embolus by pushing coils through the fistula into the ICA and thrombosis of the internal jugular vein. Both complications can be prevented by regular use of control angiography or road-mapping and with appropriate anticoagulation. A nondetachable balloon may be inflated in the ICA at the ostium to prevent coil prolapse into the ICA, the "balloon-assist technique." Series for coil embolization describe good results using the transarterial or transvenous route [56,57]. Lewis et al [58] described great success using detachable balloons.

Parent artery occlusion

In general, occlusion of a direct CCF with preservation of the ICA is preferred. In some cases, however, attempts at fistula occlusion with the techniques described previously are unsuccessful or impossible. In other cases, ICA compromise from balloon or coil prolapse may pose risks for thromboembolism such that ICA occlusion is preferred. In these cases, assessment of the patient's ability to tolerate ICA occlusion is paramount. In cases of extremely high-flow fistulas, complete diversion of ipsilateral ICA flow may already be present, with collateral flow defined from other sources with simple angiography. If the patient has tolerated this condition without ischemia, test occlusion may be unnecessary. If the posterior communicating and anterior communicating artery collaterals are patent, the safety of parent occlusion is high. Otherwise, BTO is mandatory.

Occlusion of the ICA, like direct CCF occlusion, may be performed with balloon or coil embolization. Balloon occlusion is performed using the identical access techniques as those used for CCF occlusion. In this case, however, balloon size is matched to the size of the ICA. This match is best predicted by noting the volume required to occlude the ICA during BTO. Medium- or high-detachment force balloons are preferred because of the risk of early detachment in the high-flow environment of the ICA. We prefer a multiple balloon approach, often using three balloons, to prevent distal migration of the distal balloon. In this approach, the first balloon is positioned distal to or across the fistula opening but is not detached until the proximal balloons are in position. On angiographic confirmation of fistula occlusion and safe detachment of the proximal balloon(s), the distal balloon is detached. The risk of distal balloon migration has been described in the acute and delayed settings [59]. The multiple balloon technique minimizes this risk. As mentioned in the section on balloon occlusion of CCFs, detachable balloons are currently unavailable in the United States; therefore, use of this technique with approved devices is impossible until a new product becomes available.

Fistula occlusion with coils depends somewhat more on ICA occlusion distal to the fistula than balloon embolization, because multiple coils are needed to eliminate flow. Positioning coils at the level of the fistula within the ICA may permit continued retrograde filling as the microcatheter migrates proximally. For this reason, moderately dense coil packing is needed distal and proximal to the fistula site. Coil occlusion of the ICA also risks distal migration during the procedure as well as partial fistula occlusion with loss of arterial access. Although this latter complication is less of a concern than with attempted fistula occlusion during ICA preservation, it remains possible if significant retrograde filling is present. Distal coil migration is a significant concern, however, particularly during detachment of the initial distal coils. Antegrade flow may be stopped to permit safe detachment of the coils within the ICA by temporary occlusion of the proximal ICA with a nondetachable silicone balloon. Proximal balloon occlusion may also limit the risk of thromboembolus that arises from the coils by limiting the flow through them while thrombus is developing. Accurate visualization of the distal ICA is necessary during placement of the distal coils. Therefore, road-mapping is performed before proximal balloon occlusion. After road-mapping, further control angiography is unnecessary until dense coil packing is achieved proximal to the fistula. The proximal balloon is left inflated until this is accomplished. The ease of coil delivery and the ability to retrieve coils before detachment, if necessary, make coil occlusion of the ICA a technically uncomplicated and safe procedure. Even before DSBs became unavailable, we preferred the coil occlusion technique for these reasons.

Endovascular repair: indirect carotid cavernous fistulas (types B, C, and D)

Transarterial embolization

The complex anatomy of indirect CCFs makes cure by transarterial embolization unlikely. In addition, potential complications of the transarterial approach (eg, thromboembolic stroke, cranial nerve palsies) can be virtually eliminated by use of the transvenous approach. For these reasons, the transarterial approach is typically used only to reduce arterial inflow before transvenous occlusion for high-flow indirect CCFs and after failure of transvenous attempts. Some interventionalists think that flow reduction before venous side occlusion may reduce the risk of venous hypertension that may occur before complete venous occlusion. Selection of a site for transarterial embolization requires careful selective angiography of the branches of the ECA. Typically, a 5- or 6-French guide catheter placed in the ostium of the ECA allows selective catheterization of the meningeal branches with a microcatheter using roadmap guidance. When meningeal branches feeding the CCF are identified as a potential site of embolization, provocative testing is performed to evaluate the potential for postembolization cranial nerve palsy. This evaluation can be reliably performed by lidocaine injection (1% solution, 2.5–5 mL), followed by careful examination of cranial nerve function. Development of a new cranial nerve deficit indicates a risk for cranial nerve ischemia with embolization. If permanent embolization is deemed safe, catheter position is confirmed and the embolic agent is prepared.

In general, two embolic agents are considered for use. First, polyvinyl alcohol (PVA) particles (150–250 μm) may be mixed with a dilute contrast solution and slowly injected. If a blank roadmap image is created initially, visualization of the injectate becomes easier. Visualization of arteries not opacified in the microcatheter angiogram may indicate reflux of embolic agent. This reflux must be avoided to prevent embolization to intracranial arteries or the ophthalmic artery [60–62]. PVA embolization has the advantage of easy delivery to the fistula site but may flow through the fistula or result in proximal vessel occlusion because of the difficulty in precisely matching particle size to fistula size. This discrepancy frequently leads to early recanalization.

Second, liquid embolic agents, such as N-butyl cyanoacrylate (NBCA), have an advantage in transarterial embolization because of their ability to conform to the size of the fistula and feeding artery. The viscous opacified acrylic typically does not flow to the smallest involved branches, however, preferring to polymerize in larger arteries. Permanent occlusion may also be achieved if acrylic is deposited within the fistula and into the cavernous sinus. The risk of reflux or embolization through anastomoses to more dangerous locations still exists but may be avoided with similar road-mapping and injection techniques as described for PVA injection.

For either technique, selection of the intracavernous ICA branches has limited use. In most cases, microcatheter access cannot be gained distal enough to the ICA for safe embolization with PVA or NBCA. In some cases, enlargement of the meningohypophyseal trunk permits safe access. Detachable coils may permit safe embolization when only proximal access is available. Vinuela et al [62] described some success with this technique.

Transvenous occlusion

Most interventionalists prefer the transvenous approach because of the lower likelihood of immediate complete occlusion and the ischemic risk of transarterial occlusion of indirect CCFs. Success rates with the transvenous approach are significantly higher than with the transarterial approach for indirect CCFs, as reported by Halbach et al [63]. General approaches to the cavernous sinus access and imaging are identical to the technique described for transvenous occlusion of type A CCFs. Venous side occlusion may be achieved by balloon or coil occlusion (Fig. 10). Liquid embolics and PVA may occlude distal venous pathways, leading to increased pressure within the cavernous sinus and aggravated symptoms.

Summary

CCFs are a heterogeneous group of lesions with varying anatomy and causes. Despite the

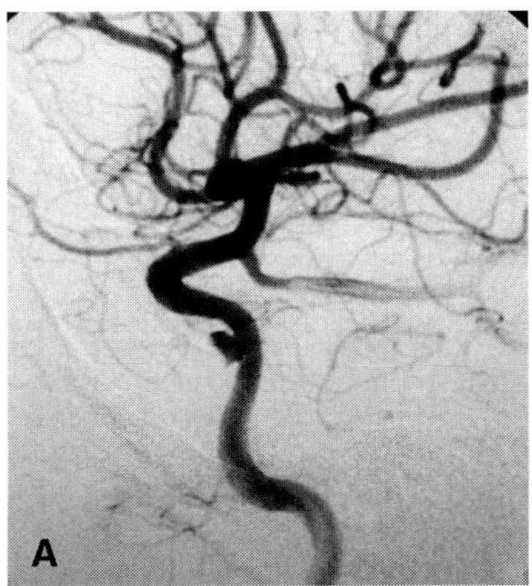

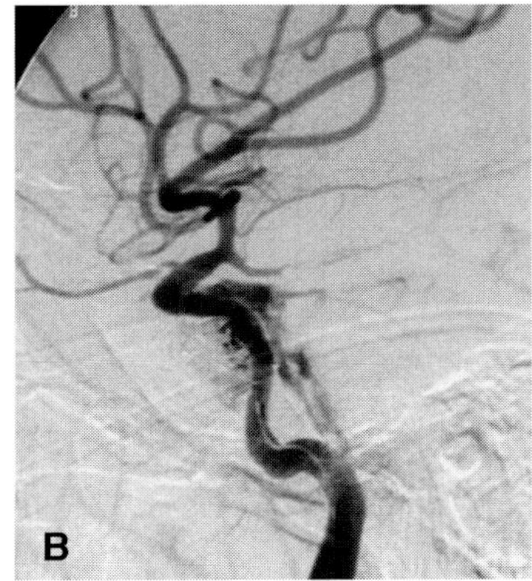

Fig. 10. Indirect (type D2) carotid cavernous fistula treated with transvenous coiling. Access to the posterior cavernous compartment was gained through the inferior petrosal sinus.

complexity of these lesions, a logical treatment plan can be derived with a good understanding of the different types of fistulas and knowledge of the relevant anatomy. Treatments tailored to the specific fistula type and anatomic considerations allow satisfactory treatment with good safety.

References

[1] Peeters FLM, Kroger R. Dural and direct cavernous fistulas. AJR Am J Roentgenol 1979;132:599–606.

[2] Connors JJ, Wojak JC. Treatment of carotid cavernous fistula. In: Interventional neuroradiology: strategies and practical techniques. Philadelphia: WB Saunders; 1999. p. 215–26.

[3] Obrador S, Gomez-Bueno J, et al. Spontaneous carotid-cavernous fistula produced by ruptured aneurysm of the meningohypophyseal branch of the internal carotid artery. Case report. J Neurosurg 1974;40:539–43.

[4] Debrun G. Treatment of traumatic carotid-cavernous fistula using detachable balloon catheters. AJNR Am J Neuroradiol 1983;4:355–6.

[5] Eggers F, Lukin R, Chambers AA. Iatrogenic carotid-cavernous fistula following Fogarty catheter thromboendarterectomy. Case report. J Neurosurg 1979;51:543–5.

[6] Pedersen RA, Troost BT, Schramm VL. Carotid cavernous sinus fistula after external ethmoid-sphenoid surgery. Clinical course and management. Arch Otolaryngol 1981;107:307–8.

[7] Kaufman HH, Lind TA, Mullin S. Spontaneous carotid cavernous fistula with fibromuscular dysplasia. Acta Neurochir (Wien) 1978;40:123–9.

[8] Hollister DW. Heritable disorders of connective tissue: Ehlers-Danlos syndrome. Pediatr Clin N Am 1978;25:575–91.

[9] Raskind R, Johnson N, Hance D. Carotid cavernous fistula in pregnancy. Angiology 1977;28:671–6.

[10] Brismar G, Brismar J. Spontaneous carotid cavernous fistulas. Phlebographic appearance and relation to thrombosis. Acta Radiol 1976;17:180–92.

[11] Toya S, Shiobara R, Izumi J. Spontaneous carotid cavernous fistula during pregnancy or in the postpartum stage: report of two cases. J Neurosurg 1981;54:252–6.

[12] Seeger JF, Gabriel TO, Giannotta SL, Lotz PR. Carotid cavernous fistulas and venous thrombosis. AJNR Am J Neuroradiol 1980;1:141–8.

[13] De Keiser RSW. Spontaneous carotid cavernous fistulas. Neuroophthalmology 1981;2:35–46.

[14] Parkinson D. A surgical approach to the cavernous portion of the carotid artery: anatomical studies and case report. J Neurosurg 1965;23:474–83.

[15] Lasjaunas P, Berenstein A. The cavernous sinus region. In: Surgical neuroangiography, vol. 1. New York: Springer-Verlag; 1987. p. 54–60.

[16] Sunderland S, Hughes ESR. The pupilloconstrictor pathway and the nerves to the ocular muscles in man. Brain 1946;69:301–9.

[17] Bouthillier A, van Loveren HR, Keller JT. Segments of the internal carotid artery: a new classification. Neurosurgery 1996;38:425–32.

[18] Harris FS, Rhoton AL. Anatomy of the cavernous sinus. J Neurosurg 1976;45:169–80.

[19] Lasjaunas P, Berenstein A. The inferolateral trunk. In: Surgical neuroangiography, vol. 1. New York: Springer-Verlag; 1987. p. 70–1.

[20] Barrow DL, Krisht A. Cavernous sinus dural arteriovenous malformations. In: Awad IA, Barrow DL, editors. Dural arteriovenous malformations. Park Ridge, IL: AANS Publications; 1993. p. 117–30.

[21] McConnell EM. The arterial blood supply of the human hypophysis cerebri. Anat Rec 1953;115: 175–203.

[22] Lasjaunas P, Berenstein A. The neuromeningeal artery. In: Surgical neuroangiography, vol. 1. New York: Springer-Verlag; 1987. p. 132–3.
[23] Barrow DL, Spector RH, Braun IF, et al. Classification and treatment of spontaneous carotid cavernous fistulas. J Neurosurg 1985;62:248–56.
[24] Ernst RJ, Tomsick TA. Classification and angiography of carotid cavernous fistulas. In: Tomsick TA, editor. Carotid cavernous fistula. Cincinnati: Digital Education Publishing; 1997. p. 13–22.
[25] Tomsick TA. Types B, C, and D (dural) CCF: etiology, prevalence, and natural history. In: Carotid cavernous fistula. Cincinnati: Digital Educational Publishing; 1997. p. 59–73.
[26] Tomsick TA. Type A CCF: etiology, prevalence, and natural history. In: Carotid cavernous fistula. Cincinnati: Digital Educational Publishing; 1997. p. 35–8.
[27] Larson JJ, Tew JM Jr, Tomsick TA, van Loveren HR. Treatment of the internal carotid artery by intravenous balloon occlusion: long-term follow-up of 58 patients. Neurosurgery 1995;36:26–30.
[28] Parkinson D. Transcavernous repair of a carotid cavernous fistula: a case report. J Neurosurg 1967; 26:420–4.
[29] Helmke K, Kruger O, et al. The direct carotid cavernous fistula: a clinical, pathoanatomical, and physical study. Acta Neurochir (Wien) 1994;127: 1–5.
[30] Friedmann G, Prowein RA, Luster G. Karotis-sinus-cavernosus-Aneurysmen. Fortschr Neurol Psychiatr 1970;38:57–79.
[31] Debrun G, Lacour P, Vinuela F, et al. Treatment of 54 carotid cavernous fistulas. J Neurosurg 1981;55: 678–92.
[32] Higashida RT, Halbach VV, Tsai FY, et al. Interventional neurovascular treatment of traumatic carotid vertebral lesions: results in 234 cases. AJR Am J Roentgenol 1989;153:577–82.
[33] Lasjaunas P, Berenstein A. Endovascular treatment of craniofacial lesions. In: Surgical neuroangiography, vol. 2. New York: Springer-Verlag; 1987. p. 176–211.
[34] Farley MK, Clark RD, Fallor MK, et al. Spontaneous carotid cavernous fistula and the Ehlers-Danlos syndrome. Ophthalmology 1983;90:1337–42.
[35] Numaguchi Y, Higashida RT, Abernathy JM, et al. Balloon embolization in carotid cavernous fistula in fibromuscular dysplasia. AJNR Am J Neuroradiol 1987;8:380–2.
[36] Taki N, Nakahara I, Nishi S, et al. Pathogenic and therapeutic considerations of carotid cavernous sinus fistulas. Acta Neurochir (Wien) 1994; 127:6–14.
[37] Grossman RI, Sergot RC, Goldberg HI, et al. Dural malformations with ophthalmic manifestations: results of particulate embolization in seven patients. AJNR Am J Neuroradiol 1985;6:809–13.
[38] Mehringer C, Heishima G, Grinnel V, et al. Improved localization of carotid cavernous fistula during angiography. AJNR Am J Neuroradiol 1982;3:82–4.
[39] Lie TA. Congenital anomalies of the carotid arteries, including the carotid-basilar and carotid-vertebral anastomoses. An angiographic study and a review of the literature. Amsterdam: Excerpta Medica; 1968.
[40] Taniguchi RM, Odom GL, et al. Spontaneous carotid cavernous shunts presenting diagnostic problems. J Neurosurg 1971;35:384–91.
[41] Newton TH, Hoyt WF. Dural arteriovenous shunts in the region of the cavernous sinus. Neuroradiology 1970;1:71–81.
[42] Walker AE, Allegre GE. Carotid-cavernous fistulas. Surgery 1956;39:415–22.
[43] Hamby WB. Signs and symptoms of carotid cavernous fistula. Carotid-cavernous fistula. Springfield, IL Charles C. Thomas; 1966. p. 64–97.
[44] Sasaki H, Nukui H, Kaneko M, et al. Long-term observations in cases with spontaneous carotid-cavernous fistulas. Acta Neurochir (Wien) 1988; 90(3–4):117–20.
[45] Halbach VV, Hieshima GB, Higashida RT, et al. Carotid cavernous fistulas: indications for urgent treatment. AJNR Am J Neuroradiol 1986;8:627–33.
[46] Meyers PM, Halbach VV, Dowd CF, et al. Dural carotid cavernous fistula: definitive endovascular management and long-term follow-up. Am J Ophthalmol 2002;134:85–92.
[47] Gamgee JS. Stab through the ear, traumatic aneurysm, death after ligature of common carotid artery. Lancet 1875;1:535.
[48] Jaeger R. Intracranial aneurysms. South Surg 1942; 15:205–17.
[49] Hamby WB. Carotid cavernous fistula. Report of 32 surgically treated cases and suggestions for definitive operation. J Neurosurg 1964;21:859–67.
[50] Parkinson D. Carotid cavernous fistula: direct repair with preservation of the carotid artery. Technical note. J Neurosurg 1973;38:99–106.
[51] Mullan S. Treatment of carotid-cavernous fistulas by cavernous sinus occlusion. J Neurosurg 1979;50: 131–44.
[52] van Loveren HR, Tauber M, Lewis AI, Tew JM. Direct surgical treatment of carotid cavernous fistula. In: Tomsick TA, editor. Carotid cavernous fistula. Cincinnati: Digital Educational Publishing; 1997. p. 83–94.
[53] Debrun G, Lacour P, Caron JP, et al. Detachable balloon and calibrated-leak balloon techniques in the treatment of cerebral vascular lesions. J Neurosurg 1978;49:635–49.
[54] Higashida RB, Halbach VV, Dromandy B, Bell JD, Hieshima GB. Endovascular treatment of intracranial aneurysms with a new silicone microballoon device: technical considerations and indications for therapy. Radiology 1990;174:687–91.

[55] Tomsick TA. Osmotic effects upon long term inflation of latex detachable balloons. Neurosurgery 1985;17:952–4.

[56] Courtheoux P, Labbe D, Hamel C, Lecog PJ, Jahara M, Theron J. Treatment of bilateral spontaneous dural carotid cavernous fistulas by coil and sclerotherapy. Neurosurgery 1987;66:468–70.

[57] Halbach VV, Higashida RT, Hieshima GB, Reicher M, Norman D, Newton TH. Dural fistulas involving the cavernous sinus: results of treatment in 30 patients. Radiology 1987;163:437–42.

[58] Lewis AI, Tomsick TA, Tew JM. Management of 100 consecutive direct carotid cavernous fistulas: results of treatment with detachable balloons. Neurosurgery 1995;36:239–45.

[59] Barrow DL, Fleischer AS, Hoffman JC. Complications of detachable balloon catheter technique in the treatment of traumatic intracranial arteriovenous fistulas. J Neurosurg 1982;56:396–403.

[60] Picard L, Bracard S, Mallet J, et al. Spontaneous dural arteriovenous fistulas. Semin Interv Radiol 1987;4:210–40.

[61] Vinuela F, Fox AL, Debrun GM, et al. Spontaneous carotid-cavernous fistulas: clinical, radiological and therapeutic considerations. Experience with 20 cases. J Neurosurg 1984;60:976–84.

[62] Vinuela F, Duckwiler G, Guglielmi G. CCF: types B, C, and D arterial embolization. In: Tomsick TA, editor. Carotid cavernous fistula. Cincinnati: Digital Educational Publishing; 1997. p. 155–62.

[63] Halbach VV, Higashida RT, Hieshima GB, Hardin CW, Pibram H. Transvenous embolization of dural fistulas involving the cavernous sinus. AJNR Am J Neuroradiol 1989;10:377–84.

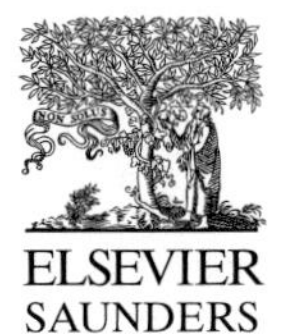

ELSEVIER
SAUNDERS

Neurosurg Clin N Am 16 (2005) 297–308

NEUROSURGERY
CLINICS
OF NORTH AMERICA

Intracranial Angioplasty and Stenting: Modern Approaches to Revascularization for Atherosclerotic Disease

Johnathan A. Engh, MD[a], Elad I. Levy, MD[b,*], Jay U. Howington, MD[c], Lee R. Guterman, PhD, MD[b]

[a]*Department of Neurosurgery, University of Pittsburgh, 200 Lothrop Street, Suite B-400, Pittsburgh, PA 15213, USA*

[b]*Department of Neurosurgery and Toshiba Stroke Research Center, School of Medicine and Biomedical Sciences, State University of New York at Buffalo, 3 Gates Circle, Buffalo, NY 14209–1194, USA*

[c]*Neurological Institute of Savannah, Memorial Health University Hospital, 4 Jackson Boulevard, Savannah, GA 31405, USA*

Atherosclerotic disease accounts for more deaths than any other disease process in the world. The United States is no exception: cardiovascular disease is the leading cause of death, and ischemic stroke is the third leading cause of death [1]. Furthermore, ischemic stroke is the primary cause of adult disability in the United States. The current incidence of combined stroke and transient ischemic attack (TIA) in the United States is approximately 1 million events per year [2,3]. Atherosclerotic disease of the intracranial arteries has been postulated as the cause of 5% to 10% of all intracranial ischemic events in the United States, approximately 50,000 to 100,000 vascular events per year [4–12]. Yet, the optimal treatment strategy for patients with this disease remains undetermined. Antiplatelet therapy, anticoagulation therapy, and interventional angioplasty with or without stenting have all been used in an effort to optimize the care of these patients. Enthusiasm regarding intracranial stent-assisted angioplasty, in particular, has increased considerably over the past decade. The efficacy of interventional therapy versus medical therapy for patients with symptomatic intracranial atherosclerosis has not been compared in a randomized prospective trial, however.

* Corresponding author.
E-mail address: elevy@buffns.com (E.I. Levy).

Epidemiology of symptomatic intracranial atherosclerosis

A multitude of retrospective studies have been performed to quantify the incidence of intracranial atherosclerosis in patients who present after a stroke or TIA. Most of these studies indicate that atherosclerotic intracranial stenosis (ie, of the carotid siphon, M1 segment of the middle cerebral artery, vertebral artery, or basilar artery) accounts for between 5% and 10% of all ischemic strokes in the United States per year. Most of these studies defined radiologically significant intracranial lesions as stenoses of more than 50% maximum vessel caliber combined with an infarction in the parent vessel territory in the absence of an embolic source of stroke. It has previously been demonstrated that there are high levels of interobserver agreement regarding the degree of intracranial stenosis in a particular patient [13]. In patients who undergo an adequate medical workup after a stroke, large vessel intracranial stenosis is the third leading etiology of ischemic cerebral events after cardioembolic stroke and extracranial carotid artery stenosis [4,5]. The Centers for Disease Control and Prevention estimate a combined incidence of TIAs and stroke in the United States of 1 million events per year; as a result, intracranial atherosclerosis accounts for roughly 50,000 to 100,000 intracranial ischemic events per year [3]. Furthermore, multiple

1042-3680/05/$ - see front matter
doi:10.1016/j.nec.2004.08.014

studies have indicated that black Americans, Asians, and Hispanics are more likely to have symptomatic intracranial stenosis than age-matched controls [9,11,14]. Men may be more likely than women to have symptomatic intracranial atherosclerotic disease, but the data are less clear on this issue [9,11,14].

The annual stroke risk for patients with significant large vessel intracranial stenosis may be particularly high. Retrospective trials have quoted a yearly stroke risk in these patients ranging from 5% to 30%, depending on location, symptomology, and severity of stenosis [12,15–23]. The only prospective trial to date regarding the incidence of ischemic stroke in such patients is the Extracranial-Intracranial (EC-IC) Bypass Study [24]. In the nonsurgical arm of this trial, 258 patients with middle cerebral artery stenosis or carotid siphon stenosis were randomized to receive a total of 1300 mg of aspirin per day as well as management of medical risk factors, such as hypertension and diabetes. This group of patients had a stroke rate of 8% to 10% per year. No such prospective data exist for stenotic disease of the posterior circulation, but retrospective data suggest an annual stroke rate of 2.5% to 5.5% in patients with asymptomatic angiographically proven stenosis exceeding 50% in the posterior circulation [18–20]. Symptomatic posterior circulation stenosis of this severity may be a far more treacherous problem: one retrospective study demonstrated an annual stroke rate of 22% in the territory of the affected vessel in 68 such patients [12]. Furthermore, these patients are at a particularly high risk of stroke recurrence after a previous ischemic event (somewhere between 7.1% and 7.9% within the first 30 days), and nearly 50% have repeat symptoms within 12 months [21,22,25]. Therefore, effective therapies for symptomatic intracranial atherosclerosis of the posterior circulation are in particularly high demand.

Medical therapy for intracranial atherosclerosis

Several antiplatelet agents have been used in an attempt to treat patients with intracranial atherosclerotic disease, including aspirin, ticlopidine, clopidogrel, and combinations of these medications. The only drug in this group that has been studied prospectively is aspirin. As mentioned, the stroke rate among patients randomized to aspirin therapy in the EC-IC Bypass Study was 8% to 10% per year [24]. Patients randomized to the surgical arm of the study underwent bypass surgery, and no placebo arm was created. Therefore, no data exist regarding the absolute or relative stroke risk reduction associated with aspirin therapy in patients with known large vessel intracranial stenosis. Furthermore, the use of a radiographic standard instead of a physiologic standard (eg, stroke symptoms attributable to the stenotic vessel with insufficient blood flow demonstrated by radiographic studies) for the enrollment of patients into this trial creates uncertainty as to the applicability of the data to patients with symptomatic intracranial stenosis. Nonetheless, the high stroke rate among patients receiving aspirin in this study underscores the tremendous need for more effective treatments for this disease in general.

Several studies provide insight with respect to the relative efficacy of aspirin versus other antithrombotic agents in the prevention of stroke. In the Ticlopidine Aspirin Stroke Study, 3069 patients with extracranial and intracranial atherosclerotic disease were randomized to receive aspirin (1300 mg daily) or ticlopidine (500 mg daily; a platelet-aggregation inhibitor) after the occurrence of a noncardioembolic TIA [4,26]. The results showed that ticlopidine was more effective than aspirin in stroke prevention (21% relative risk reduction). Ticlopidine has been linked to multiple blood dyscrasias, however, most notably thrombocytopenia and neutropenia. As a result, clopidogrel, a platelet-aggregation inhibitor that is closely related to ticlopidine, gained increased popularity in stroke prevention. In the Clopidogrel versus Aspirin in Patients at Risk of Ischemic Events trial, more than 19,000 patients with documented cardiovascular, cerebrovascular, or other vascular disease were randomized to medical therapy with clopidogrel (75 mg daily) or aspirin (325 mg daily) [4,27]. Of these patients, 6431 were enrolled as the result of a stroke. In this group, the relative risk reduction for recurrent stroke was 8.7% in favor of clopidogrel.

Another important trial addressing medical therapy for the prevention of recurrent stroke among patients with multiple causes of stroke is the second European Stroke Prevention Study, in which a combination of extended-release dipyridamole (400 mg daily) and aspirin (50 mg daily) was compared with either drug alone and with placebo over a 2-year period [28]. The combination was found to be significantly more effective than either drug, providing a 37% relative stroke risk reduction versus 16% for dipyridamole alone and 18% for aspirin alone [4,28,29]. No specific comparison was made between extended-release dipyridamole and aspirin in the management of primary atherosclerotic cerebrovascular disease, however. Although multiple studies have proven that other antiplatelet agents are superior to aspirin in the prevention of stroke recurrence, no study to date has demonstrated that any other antiplatelet agent is superior to aspirin alone in the prevention of primary or recurrent stroke secondary to atherosclerotic intracranial stenosis.

The major medical alternative to antiplatelet therapy is anticoagulation, typically with warfarin. Warfarin therapy is the current standard of care for the management of patients with cardioembolic stroke as well as for the prevention of cardioembolic stroke in patients with known atrial fibrillation [30]. This drug has never been shown to be superior to antiplatelet therapy in the prevention of noncardioembolic stroke, however. In a recent randomized, multicenter, double-blind trial, 2206 patients with a previous noncardioembolic ischemic stroke were assigned to receive warfarin (with a target international normalized ratio [INR] of 1.4–2.8) or aspirin (325 mg daily) [31]. At a 2-year follow-up interval, no significant differences were found in the rates of stroke, death, or major hemorrhage in the two groups. Another randomized, prospective, multicenter trial in which the effectiveness of aspirin and warfarin was compared with respect to noncardioembolic stroke was the Stroke Prevention in Reversible Ischemia Trial [32]. Patients with intracranial or extracranial arterial stenoses were included in this trial. A total of 1316 patients with a history of noncardioembolic TIA or minor ischemic stroke were randomized to receive aspirin (30 mg daily) or warfarin (target INR of 3–4.5). There was an excess of hemorrhagic complications in the warfarin group, and the trial was stopped at the first interim analysis. Critics of the study thought that a higher aspirin dose and a lower INR range would have been more reasonable in the comparison of the two medications.

Despite the lack of benefit of warfarin in the treatment of patients with noncardioembolic stroke, the results of a few retrospective trials suggest the superiority of warfarin to aspirin in the management of patients with isolated symptomatic intracranial stenosis (extracranial carotid artery disease excluded). The most important of these trials is the retrospective Warfarin-Aspirin Symptomatic Intracranial Disease (WASID) study, a multicenter trial that assessed the outcomes of 151 patients receiving warfarin or aspirin for the treatment of symptomatic 50% to 99% intracranial stenosis [7]. In this study, warfarin provided a 46% relative risk reduction of a major vascular event compared with aspirin. The stroke rate among the aspirin-treated patients was approximately 10% per year.

Building on the findings of their retrospective study, the same group of physicians embarked on a prospective WASID study comparing the effectiveness of warfarin (target INR of 2–3) versus aspirin (1300 mg daily) for patients with symptomatic stenosis of an intracranial vessel [5,10,33]. Once complete, the prospective WASID study will be the most important study of its kind. This study is a prospective, randomized, double-blind multicenter trial for patients with symptomatic and significant (angiographically proven ≥50%) intracranial stenosis. Primary end points are stroke or other vascular death. Exclusion criteria include tandem stenoses, cardiac source of embolism, contraindications to medical therapy, severe neurologic deficit, and dementia. Inclusion criteria are listed in Box 1 [33]. The WASID trial will have substantial implications for neurosurgeons. Of primary importance, the results of this trial will

Box 1. Inclusion criteria for the Warfarin versus Aspirin for Symptomatic Intracranial Disease (WASID) trial

- TIA or minor stroke (Rankin score ≤3) within 90 days before randomization
- Stenosis of 50% to 99% of a major intracranial artery (carotid artery, M1 branch of the middle cerebral artery, vertebral artery, or basilar artery) proven by conventional angiography within 90 days before randomization
- TIA or stroke attributed to high-grade intracranial stenosis
- Patient at least 40 years old
- Patient willing and able to follow an outpatient protocol of monthly blood tests and triennial clinic visits and available by telephone
- Patient provided informed consent

From WASID inclusion criteria. Emory University. Available at: www.sph.emory.edu/WASID. Accessed January 16, 2004.

provide an incidence of vascular events in general for patients receiving the best medical therapy; this incidence must be lower than the incidence of such events combined with complication rates associated with intracranial angioplasty with or without stenting for such interventions to be feasible as a primary treatment for symptomatic intracranial stenosis. In addition, the trial will identify which patients have an especially high incidence of vascular events and which vessels are less responsive to medical therapy; such data will help physicians to decide which patients should undergo endovascular interventions rather than medical therapy with aspirin or warfarin [5]. By using this information, a trial comparing the best medical therapy with intracranial angioplasty with or without stenting can then be performed. The original protocol of the WASID study involved the enrollment and randomization of 806 patients; however, the study was prematurely halted at approximately 600 patients. The results of the study are pending publication. Regardless of the outcome of the trial, the high stroke rate among patients with intracranial atherosclerosis who are receiving the best medical therapy necessitates a better treatment option for this disease.

Evolution of intracranial angioplasty and stenting

Intracranial angioplasty was born in 1980 with the performance of a successful basilar artery angioplasty on two patients by Sundt et al [34]. As more experience was gained with such procedures, the morbidity and mortality rates were thought to be too high to justify this procedure as a reasonable intervention at that time. The techniques of intracranial angioplasty and stenting have improved remarkably, however, particularly over the past 5 years, and the instrumentation is far more advanced as well. Microcatheters and balloons are more pliable and supple than they were during the early pilot studies. Furthermore, sizing of the catheters and balloons is now more appropriate to the intracerebral vasculature, which consists of a smaller caliber vascular bed with thinner vessels than the corresponding coronary vasculature. Nevertheless, intracranial angioplasty remains an uncommon procedure: only 42% of major medical centers in the United States are performing angioplasty of the cerebral vessels, and the mean number of intracranial stenoses treated at these centers per year is 12, or 1 per month [35].

Percutaneous transluminal angioplasty for intracranial atherosclerotic disease has been subject to a tremendous learning curve since its inception more than 20 years ago. The biggest change over this period is an increased understanding of the differences between the architecture of cerebral vessels compared with that of coronary vessels. This understanding developed as a result of a high incidence of vessel rupture and dissection; early complication rates ranged from 5% to as high as 50% in small retrospective studies [36–46]. A grouping of these studies, with their enrollment and complication data, is provided in Table 1.

The largest retrospective study of intracranial angioplasty to date is the series of 70 patients spanning a 9-year period reported by Connors and Wojak [47]. This study illustrates the learning curve involved in the application of intracranial angioplasty to the cerebral vasculature: because intracranial vessels are smaller and more friable than coronary vessels, angioplasty must be performed in a more gradual and less aggressive fashion to be successful. Over the course of the study, these authors' technique evolved, and their outcomes improved as a result (Table 2). Grouping of the patients in this study was determined by two variables: rate of balloon inflation and balloon size. After their relative success with group 1, these authors adopted a more aggressive technique that involved oversizing of the treated vessel (group 2). Unfortunately, this approach led to an increase in the dissection rate and even to abrupt vessel occlusion and death in 1 patient. As a result, they began to use an undersized balloon and an extremely slow inflation technique (group 3). This technical adjustment was of tremendous value: although 14% of patients suffered a dissection in the treated vessel, none of the patients suffered a stroke consequently [47]. Furthermore, microangioplasty balloon catheters and postprocedural abciximab therapy were technologic advances available to most patients in group 3 and likely contributed to the improved outcomes [47]. Although these authors did not provide long-term follow-up data on recurrent stenosis rates, their data were promising because, despite a larger patient population, their complication rates were lower than those in most contemporary intracranial angioplasty studies.

Connors and Wojak [47] noted the implications of a less aggressive approach in achieving adequate intracranial flow. According to Poiseuille's law, flow is directly proportional to the

Table 1
Retrospective studies of angioplasty alone for intracranial atherosclerotic disease with associated complication rates

Study	Intracranial vessels treated	Initial success rate (%)	Immediate complication rate (%)
Alazzaz et al, 2000 [36]	16	75	13
Callahan and Berger, 1997 [37]	15	100	13
Clark et al, 1995 [38]	22	82	12
Higashida et al, 1993 [39]	8	75	38
Marks et al, 1999 [40]	23	91	9
McKenzie et al, 1996 [41]	12	92	8
Mori et al, 1997 [42]	35	77	9
Nahser et al, 2000 [43]	20	95	5
Takis et al, 1997 [44]	10	80	40
Terada et al, 1996 [45]	12	67	33
Touho, 1995 [46]	19	68	N/A

Abbreviation: N/A, not available.

Success rate is defined as the percentage of patients with decreased stenosis of the treated vessel immediately after angioplasty who did not develop an acute complication. Complication rate includes the occurrence of stroke attributed to the treated vessel, vessel rupture, and periprocedural death. Asymptomatic dissections and TIAs are not included. Complication rate is listed per vessel treated. Restenosis rates are not included because of the variance in follow-up intervals and criteria.

fourth power of the radius of the vessel lumen in a laminar flow system:

$$\text{Flow} = \Delta P \pi r^4 / 8(\text{Viscosity})(\text{Vessel length})$$

Multiple aspects of this law are manipulated in the clinical setting in an attempt to improve cerebral blood flow in patients with atherosclerotic intracranial cerebrovascular disease. For example, vasopressor therapy and volume expansion help to improve the pressure differential, and mild hemodilution therapy helps to decrease blood viscosity. None of these therapies has been shown to be as effective as an increase in vessel lumen caliber, however; in fact, a small change in vessel caliber yields a tremendous relative increase in flow. For example, a 10 mm vessel with 75% stenosis (on conventional angiography) has a lumen radius of only 1.25 mm. Achieving a partial resolution of this stenosis to only 50% provides a lumen radius of 2.5 mm. As a result of this change, vessel flow increases by a factor of 16.

Another important principle illustrated by the experience of Connors and Wojak [47] is that intracranial vessels are less resistant to dilation than coronary vessels or even extracranial cerebral vessels. Intracranial vessels lack the external

Table 2
Patient groups and outcomes for intracranial angioplasty in a retrospective study from Connors and Wojak

Patient group	1	2	3
Patients	8	12	50
Balloon size	Approximate to vessel diameter but always smaller than treated vessel	Equal to vessel diameter, with oversizing up to 0.25 mm allowed	Always undersized by 0.2–0.7 mm
Inflation period	15–30 seconds	A few seconds	Several minutes
Patient dissection rate (%)	50	75	14
Patient stroke rate (%)[a]	0	8	0
Patient death rate (%)	0	8	2

[a] Stroke rate refers to infarctions within the territory of the treated vessel.

Data from Connors JJ III, Wojak JC. Percutaneous transluminal angioplasty for intracranial atherosclerotic lesions: evolution of technique and short-term results. J Neurosurg 1999;91(3):415–23.

elastic lamina and the extensive adventitia of the extracranial carotid and vertebral arteries. Furthermore, the muscular tunica media of the coronary vessels is essentially absent in the intracranial vessels. As a result, aggressive dilation of intracranial vessels via excessive balloon size or rapid balloon inflation often leads to dissection and thrombosis or, even worse, rupture and hemorrhage [47].

Early lessons learned about the anatomy of intracranial vessels and plaques are recapitulated by the work of Mori et al [48], who developed a classification system of intracranial plaques on the basis of plaque length, stenosis degree, and lesion eccentricity (Table 3). This histopathologic classification scheme is predictive of periprocedural complication rates and subsequent restenosis rates. Using this system, Mori et al [48] found that type A lesions had a 92% immediate success rate and a 0% restenosis rate at 1 year of follow-up. Type B lesions had an 86% immediate success rate and a 33% restenosis rate at 1 year of follow-up. Type C lesions had a 33% immediate success rate and a 56% restenosis rate at 1 year of follow-up. On the basis of these data, this group recommended percutaneous transluminal angioplasty only for type A and B lesions of the posterior circulation in patients experiencing crescendo TIAs [48]. Most patients with symptomatic intracranial atherosclerotic disease do not harbor Mori type A intravascular lesions, however, and their symptoms are more likely to be refractory to medical management. Mori type C lesions are associated with an 87% combined risk of stroke or death versus an 8% combined risk of stroke or death with Mori type A lesions [48,49]. Clearly, technologic refinements of intracranial angioplasty were required for the benefit of those patients in greatest need. Furthermore, the risk of major complications, such as vessel dissection, distal embolization, and arterial rupture, underscored the need for an adjunct technology to improve outcomes. Finally, some reports of angioplasty alone for intracranial atherosclerosis have demonstrated more than 40% postprocedural stenosis [38,40]. The emerging solution to these challenges is intracranial stenting, a technique that has appeared only in the past 5 years. The concept is relatively simple: a permanent device is placed in the vessel to maintain lumen patency after angioplasty, helping to decrease restenosis rates as well as to increase short-term lumen patency rates by preventing vessel recoil. Like intracranial angioplasty, stenting is a technique originally pioneered by interventional cardiologists and subsequently applied to the intracranial circulation. Stents have been proven to decrease dissection risk and improve long-term patency rates in coronary vessels and the extracranial carotid vessels in multiple studies [50,51].

Table 3
Classification of intracranial atherosclerotic plaques

Lesion type	Length	Stenosis	Eccentricity
A	<5 mm	Not totally occluded	Concentric or moderately eccentric
B	5–10 mm	If occluded, for <3 months	Very eccentric or totally occluded
C	>10 mm	Occluded for >3 months	Angulated >90° with excessive proximal segment tortuosity or totally occluded

Data from Mori T, Fukuoka M, Kazita K, Mori K. Follow-up study after intracranial percutaneous transluminal cerebral balloon angioplasty. AJNR Am J Neuroradiol 1998;19(8):1525–33.

Most reports of intracranial angioplasty with stenting include even fewer patients than do reports of angioplasty alone. Nevertheless, they provide promising data for the treatment of patients with symptoms caused by medically refractory intracranial stenosis, particularly of the posterior circulation. In 1999, Phatouros et al [52] successfully treated a thrombotic occlusion of the basilar artery via angioplasty with stenting. In 2000, Rasmussen et al [53] published the results of stent-assisted angioplasty of the intracranial vertebral or basilar artery in eight patients with medically refractory posterior circulation TIAs. Successful vessel revascularization with a mean residual stenosis of 17% was achieved in all patients. One patient died of a subarachnoid hemorrhage that occurred the evening of the procedure, however, for a mortality rate of 12.5% [53].

Gomez et al [54] reported the treatment of medically refractory basilar stenosis via angioplasty and stenting in 12 patients. The mean degree of stenosis in these patients changed from 71.4% before the procedure to 10.3% after the procedure. At a mean follow-up of 6 months, there were no deaths, restenoses, or strokes. Angiographic follow-up was available for only 2 patients, however. The same group also reported a single middle cerebral artery stenosis successfully treated with angioplasty and stenting [55]. Over a similar period, Levy et al [56] described 11 patients with medically refractory intracranial basilar or vertebral artery stenosis treated with transluminal angioplasty and stenting. Four (36%) of 11 patients died. The stented vessel was patent in only 5 (71%) of the 7 surviving patients at the time of angiographic follow-up. These findings emphasize the potentially devastating complications of this procedure, particularly in the posterior circulation. Lylyk et al [57] treated 34 successive patients with more than 50% intracranial stenosis secondary to atherosclerosis or dissection via a combination of direct stenting (ie, stenting without prior balloon dilation on a separate catheter) and conventional stent placement (ie, stenting after prior balloon dilation of the treated vessel). Successful stent deployment occurred in all but 2 patients, and 2 patients died as a result of the procedure, but the remaining results were favorable. Mori et al [58] successfully treated 8 of 10 patients with vertebrobasilar or distal internal carotid artery stenosis via flexible coronary stents. Fifteen patients with intracranial carotid or vertebrobasilar stenosis were treated via conventional angioplasty with or without stenting by Ramee et al [49]. The 5 patients who received stents had no complications, although 1 patient for whom stent placement was intended had an extremely tortuous carotid siphon that the authors were unable to traverse with the stent. In addition, multiple case series of successful stent-assisted angioplasty with 3 or fewer patients each have been reported [59–61]. A summary of these studies is delineated in Table 4.

To date, the only prospective clinical trial regarding the safety and efficacy of stenting for intracranial atherosclerosis is the Stenting of Symptomatic Atherosclerotic Lesions in the Vertebral or Intracranial Arteries (SSYLVIA) trial [62]. Unlike the previous stenting trials discussed in this review, the results of direct (or primary) stenting performed in 43 patients with intracranial arterial stenosis and 18 patients with extracranial vertebral artery stenosis were evaluated in this trial. Although the SSYLVIA trial was a prospective multicenter trial, the study patients were not randomized. Nevertheless, this trial provides an assessment of the usefulness of a stent system specifically designed for intracranial atherosclerosis (NEUROLINK; Guidant Corporation, Menlo Park, California). All patients were enrolled within 7 days of a stroke or a TIA, and none developed new symptoms within 24 hours of the procedure. The stroke or TIA had to be ascribed to the stenotic vessel, and the degree of vessel stenosis had to be at least 50% to be considered adequate for treatment. Initial stent deployment was successful in 95% of patients, and the stroke rate in the territory of the treated vessel at 1 year of follow-up was 13.2%. Unfortunately, these results are an amalgamation of data for extracranial and intracranial lesions, which precludes an assessment of the effectiveness of direct stenting for intracranial arterial stenosis alone. Of greater concern are the angiographic follow-up data: 49 patients have undergone follow-up angiography 6 months after the intervention, and 18 (37%) of these patients demonstrated more than 50% restenosis of the treated vessel at that time. The high restenosis rate implies that bare metal stents are not the definitive answer in the long-term maintenance of vessel patency after intracranial angioplasty, and it underscores the need for more effective stents.

Future directions

Recent advances in the evolution of stent-assisted angioplasty for intracranial atherosclerosis are staged stenting and drug-coated stents. Staged stenting involves angioplasty followed by repeat angioplasty and stent placement at a later time (Fig. 1). The technique was originally developed to improve the treatment of eccentric high-grade (Mori type C) stenoses. In 2002, Levy et al [63] performed a retrospective review of a consecutive series of eight patients treated for medically refractory intracranial vertebrobasilar stenosis. All patients had eccentric high-grade stenoses. The procedure planned for these patients was angioplasty followed by repeat angioplasty and stent placement 1 month or more after the original procedure. The time interval was chosen because experimental data in animal models suggest that the process of remodeling in an atherosclerotic vessel injured by balloon angioplasty lasts for up to 1 month and that the healing lesion is particularly fragile during this period [64,65]. One patient suffered a periprocedural dissection requiring immediate stent placement [63]. The vessel was too tortuous to navigate in one patient, and it was widely patent at follow-up after angioplasty alone in another patient. Stent placement was accomplished successfully in the remaining patients. No deaths or permanent neurologic morbidity occurred.

Table 4
Outcomes and complications associated with stent-assisted angioplasty for intracranial atherosclerotic stenosis

Study	Intracranial vessels treated	Initial success rate (% of patients)	Major complication rate (% of patients)
Gomez et al, 2000 [55] (middle cerebral artery only)	1	100	0
Gomez et al, 2000 [54] (basilar artery only)	12	100	0
Levy et al, 2001 [56]	11	64	36
Lylyk et al, 2002 [57] (these patients had dissections as well as atherosclerotic lesions)	34	100	6
Mori et al, 1999 [59]	1	100	0
Mori et al, 2000 [58]	12	83	0
Morris et al, 1999 [60]	3	100	0
Nakahara et al, 2002 [61]	2	100	0
Ramee et al, 2001 [49] (10 additional patients were treated with angioplasty alone)	5	100	0
Rasmussen et al, 2000 [53]	8	88	13

Success is defined as decreased stenosis of the treated vessel immediately after angioplasty and stenting without the development of an acute complication. Major complications include stroke attributed to the treated vessel, vessel rupture, and periprocedural death. Asymptomatic dissection and TIA are not included. Complication rate is listed per vessel treated. Restenosis rates are not included because of the variance in follow-up intervals and criteria.

Early successes with intracranial stenting led many physicians to question whether angioplasty was necessary before stenting of stenotic vessels. The SSYLVIA trial and a few retrospective intracranial studies had demonstrated success with intracranial stenting [49,57,62]; furthermore, multiple prospective studies of coronary stenting demonstrated that direct stenting was equally safe and more cost-effective than conventional stent-assisted angioplasty [66–68]. Levy et al [69] evaluated this approach in patients with medically refractory basilar artery stenosis. Four patients were treated with direct stent placement; two of these patients developed pontine infarctions manifested by dense postprocedural quadriparesis. The authors thought that an "embolic shower" was probably responsible for the events, and they suggested the avoidance of direct stent placement into the basilar artery. Unlike the coronary circulation, which can be forgiving of small embolic infarctions, the cerebral circulation is extremely sensitive to perforator infarctions, particularly in the posterior circulation; thus, direct stenting is unlikely to be the safest approach in this vascular bed.

An increasing number of randomized prospective trials have demonstrated the efficacy of drug-coated stents in the coronary circulation. Antiproliferative and immunosuppressive agents have been used. For example, the sirolimus-eluting stent was compared with a standard stent in 1058 patients with newly diagnosed coronary stenosis; at a 270-day follow-up interval, the stent failure rate in the target vessel was 21% for bare metal stents versus 8.6% for the sirolimus stent [70]. Furthermore, the results of the Randomized Study with the Sirolimus-Eluting Bx Velocity Balloon-Expandable Stent (RAVEL) showed that sirolimus-eluting stents prevent neointimal proliferation, regardless of vessel diameter [71]. Neither of these trials demonstrated any adverse effects of the sirolimus-eluting stent [70,71]. Another stent that has been studied is the polymer-based paclitaxel-eluting stent. In a prospective, randomized, multicenter trial of 536 patients, paclitaxel-eluting stents reduced neointimal propagation as well as restenosis rates at 6 months of follow-up [72]. Other agents that have been used for stent coating or elution include QP-2, rapamycin, actinomycin D, dexamethasone, tacrolimus, and everolimus [73]. Although the active agents differ, the message is clear: drug-coated stents yield lower restenosis rates than bare metal stents.

Because coronary vessels are generally of larger caliber than cerebral vessels and their vessel wall histology is different, there is a tremendous need for a randomized clinical trial of the efficacy

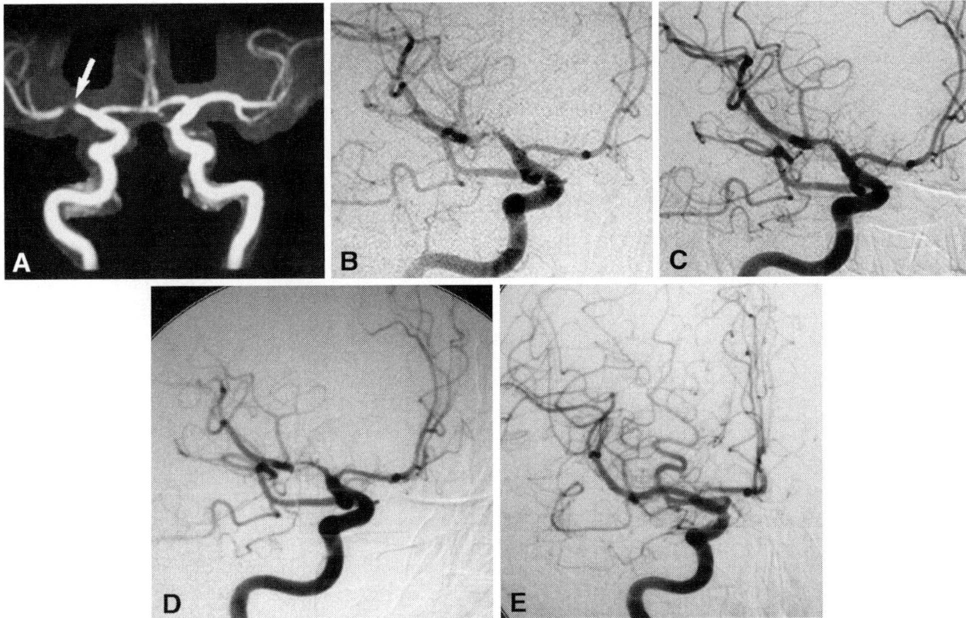

Fig. 1. (*A*) Magnetic resonance angiogram of the intracranial circulation in a 64-year-old woman with recurring transient ischemic attacks demonstrating focal, high-grade, middle cerebral artery (MCA) stenosis. (*B*) Digital subtraction angiogram (DSA) in the same patient demonstrating the focal stenosis in the MCA proximal to the bifurcation. (*C*) DSA after the initial angioplasty. This angioplasty is suboptimal, as evidenced by the residual stenosis. (*D*) DSA 6 weeks after the initial angioplasty. The residual stenosis is now more prominent, but the healed lesion is theoretically more stable than in the period immediately after the initial angioplasty. This lesion was then treated with repeat angioplasty and stent placement. (*E*) DSA 3 months after the original angiogram demonstrates continued complete resolution of the stenosis.

of drug-coated stents within the intracranial circulation. The purpose of the Stenting in Small Coronary Arteries trial was to assess the effects of stenting in smaller vessels [74]. A total of 145 patients were randomized to receive angioplasty alone or angioplasty combined with a heparin-coated stent. Among the heparin-coated stent group, not only was the event-free survival rate higher, but the 6-month angiographic results were superior. This study confirms the finding of the RAVEL study that small-caliber vessels respond favorably to drug-coated stents [71].

No drug-coated stents are currently approved by the US Food and Drug Administration for intracranial use; however, many seem to be on the way. Experimental data indicate that such stents may yield lower rates of long-term restenosis than bare metal stents: a recent study using heparin-coated stents versus bare metal stents in a canine basilar artery model demonstrated an average of 12% luminal stenosis in the drug-coated stents at 12 weeks of follow-up versus 22% in the bare metal stent group [75]. Further study is needed to determine the safety, efficacy, ideal dosing parameters, and durability of these devices. Nonetheless, it is essential that a safe and effective drug-coated stent be developed to maintain the patency of intracranial arteries after angioplasty.

The future of evidence-based treatment of intracranial atherosclerotic disease will involve the conclusion of the WASID trial and the initiation of other clinical trials to evaluate the safety and efficacy of drug-coated stents in the cerebral vasculature. Finally, a randomized multicenter trial comparing angioplasty and stenting with medical management alone must be performed. Until the results of such a trial are published, it may be reasonable to recommend intracranial angioplasty and stenting only for patients with symptomatic intracranial stenosis who have symptoms that are refractory to medical therapy. A therapy superior to antithrombotic medications is sorely needed for the many patients with medically refractory intracranial stenosis.

Summary

The tremendous importance of intracranial atherosclerotic disease cannot be overestimated. Traditionally, patients with this condition have been managed by neurologists and internists. As the inadequacy of medical therapy has come to light, neurosurgeons and neurointerventionists have begun to pay more attention to this highly prevalent problem. The newfound interest in this disease is well justified: intracranial atherosclerotic stenosis is more prevalent and more dangerous than unruptured cerebral aneurysms and arteriovenous malformations put together [15]. It is essential that we maintain our focus regarding the relative frequency and importance of the diseases that we treat as physicians so as to deliver the best therapies to the largest number of patients. Over the next few years, a rigorous assessment of the efficacy of coated stents compared with medical therapy for the treatment of intracranial atherosclerotic disease will provide another step toward the goal of adequately managing this difficult problem.

References

[1] Williams GR, Jiang JG, Matchar DB, Samsa GP. Incidence and occurrence of total (first-ever and recurrent) stroke. Stroke 1999;30(12):2523–8.

[2] Ovbiagele B, Kidwell CS, Saver JL. Epidemiological impact in the United States of a tissue-based definition of transient ischemic attack. Stroke 2003;34(4): 919–24.

[3] Williams GR. Incidence and characteristics of total stroke in the United States. BMC Neurol 2001;1(1): 2523–8.

[4] Albers GW, Amarenco P, Easton JD, Sacco RL, Teal P. Antithrombotic and thrombolytic therapy for ischemic stroke. Chest 2001;119(1 Suppl): 300S–20S.

[5] Benesch CG, Chimowitz MI. Best treatment for intracranial arterial stenosis? 50 years of uncertainty. The WASID Investigators. Neurology 2000;55(4): 465–6.

[6] Chimowitz MI. Angioplasty or stenting is not appropriate as first-line treatment of intracranial stenosis. Arch Neurol 2001;58(10):1690–2.

[7] Chimowitz MI, Kokkinos J, Strong J, et al. The Warfarin-Aspirin Symptomatic Intracranial Disease Study. Neurology 1995;45(8):1488–93.

[8] Executive Committee for the Asymptomatic Carotid Atherosclerosis Study. Endarterectomy for asymptomatic carotid artery stenosis. JAMA 1995; 273(18):1421–8.

[9] Gorelick PB. Distribution of atherosclerotic cerebrovascular lesions. Effects of age, race, and sex. Stroke 1993;24(12 Suppl):I16–21.

[10] Major ongoing stroke trials. Warfarin versus aspirin for intracranial disease. Stroke 1999;30(8): 2256–61.

[11] Sacco RL, Kargman DE, Gu Q, Zamanillo MC. Race-ethnicity and determinants of intracranial atherosclerotic cerebral infarction. The Northern Manhattan Stroke Study. Stroke 1995;26(1):14–20.

[12] Warfarin-Aspirin Symptomatic Intracranial Disease (WASID) Study Group. Prognosis of patients with symptomatic vertebral or basilar artery stenosis. Stroke 1998;29(7):1389–92.

[13] Samuels OB, Joseph GJ, Lynn MJ, Smith HA, Chimowitz MI. A standardized method for measuring intracranial arterial stenosis. AJNR Am J Neuroradiol 2000;21(4):643–6.

[14] Wityk RJ, Lehman D, Klag M, Coresh J, Ahn H, Litt B. Race and sex differences in the distribution of cerebral atherosclerosis. Stroke 1996;27(11): 1974–80.

[15] Angioplasty and stenting of extracranial brachiocephalic stenoses (other than the cervical carotid bifurcation) and intracranial stenoses. AJNR Am J Neuroradiol 2001;22(8 Suppl):S31–3.

[16] Bogousslavsky J, Barnett HJ, Fox AJ, Hachinski VC, Taylor W. Atherosclerotic disease of the middle cerebral artery. Stroke 1986;17(6):1112–20.

[17] Marzewski DJ, Furlan AJ, St. Louis P, Little JR, Modic MT, Williams G. Intracranial internal carotid artery stenosis: long-term prognosis. Stroke 1982;13(6):821–4.

[18] Moufarrij NA, Little JR, Furlan AJ, Leatherman JR, Williams GW. Basilar and distal vertebral artery stenosis: long-term follow-up. Stroke 1986;17(5): 938–42.

[19] Pessin MS, Gorelick PB, Kwan ES, Caplan LR. Basilar artery stenosis: middle and distal segments. Neurology 1987;37(11):1742–6.

[20] Pessin MS, Kwan ES, DeWitt LD, Hedges TR III, Gale D, Caplan LR. Posterior cerebral artery stenosis. Ann Neurol 1987;21(1):85–9.

[21] Rundek T, Elkind M, Chen X, et al. Increased early stroke recurrence among patients with extracranial and intracranial atherosclerosis: the Northern Manhattan Stroke Study [abstract]. Neurology 1998; 50(Suppl 4):A75.

[22] Sacco RL, Foulkes MA, Mohr JP, Wolf PA, Hier DB, Price TR. Determinants of early recurrence of cerebral infarction. The Stroke Data Bank. Stroke 1989;20(8):983–9.

[23] Wechsler LR, Kistler JP, Davis KR, Kaminski MJ. The prognosis of carotid siphon stenosis. Stroke 1986;17(4):714–8.

[24] EC/IC Bypass Study Group. Failure of extracranial-intracranial arterial bypass to reduce the risk of ischemic stroke. Results of an international randomized trial. N Engl J Med 1985;313(19):1191–200.

[25] Thijs VN, Albers GW. Symptomatic intracranial atherosclerosis: outcome of patients who fail antithrombotic therapy. Neurology 2000;55(4):490–7.

[26] Hass WK, Easton JD, Adams HP Jr, et al. A randomized trial comparing ticlopidine hydrochloride with aspirin for the prevention of stroke in high-risk patients. Ticlopidine Aspirin Stroke Study Group. N Engl J Med 1989;321(8):501–7.
[27] CAPRIE Steering Committee. A randomised, blinded, trial of clopidogrel versus aspirin in patients at risk of ischaemic events (CAPRIE). Lancet 1996; 348(9038):1329–39.
[28[Diener HC, Cunha L, Forbes C, Sivenius J, Smets P, Lowenthal A. European Stroke Prevention Study. 2. Dipyridamole and acetylsalicylic acid in the secondary prevention of stroke. J Neurol Sci 1996;143(1–2): 1–13.
[29] Wilterdink JL, Easton JD. Dipyridamole plus aspirin in cerebrovascular disease. Arch Neurol 1999; 56:1087–92.
[30] Hart RG, Halperin JL. Atrial fibrillation and thromboembolism: a decade of progress in stroke prevention. Ann Intern Med 1999;131(9):688–95.
[31] Mohr JP, Thompson JL, Lazar RM, et al. A comparison of warfarin and aspirin for the prevention of recurrent ischemic stroke. N Engl J Med 2001; 345(20):1444–51.
[32] Stroke Prevention in Reversible Ischemia Trial (SPIRIT) Study Group. A randomized trial of anticoagulants versus aspirin after cerebral ischemia of presumed arterial origin. Ann Neurol 1997;42(6): 857–65.
[33] WASID inclusion criteria. Emory University. Available at: www.sph.emory.edu/WASID. Accessed November 2, 2004.
[34] Sundt TM Jr, Smith HC, Campbell JK, Vlietstra RE, Cucchiara RF, Stanson AW. Transluminal angioplasty for basilar artery stenosis. Mayo Clin Proc 1980;55(11):673–80.
[35] Chaturvedi S, St. Pierre ME, Bertasio B. Cerebral angioplasty practice at major medical centers in the United States. Neuroradiology 2000;42(3):218–20.
[36] Alazzaz A, Thornton J, Aletich VA, Debrun GM, Ausman JI, Charbel F. Intracranial percutaneous transluminal angioplasty for arteriosclerotic stenosis. Arch Neurol 2000;57(11):1625–30.
[37] Callahan AS III, Berger BL. Balloon angioplasty of intracranial arteries for stroke prevention. J Neuroimaging 1997;7(4):232–5.
[38] Clark WM, Barnwell SL, Nesbit G, O'Neill OR, Wynn ML, Coull BM. Safety and efficacy of percutaneous transluminal angioplasty for intracranial atherosclerotic stenosis. Stroke 1995;26(7): 1200–4.
[39] Higashida RT, Tsai FY, Halbach VV, et al. Transluminal angioplasty for atherosclerotic disease of the vertebral and basilar arteries. J Neurosurg 1993; 78(2):192–8.
[40] Marks MP, Marcellus M, Norbash AM, Steinberg GK, Tong D, Albers GW. Outcome of angioplasty for atherosclerotic intracranial stenosis. Stroke 1999;30(5):1065–9.
[41] McKenzie JD, Wallace RC, Dean BL, Flom RA, Khayata MH. Preliminary results of intracranial angioplasty for vascular stenosis caused by atherosclerosis and vasculitis. AJNR Am J Neuroradiol 1996; 17(2):263–8.
[42] Mori T, Mori K, Fukuoka M, Arisawa M, Honda S. Percutaneous transluminal cerebral angioplasty: serial angiographic follow-up after successful dilatation. Neuroradiology 1997;39(2):111–6.
[43] Nahser HC, Henkes H, Weber W, Berg-Dammer E, Yousry TA, Kuhne D. Intracranial vertebrobasilar stenosis: angioplasty and follow-up. AJNR Am J Neuroradiol 2000;21(7):1293–301.
[44] Takis C, Kwan ES, Pessin MS, Jacobs DH, Caplan LR. Intracranial angioplasty: experience and complications. AJNR Am J Neuroradiol 1997;18(9): 1661–8.
[45] Terada T, Higashida RT, Halbach VV, et al. Transluminal angioplasty for arteriosclerotic disease of the distal vertebral and basilar arteries. J Neurol Neurosurg Psychiatry 1996;60(4):377–81.
[46] Touho H. Percutaneous transluminal angioplasty in the treatment of atherosclerotic disease of the anterior cerebral circulation and hemodynamic evaluation. J Neurosurg 1995;82(6):953–60.
[47] Connors JJ III, Wojak JC. Percutaneous transluminal angioplasty for intracranial atherosclerotic lesions: evolution of technique and short-term results. J Neurosurg 1999;91(3):415–23.
[48] Mori T, Fukuoka M, Kazita K, Mori K. Follow-up study after intracranial percutaneous transluminal cerebral balloon angioplasty. AJNR Am J Neuroradiol 1998;19(8):1525–33.
[49] Ramee SR, Dawson R, McKinley KL, et al. Provisional stenting for symptomatic intracranial stenosis using a multidisciplinary approach: acute results, unexpected benefit, and one-year outcome. Catheter Cardiovasc Interv 2001;52(4):457–67.
[50] George CJ, Baim DS, Brinker JA, et al. One-year follow-up of the Stent Restenosis (STRESS I) Study. Am J Cardiol 1998;81(7):860–5.
[51] Roubin GS, Yadav S, Iyer SS, Vitek J. Carotid stent-supported angioplasty: a neurovascular intervention to prevent stroke. Am J Cardiol 1996;78(3A):8–12.
[52] Phatouros CC, Higashida RT, Malek AM, et al. Endovascular stenting of an acutely thrombosed basilar artery: technical case report and review of the literature. Neurosurgery 1999;44(3):667–73.
[53] Rasmussen PA, Perl J II, Barr JD, et al. Stent-assisted angioplasty of intracranial vertebrobasilar atherosclerosis: an initial experience. J Neurosurg 2000;92(5):771–8.
[54] Gomez CR, Misra VK, Liu MW, et al. Elective stenting of symptomatic basilar artery stenosis. Stroke 2000;31(1):95–9.
[55] Gomez CR, Misra VK, Campbell MS, Soto RD. Elective stenting of symptomatic middle cerebral artery stenosis. AJNR Am J Neuroradiol 2000;21(5): 971–3.

[56] Levy EI, Horowitz MB, Koebbe CJ, et al. Transluminal stent-assisted angioplasty of the intracranial vertebrobasilar system for medically refractory, posterior circulation ischemia: early results. Neurosurgery 2001;48(6):1215–23.

[57] Lylyk P, Cohen JE, Ceratto R, Ferrario A, Miranda C. Angioplasty and stent placement in intracranial atherosclerotic stenoses and dissections. AJNR Am J Neuroradiol 2002;23(3):430–6.

[58] Mori T, Kazita K, Chokyu K, Mima T, Mori K. Short-term arteriographic and clinical outcome after cerebral angioplasty and stenting for intracranial vertebrobasilar and carotid atherosclerotic occlusive disease. AJNR Am J Neuroradiol 2000;21: 249–54.

[59] Mori T, Kazita K, Mori K. Cerebral angioplasty and stenting for intracranial vertebral atherosclerotic stenosis. AJNR Am J Neuroradiol 1999; 20(5):787–9.

[60] Morris PP, Martin EM, Regan J, Braden G. Intracranial deployment of coronary stents for symptomatic atherosclerotic disease. AJNR Am J Neuroradiol 1999;20(9):1688–94.

[61] Nakahara T, Sakamoto S, Hamasaki O, Sakoda K. Stent-assisted angioplasty for intracranial atherosclerosis. Neuroradiology 2002;44(8):706–10.

[62] Lutsep HL, Barnwell SL, Mawad M, et al. Stenting of Symptomatic Atherosclerotic Lesions in the Vertebral or Intracranial Arteries (SSYLVIA): study results [abstract P83A]. Stroke 2003;34:253.

[63] Levy EI, Hanel RA, Bendok BR, et al. Staged stent-assisted angioplasty for symptomatic intracranial vertebrobasilar artery stenosis. J Neurosurg 2002; 97(6):1294–301.

[64] Tanaka H, Sukhova GK, Swanson SJ, et al. Sustained activation of vascular cells and leukocytes in the rabbit aorta after balloon injury. Circulation 1993;88(4 Part 1):1788–803.

[65] Wainwright CL, Miller AM, Wadsworth RM. Inflammation as a key event in the development of neointima following vascular balloon injury. Clin Exp Pharmacol Physiol 2001;28(11):891–5.

[66] Airoldi F, Di Mario C, Gimelli G, et al. A randomized comparison of direct stenting versus stenting with predilatation in native coronary artery disease: results from the multicentric Crosscut study. J Invasive Cardiol 2003;15(1):1–5.

[67] Ijsselmuiden AJ, Tangelder GJ, Cotton JM, et al. Direct coronary stenting compared with stenting after predilatation is feasible, safe, and more cost-effective in selected patients: evidence to date indicating similar late outcomes. Int J Cardiovasc Intervent 2003;5(3):143–50.

[68] Taylor AJ, Broughton A, Federman J, et al. Efficacy and safety of direct stenting in coronary angioplasty. J Invasive Cardiol 2000;12(11):560–5.

[69] Levy EI, Hanel RA, Boulos AS, et al. Comparison of periprocedure complications resulting from direct stent placement compared with those due to conventional and staged stent placement in the basilar artery. J Neurosurg 2003;99(4):653–60.

[70] Moses JW, Leon MB, Popma JJ, et al. Sirolimus-eluting stents versus standard stents in patients with stenosis in a native coronary artery. N Engl J Med 2003;349(14):1315–23.

[71] Regar E, Serruys PW, Bode C, et al. Angiographic findings of the multicenter Randomized Study With the Sirolimus-Eluting Bx Velocity Balloon-Expandable Stent (RAVEL): sirolimus-eluting stents inhibit restenosis irrespective of the vessel size. Circulation 2002;106(15):1949–56.

[72] Colombo A, Drzewiecki J, Banning A, et al. Randomized study to assess the effectiveness of slow- and moderate-release polymer-based paclitaxel-eluting stents for coronary artery lesions. Circulation 2003; 108(7):788–94.

[73] Grube E, Bullesfeld L. Initial experience with paclitaxel-coated stents. J Interv Cardiol 2002; 15(6):471–5.

[74] Moer R, Myreng Y, Molstad P, et al. Stenting in small coronary arteries (SISCA) trial. A randomized comparison between balloon angioplasty and the heparin-coated beStent. J Am Coll Cardiol 2001; 38(6):1598–603.

[75] Levy EI, Boulos AS, Hanel RA, et al. In vivo model of intracranial stent implantation: a pilot study to examine the histological response of cerebral vessels after randomized implantation of heparin-coated and uncoated endoluminal stents in a blinded fashion. J Neurosurg 2003;98(3):544–53.

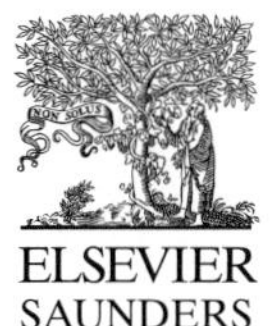
ELSEVIER
SAUNDERS

Neurosurg Clin N Am 16 (2005) 309–312

NEUROSURGERY
CLINICS
OF NORTH AMERICA

Neuroepidemiology of Unruptured Intracranial Aneurysms: Implications for Decision Making Regarding Patient Management

David O. Wiebers, MD

Department of Neurology, Mayo Medical School, Mayo Clinic, 200 First Street SW, Rochester, MN 55905, USA

Unruptured intracranial aneurysms (UIAs) are relatively common, affecting up to 2–5% of the population at some point in life. These lesions are not congenital but rather develop with increasing age. Epidemiologic data from many vantage points suggest that most of these lesions do not rupture. Consequently, it is desirable to identify which unruptured aneurysms are at the greatest risk of subsequent rupture when considering which ones to repair. Optimal management of patients with UIAs also involves predicting which individuals have the greatest likelihood of success and lowest likelihood of complications from repairing their UIA and reconciling these data with natural history data involving these lesions.

It is important to recognize that ruptured intracranial aneurysms and UIAs constitute distinctly different clinical entities and need to be considered and managed accordingly. If it were possible to extrapolate the natural history of UIAs by studying series of patients with ruptured aneurysms, there would have been no need for natural history studies involving UIA patients. The findings of the International Study of Unruptured Intracranial Aneurysms (ISUIA) [1,2] and other natural history studies reinforce the fact that UIAs and ruptured aneurysms are different entities and that their natural histories are distinct from one another.

In the debate about the natural history of UIAs, some investigators have cited circumstances of patients with small unruptured aneurysms diagnosed after subarachnoid hemorrhage (SAH) and have argued on this basis that small unruptured aneurysms may have substantial rupture rates, even among patients with no history of SAH [3]. Others have also attempted to extrapolate the natural history of UIAs by considering incidence rates of SAH and inferred prevalences of UIAs in the population [4]. Considerable confusion has been added to the field by not recognizing the difference between the following two questions:

1. What is the probability of a ruptured aneurysm being a certain size?
2. What is the probability of future rupture of a given sized aneurysm discovered before rupture?

The second of these questions is relevant to the clinical management of patients with UIAs. This principle graphically applies not only to aneurysm size but to aneurysm location. The bottom line is that one does not learn about the natural history of UIAs by studying characteristics of patients or populations with ruptured aneurysms [5]. Available information suggests that most aneurysms that are going to rupture do so at the time of, or relatively soon after, they form and that the critical size for rupture is lower for those aneurysms that rupture early.

In contrast to the situation of patients with ruptured intracranial aneurysms, where one is attempting to repair virtually all aneurysms and an early focus involves which mode of treatment fits the particular situation at hand, patients with UIAs evoke much more emphasis on the

E-mail address: wiebers.david@mayo.edu

1042-3680/05/$ - see front matter
doi:10.1016/j.nec.2004.08.018

Table 1
Five-year cumulative rupture rates according to size and location of unruptured aneurysm and according to patient group among patients in the unoperated cohort

Aneurysm location	Aneurysm size/group				
	<7 mm group 1[a]	<7 mm group 2[b]	7–12 mm	13–24 mm	>25 mm
Cavernous (n = 210)	0%	0%	0%	3 (0%)	6 (4%)
AC/MC/IC (n = 1037)	0%	1 (5%)	2 (6%)	14 (5%)	40%
Post-P comm (n = 445)	2 (5%)	3 (4%)	14 (5%)	18 (4%)	50%

Abbreviations: AC, anterior communicating or anterior cerebral artery; Cavernous, cavernous carotid artery; IC, internal carotid artery (not cavernous carotid artery); MC, middle cerebral artery; Post-P comm, vertebrobasilar, posterior cerebral arterial system, or posterior communicating artery.

[a] Patients in group 1 had no history of SAH.

[b] Patients in group 2 had a history of SAH from a separate aneurysm.

(*Reprinted from* International Study of Unruptured Intracranial Aneurysms Investigators. Unruptured intracranial aneurysms: natural history, clinical outcome, and risks of surgical and endovascular treatment. Lancet 2003;362;103–10.)

consideration of whether or not aneurysmal repair is warranted. This applies to UIAs of all sizes and locations, because many higher natural history risk patients are also at higher risk with regard to treatment morbidity and mortality.

The latest and most robust data regarding natural history and treatment morbidity and mortality among patients with UIAs emanating from the ISUIA allow a more individualized and detailed assessment of the risks of natural history versus the risk of surgical or endovascular repair based on much more than aneurysm size. It continues to be a general principle, however, that for group 1 patients (no history of SAH from another aneurysm) with aneurysms less than 7 mm in diameter, it is unlikely that one will improve on the natural history of these lesions, particularly in older patients and those with aneurysms in the anterior circulation. It must be kept in mind, however, that available natural history studies, including the ISUIA, include few asymptomatic patients with small UIAs, particularly those with acute or changing symptoms or observed aneurysmal growth; thus, these rare circumstances may constitute exceptions to the previously stated principle. Current data do not allow one to establish that a positive family history of intracranial aneurysm or SAH increases the risk of future rupture of an unruptured aneurysm.

For group 1 patients with aneurysms 7 mm or greater in diameter and group 2 patients, rupture rates are more substantial than for group 1 patients with aneurysms less than 7 mm in diameter and generally vary according to aneurysmal size and location. It is now possible to be more sophisticated in making comparisons between natural history and treatment morbidity and mortality on the basis of more than aneurysmal size, and it is important that one considers size-, site-, and group-specific natural history rates for comparison with size, site, and age treatment morbidity and mortality rates (Table 1, Figs. 1–3). The age of the patient has emerged as a crucial decision-making element, largely because age has a major impact on operative morbidity and mortality but relatively little impact on natural history. The age range in which impact is greatest begins at approximately 50 years and older for open surgery and at approximately 70 years and older for endovascular procedures.

Overall, the rupture risk is lowest for asymptomatic group 1 patients with UIAs less than 7 mm in diameter in the anterior circulation. Surgical morbidity and mortality are most favorable for asymptomatic patients less than 50 years of age with UIAs less than 24 mm in diameter in the anterior circulation and no history of cerebrovascular ischemic events. Endovascular morbidity and mortality seem to be less age dependent, and this could favor endovascular procedures, particularly in those patients between 50 and 70 years of age. Another issue of major importance, however, involves the question of immediate versus long-term risk with regard to treatment effectiveness and durability. This issue emphasizes the importance of long-term follow-up in patients after surgical and endovascular procedures so as to assess not only the immediate and short-term complications but the long-term effectiveness.

In circumstances in which repair of UIAs is considered, it is important to recognize that available data suggest substantially lower

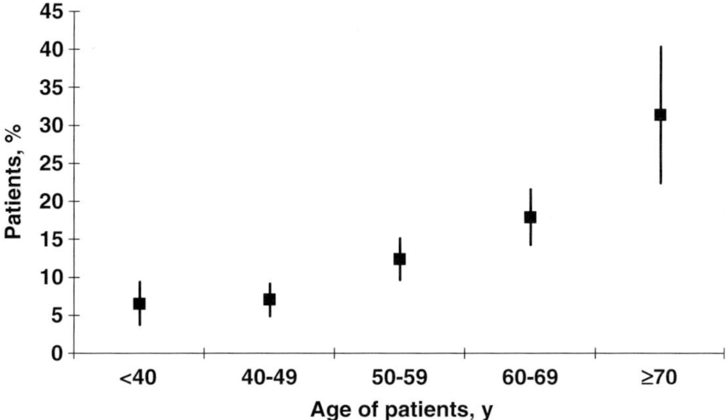

Fig. 1. Poor outcome at 1 year in the surgical cohort by age. Poor outcome is death, a Rankin score between 3 and 5, or impaired cognitive status. Bars show 95% confidence intervals. (*Reprinted from* International Study of Unruptured Intracranial Aneurysms Investigators. Unruptured intracranial aneurysms: natural history, clinical outcome, and risks of surgical and endovascular treatment. Lancet 2003;362;103–10.)

complication rates are associated with institutions and individuals treating large numbers of patients with cerebral aneurysms on an ongoing basis [3,6–8]. It is therefore of great importance to seek out individuals and institutions with substantial ongoing experience with treatment procedures.

Whether or not the patients with UIAs undergo aneurysmal repair, it is important to emphasize that patients avoid smoking (including passive smoke). In situations in which UIAs are left alone and monitored, it also seems advisable to suggest that patients avoid heavy alcohol consumption and that they avoid stimulant medications and drugs as well as excessive straining and Valsalva maneuvers resulting in major increases in blood pressure. It is not generally necessary to alter daily physical activities. Although there are many other medical reasons to treat chronic hypertension, data from the ISUIA and other studies indicate that chronic hypertension may have little or no effect on aneurysmal

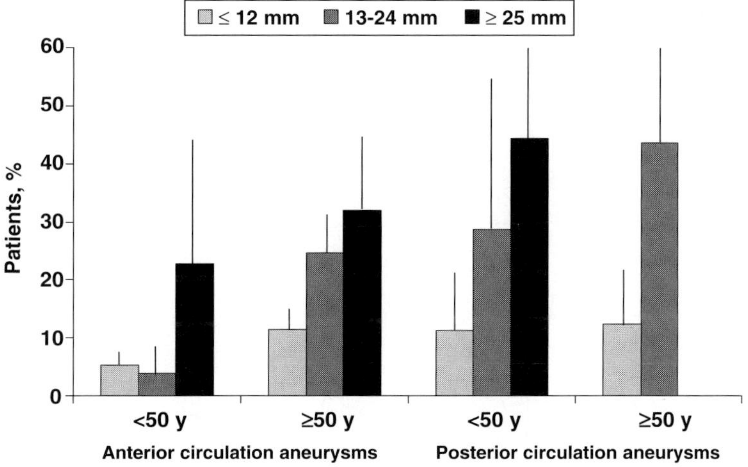

Fig. 2. Poor surgical outcome at 1 year by age, site, and size of aneurysm. Poor outcome is death, a Rankin score between 3 and 5, or impaired cognitive status. Bars show 95% confidence intervals. (*Reprinted from* International Study of Unruptured Intracranial Aneurysms Investigators. Unruptured intracranial aneurysms: natural history, clinical outcome, and risks of surgical and endovascular treatment. Lancet 2003;362;103–10.)

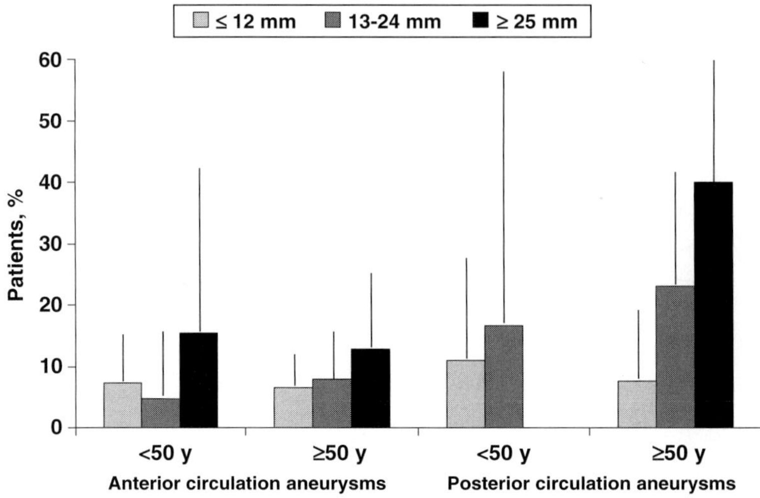

Fig. 3. Poor endovascular outcome at 1 year by age, site, and size of aneurysm. Poor outcome is death, a Rankin score between 3 and 5, or impaired cognitive status. Bars show 95% confidence intervals. (*Reprinted from* International Study of Unruptured Intracranial Aneurysms Investigators. Unruptured intracranial aneurysms: natural history, clinical outcome, and risks of surgical and endovascular treatment. Lancet 2003;362;103–10.)

development or future rupture of UIAs. For situations in which UIAs are not repaired, patients are often monitored annually with magnetic resonance angiography (MRA) or CT angiography for 2 to 3 years and then every 2 to 5 years thereafter if they are stable clinically and radiographically.

References

[1] International Study of Unruptured Intracranial Aneurysms Investigators. Unruptured intracranial aneurysms—risk of rupture and risks of surgical intervention. N Engl J Med 1998;339:1725–33.

[2] International Study of Unruptured Intracranial Aneurysms Investigators. Unruptured intracranial aneurysms: natural history, clinical outcome, and risks of surgical and endovascular treatment. Lancet 2003;362:103–10.

[3] Weir B. Unruptured intracranial aneurysms: a review. J Neurosurg 2002;96:3–42.

[4] Winn H, Jane J, Taylor J, Kaiser D, Britz G. Prevalence of asymptomatic incidental aneurysms: a review. J Neurosurg 2002;96:43–9.

[5] Wiebers DO, Piepgras DG, Meyer FB, et al. Unruptured intracranial aneurysms: pathogenesis, natural history, treatment and patient management considerations. Mayo Clin Proc, in press.

[6] Johnston SC, Zhao S, Dudley RA, et al. Treatment of unruptured cerebral aneurysms in California. Stroke 2001;32:597–605.

[7] Solomon RA, Fink ME, Pile-Spellman J. Surgical management of unruptured intracranial aneurysms. J Neurosurg 1994;80:440–6.

[8] Taylor CL, Yuan Z, Selman WR, et al. Mortality rates, hospital length of stay, and the cost of treating subarachnoid hemorrhage in older patients: institutional and geographical differences. J Neurosurg 1997;86:583–8.

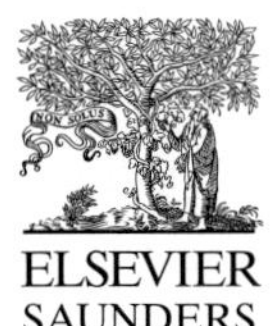
ELSEVIER
SAUNDERS

Neurosurg Clin N Am 16 (2005) 313–316

NEUROSURGERY
CLINICS
OF NORTH AMERICA

Indications for Treatment of Cerebral Aneurysms from an Endovascular Perspective: The Creation of an Evidence Base for Interventional Techniques

Andrew J. Molyneux, MB, BChir, FRCR*

Department of Neuroradiology, Neurovascular Research Unit, Radcliffe Infirmary, University of Oxford, Woodstock Road, Oxford OX2 6HE, United Kingdom

Since the first use of the Guglielmi detachable platinum coil (GDC) to treat an intracranial aneurysm in 1990 by the University of California at Los Angeles group [1], the treatment of intracranial aneurysm disease has been revolutionized. The GDC device opened the prospect of a completely new approach to the treatment of cerebral aneurysms. No longer is the treatment of cerebral aneurysms exclusively the province of a neurosurgeon by a direct approach at craniotomy. The endovascular techniques that have been developed in the last 14 years and are described in this issue have fundamentally changed the treatment approach and are likely to continue to do so.

The results of the International Subarachnoid Aneurysm Trial (ISAT) [2] have shown that for that group of patients with ruptured cerebral aneurysms suitable for endovascular coil treatment, there is a 7.4% (95% confidence interval [CI], 3.6–11.1) absolute reduction in the risk of death or dependency at 1 year and a 24% (95% CI, 12–33) relative risk reduction (modified Rankin score of 3–6, 23.5% after endovascular allocation and 30.9% after neurosurgical allocation) at 1 year [3]. Thus, short-term safety and efficacy of the technique have been proven to a grade 1 evidence level. This has been done within less than 10 years of the first use of the device in Europe and only 7 years after approval of the device by the US Food and Drug Administration (FDA). The speed of obtaining such grade 1 evidence for the use of a new technique has probably never been achieved before. Challenges remain for the endovascular community and device manufacturers in two areas, however: improving the long-term angiographic results and widening the range of aneurysms that can be dealt with by endovascular techniques.

An endovascular approach to cerebral aneurysms will always be potentially more elegant than an exovascular approach by craniotomy provided that it can be achieved as safely or more safely and with a similar degree of efficacy. The definition of efficacy is ultimately clinical, namely, survival free of symptoms from the aneurysm. In most cases, this means prevention of rupture or rerupture from the aneurysm. To establish this will take many years of complete and systematic follow-up of substantial cohorts of patients. The short- and medium-term results of angiographic occlusion are regarded as a reasonable surrogate marker; however, they should be recognized as such, and it remains to be confirmed in large patient cohorts what the significance of angiographic findings are relative to this clinical outcome. The present challenge for the community is how and in what manner to assess the existing and new devices that are becoming available. It is essential that new devices be introduced in a systematic and responsible manner and that they undergo systematic assessment. We need to ensure that increasing procedural complexity does not introduce an

* Correspondence. Department of Neuroradiology, Radcliffe Infirmary, University of Oxford, Woodstock Road, Oxford OX2 6HE, United Kingdom.

E-mail address: andy.molyneux@radiology.ox.ac.uk

1042-3680/05/$ - see front matter
doi:10.1016/j.nec.2004.08.015

unacceptable increased risk to patients in exchange for no proven additional benefit.

Indications for detachable platinum coil treatment

What the International Subarachnoid Aneurysm Trial says and what it does not say

Much has been written by specialist societies [4–6], and there have been many discussions at meetings after the first publication of the initial ISAT results. It is important to understand the applicability of the results. First and foremost, the trial tested the technology and clinical experience available during the period of recruitment (1994–2002). During that time, endovascular techniques and experience evolved considerably, and neurosurgical techniques probably did not change much. Second, it is important to recognize that in any large clinical trial of a technique(s), there will be some differences between specialists in the patterns of enrollment and patient eligibility. Not every surgeon or interventionist necessarily regards the same patients as suitable for both treatments. Certainly, some endovascular operators are more comfortable treating aneurysms in different locations and with different anatomic configurations just as neurosurgeons are more comfortable clipping certain aneurysms, and individual skill varies. Thus, the exact suitability of any individual patient will and must remain the balanced judgment of the neurosurgeon and neurointerventionist, bearing in mind all the factors for that patient. These include the anatomy of the aneurysm, the clinical state and age of the patient, the skill and experience of the neurosurgeon and interventionist, the facilities available to them, and the timeliness with which treatment can be performed. Therefore, inevitably and quite correctly, there will be variations in the proportions of patients treated by the two techniques between neurosurgical centers. Nevertheless, for most patients with ruptured aneurysms, endovascular treatment will be anatomically feasible for the average trained interventionist and will be the safer treatment recommendation for the patient.

Application of newer techniques

Balloon-assisted coil treatment

This technique has been increasingly used by experienced practitioners and undoubtedly widens the anatomic range of aneurysms suitable for coiling. Its use was included in the ISAT. An operator needs to be familiar with the use of balloons, and their use undoubtedly carries a risk of vessel damage; however, the technique allows a wider anatomic range of aneurysms to be treated and widens the proportion of aneurysms treatable by endovascular techniques.

Use of intracranial stents

The approval by the FDA of the Neuroform Microdelivery Stent System (Boston Scientific, Natick, Massachusetts) has been greeted with enthusiasm by many practitioners. The availability of a self-expanding stent that can now be placed with reasonable ease in the intracranial vessels is a major advance, and there is no doubt that other similar devices will become available [7]. This device was not available or used during the ISAT. The main application of this device is improving angiographic outcomes in broad-necked aneurysms in combination with coils. Many practitioners use it as an alternative to balloon assistance. Nevertheless, one must sound a note of caution; particularly with the use of this device in the acute situation, the thromboembolic risk is increased with the use of stents, and the use of powerful antiplatelet drugs is usually required with the device. In the acute situation after subarachnoid hemorrhage (SAH), this presents its own risks. When standard platinum coils and balloon assistance can achieve good short-term results in prevention of rerupture, then, in my view, their use should be predominantly in the nonacute situation. It may be safer to confine them to retreatment, when necessary, of broad-necked internal carotid or basilar aneurysms, which is likely to be their most appropriate application. There is always a danger of over-enthusiasm with such a device; that is, "when you have a hammer, everything looks like a nail."

Use of bioactive and coated coils

Animal studies indicate that the reaction to implanted suture material, such as polyglycolic acid/lactide incorporated into or on a platinum coil, induces significantly more tissue response than bare platinum in experimental aneurysms with a thickened tissue layer at the neck [8]. On this basis, there is the hope that this will improve angiographic outcomes in patients, ultimately, with a lower risk of rebleeding. The latter will be impossible to prove, because the frequency of late rerupture after treatment with bare platinum coils is extremely low and any systematic study to demonstrate a significant difference would need to be so large and take so long as to be impossible to perform. It may be possible to demonstrate a difference in angiographic outcome provided that systematic and preferably randomized studies are performed (anecdotal case reports will not suffice). Such data will not be forthcoming without proper systematic studies, as in the field of cardiology, where the introduction of new stent technology (eg, drug-eluting stents) is routinely accompanied by data from systematic and usually randomized studies. This should certainly be the case if there is increased cost or any change to the safety profile of the device. Such studies should be demanded by the clinical community in the neurointerventional field.

Hydrogel-coated coils

Expanding hydrogel coatings on detachable platinum coils (Microvention, Aliso Viejo, California) [9] have been introduced into clinical use and have some attractions. They provide more complete filling of the aneurysm with a biocompatible material, which not only allows greater volume filling of the aneurysm but has two potential advantages: provision of a better scaffold at the aneurysm neck to allow endothelialization and reduction of the number of coils required to occlude an aneurysm, thus potentially reducing cost or at least not increasing it.

Onyx liquid embolic system

The Onyx system, which is composed of the liquid embolic agent ethylene vinyl alcohol copolymer dissolved in dimethyl sulfoxide, all of which seems to induce a vascular response, is starting to be used to treat intracranial aneurysms with the object of producing a healing reaction in the arterial wall. There have been many skeptical reactions to the use of this material, and it use is still limited to a fairly small number of physicians. The publication of the results of the multicenter European study showed some encouraging results in highly selected cases, however [10]. Recent experience has suggested that occlusion rates in the treatment of large and giant aneurysms are significantly better than those achieved with coil techniques, particularly when Onyx is used in association with stents. It may have a role to play in the management of large and giant aneurysms and recurrences after coiling, where the alternative treatment strategies are limited [11].

Summary

An approved device for endovascular treatment of intracranial aneurysms has only been available in the United States for less than 10 years. In that time, a revolution in the treatment of cerebral aneurysms has started and continues. The elegance and attraction of an endovascular approach for patients and physicians, if it matches open surgery in its safety and efficacy, cannot be argued. We now have grade 1 evidence for superior safety and efficacy at 1 year, and data are starting to accumulate of follow-up over 5- to 8-year time scales, which are reassuring that this benefit continues. Presently, in some experienced centers with access to a full range of devices, in excess of 90% of all intracranial aneurysms presented for treatment are being treated by endovascular techniques; however, a proportion of 75% to 80% is realistically achievable. What is beyond doubt and widely agreed is that patients should be managed in centers where both techniques are available. In this way, patients will receive the best possible care. It is thus difficult to argue with the conclusion of the American Society of Neuroradiology and American Society of Interventional and Therapeutic Neuroradiology position statement published in 2003 that "The study data allow us to conclude that patients with SAH and aneurysm anatomy indicating a high likelihood of success by endovascular techniques should be offered that option. This conclusion must be tempered by the limited data for long-term durability beyond 1 year" [6]. We hope that this latter statement will be addressed, at least in part, by the data that will shortly emerge from the medium-term follow-up to 5 years in the ISAT cohort.

References

[1] Guglielmi G, Vinuela F, Dion J, Duckwiler G. Electrothrombosis of saccular aneurysms via endovascular approach. Part 2: preliminary clinical experience. J Neurosurg 1991;75:8–14.

[2] International Subarachnoid Aneurysm Trial Collaborative Group. International Subarachnoid Aneurysm Trial (ISAT) of neurosurgical clipping versus endovascular coiling in 2143 patients with ruptured intracranial aneurysms: a randomized trial. Lancet 2002;360:1267–74.

[3] Harbaugh RE, Heros RC, Hadley MN. More on ISAT. Lancet 2003;361:783–4.

[4] American Association of Neurological Surgeons. CNS and AANS/CNS Section on Cerebrovascular Surgery: International Subarachnoid Aneurysm Trial: position statement. American Association of Neurological Surgeons Bulletin 2002;11. Available at: http://www.aans.org/library/article.aspx?articleid=9989. Accessed November 12, 2004.

[5] Raabe A, Schmiedek P, Seifert V, Stolke D. German Society of Neurosurgery Section on Vascular Neurosurgery: position statement on the International Subarachnoid Aneurysm Trial (ISAT). Zentralbl Neurochir 2003;64:99–103.

[6] The International Subarachnoid Aneurysm Trial (ISAT). A position statement from the Executive Committee of the American Society of Neuroradiology and American Society of Interventional and Therapeutic Neuroradiology. AJNR Am J Neuroradiol 2003;24:1404–8.

[7] Vanninen R, Manninen H, Ronkainen A. Broad based intracranial aneurysms: thrombosis induced by stent placement. AJNR Am J Neuroradiol 2003;24:263–6.

[8] Muryama Y, Tateshima S, Gonzalez NR, Vinuela F. Matrix and bioabsorbable polymeric coils accelerate healing intracranial aneurysms: long-term experimental study. Stroke 2003;34:2031–7.

[9] Kallmes DF, Fujiwara NH. New expandable hydrogel-platinum coil hybrid device for aneurysm embolisation. AJNR Am J Neuroradiol 2002;23:1580–8.

[10] Molyneux AJ, Cekirge S, Saatchi I, Gal G. Cerebral Aneurysm Multicenter European Onyx (CAMEO) trial: results of a prospective observational study in 20 European centers. AJNR Am J Neuroradiol 2004;25:39–51.

[11] Sluzewski M, Menovsky T, van Rooij WJ, Wijnada D. Coiling of very large or giant aneurysm: long-term clinical and serial angiographic results. AJNR Am J Neuroradiol 2003;24:257–62.

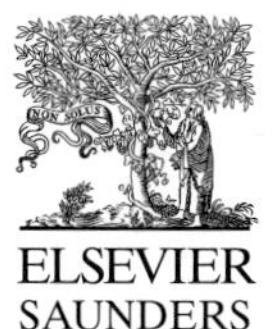

ELSEVIER
SAUNDERS

Neurosurg Clin N Am 16 (2005) 317–353

NEUROSURGERY
CLINICS
OF NORTH AMERICA

Endovascular Treatment of Intracranial Aneurysms and Vasospasm After Aneurysmal Subarachnoid Hemorrhage

Ricardo A. Hanel, MD[a,*], Demetrius K. Lopes, MD[b], J. Christopher Wehman, MD[a], Eric Sauvageau, MD[a], Elad I. Levy, MD[a], Lee R. Guterman, PhD, MD[a], L. Nelson Hopkins, MD, FACS[a]

[a]*Department of Neurosurgery and Toshiba Stroke Research Center, School of Medicine and Biomedical Sciences, University at Buffalo, State University of New York, 3 Gates Circle, Buffalo, NY 14209, USA*
[b]*Departments of Neurosurgery and Radiology, Rush-Presbyterian–St. Luke's Hospital, 1725 West Harrison Street, Suite 970, Chicago, IL 60612, USA*

Over the past decade, dramatic advances have occurred in endovascular technology and techniques for the treatment of intracranial aneurysms. The introduction of the Guglielmi detachable coil (GDC; Boston Scientific Target, Fremont, California) in 1991 for endosaccular aneurysm occlusion [1] has revolutionized the field. Subsequent development of soft and three-dimensional (3D) coil technology has expanded the application of the basic coil occlusion technique. Although endosaccular coiling seems to work best for small to medium-sized aneurysms with narrow necks, successful endovascular treatment of aneurysms with wide necks is now possible because of the addition of balloons and stents to the endovascular armamentarium. In this article, we review the evidence to support endovascular approaches for the treatment of intracranial aneurysms, basic treatment techniques, and complication avoidance and management from the perspective of surgeons who use endovascular and surgical approaches. The importance of adequate management of vasospasm in the overall outcome of patients with ruptured cerebral aneurysms and aneurysmal subarachnoid hemorrhage (SAH) is discussed.

* Corresponding author.
E-mail address: rhanel@buffns.com (R.A. Hanel).

Patient selection for endovascular treatment of intracranial aneurysms

Proper selection of patients for endovascular treatment of intracranial aneurysms requires a careful assessment of the factors influencing the risks of the various therapeutic options. The assessment of risks and benefits ultimately affects the decision whether to proceed with endovascular embolization, craniotomy, and arterial reconstruction by direct clipping, proximal artery occlusion, or a conservative management approach. Until recently, endovascular coil embolization was reserved for patients with SAH who were in poor condition and those for whom craniotomy with aneurysm clipping was considered to present a high risk. With the continuing evolution of technology and techniques, the safety and efficacy of endovascular treatment have improved to the extent that coil embolization has been projected to surpass craniotomy and clipping for aneurysms in terms of the number of aneurysms treated per year in the United States for the year 2004 (Boston Scientific Target, unpublished data, 2004). The operator should be mindful of existing therapeutic options to determine which provides the greatest benefit for the individual patient. Not infrequently, we encounter a case in which a given aneurysm cannot be safely secured by one therapeutic modality and where it is wiser to abort the

1042-3680/05/$ - see front matter
doi:10.1016/j.nec.2004.09.001

procedure and entertain other treatment options rather than to assume the risk of a potentially devastating complication.

A description of the clinical and anatomic considerations guiding the authors' decision-making process in the treatment of cerebral aneurysms follows.

Clinical considerations

One of the most evident advantages of endovascular approaches to cerebral aneurysm treatment is the lower cardiovascular stress (ie, shorter procedure, less tissue manipulation) placed on the patient and the possible avoidance of general anesthesia altogether in patients who are poor surgical candidates. In addition, endovascular approaches may be preferable for the subset of patients who are high-risk candidates for craniotomy because of their age [2] and medical comorbidities. By eliminating the necessity for brain tissue manipulation, especially in a brain that is swollen as the result of SAH, endovascular embolization can result in improved short-term functional outcomes when compared with craniotomy [3].

Conversely, surgical clipping is the mainstay for other patient subgroups. For example, patients with large intraparenchymal hemorrhages in addition to SAH are typically better treated by craniotomy, during which the mass effect of the lesion can be addressed while the aneurysm is being secured.

Anatomic considerations

Each aneurysm responds uniquely to embolic devices, but there are common anatomic characteristics that can help in the selection of the optimal therapeutic modality. Knowledge of the anatomic features of the aneurysm can guide the selection of devices and the subsequent embolization techniques that can yield the optimal result.

A comprehensive four-vessel diagnostic cerebral angiogram should be performed with careful attention paid to access routes to the aneurysm (access anatomy) as well as to the definition of the aneurysm neck from the aneurysm dome and parent vessel. Clear resolution of the neck, dome, and parent vessel of some aneurysm locations and configurations is not possible with conventional digital subtraction angiography. In such cases, the acquisition of a 3D rotational angiogram or a 3D CT angiogram can be extremely helpful in therapeutic planning. Measurement of the aneurysm dimensions and neck size in multiple projections allows selection of the appropriate types and sizes of coils and adjunctive devices (eg, stents, balloons). The dome-to-neck ratio (aspect ratio [ie, the maximum dimension of the aneurysm dome/the width of the aneurysm neck]) and neck size are parameters that can significantly affect the treatment approach decision and, in the case of an endovascular approach, aid in the selection of types and sizes of coils and adjunctive devices that may be necessary. Calcification of the neck region is another angiographic feature that should be evaluated, because this can indicate problems for aneurysm clipping. In such cases, we favor endovascular approaches over microsurgical approaches. In addition, the presence of intra-aneurysmal thrombus should be noted, because this can result in a delay in coil settling and an increase in the chance of aneurysm recanalization.

Aneurysm location

The location of an aneurysm may favor endovascular embolization or surgical clipping. The degree of difficulty encountered with microsurgical and endovascular approaches is altered by variations in individual anatomy. Consideration of exactly which features or characteristics should guide treatment approach decisions has sparked ongoing debate between cerebrovascular neurosurgeons and neuroendovascular surgeons.

The following summary is derived from the authors' experience with surgical and endovascular methods for the treatment of various types of intracranial aneurysms plus the interpretation of available evidence to support such decisions. The decision to treat each lesion should be individualized for each patient according to the configuration of the aneurysm, comorbidities of the patient, and experience of the operator. Ultimately, the operator should assist the patient to make an informed decision regarding the best treatment modality for his or her condition.

Many basilar apex aneurysms have ideal configurations for endovascular placement of coils and adjunctive devices. In such cases, the parent artery points directly into the aneurysm. Such a configuration facilitates access with the microcatheter and increases the likelihood of the coil mass remaining stable within the aneurysm. Although adjunctive devices may be required to obtain a successful result, endovascular treatment of these aneurysms presents less morbidity and mortality [4–8] and is less invasive than craniotomy [9–11]. Some basilar apex aneurysms have favorable anatomy for clipping (anteriorly pointing, located above the posterior clinoid process), but even in carefully selected surgical series, the risks of morbidity and mortality are higher with craniotomy [4–13].

Aneurysms of the superior cerebellar artery are more straightforward to treat surgically than are basilar apex aneurysms. Endovascular treatment of these lesions often requires stent or balloon assistance to obtain ideal occlusion of the aneurysm with preservation of the parent vessel [14].

Proximal posterior inferior cerebellar artery (PICA) aneurysms are often easily accessible by endovascular means but generally require a far lateral craniotomy approach for clipping. Endovascular treatment in this setting represents a less invasive solution to these aneurysms [15], but the choice in this case is more dependent on the configuration of the particular aneurysm and the comfort level of the surgeon with the skull base approach.

Although distal PICA aneurysms are readily accessible to surgical treatment with minimal brain retraction via a suboccipital approach, the endovascular approach is also an option [16]. Even though these lesions are difficult to treat with endovascular embolization without sacrificing the parent vessel, PICA occlusion distal to the tonsillomedullary segment of the PICA is often well tolerated by patients [17].

Treatment of cavernous aneurysms of the internal carotid artery (ICA) should be limited to symptomatic lesions or those at risk for rupture (eg, lesions with carotid-cavernous fistula, thromboembolism, mass effect, subarachnoid extension beyond the dural ring) [2]. Treatment of such lesions depends on whether the artery can be reconstructed or would require sacrifice after successful balloon test occlusion (BTO). The treatment of these aneurysms is almost exclusively endovascular because of the morbidity associated with surgical approaches to the cavernous ICA region.

Treatment of paraclinoid aneurysms of the ICA varies, depending on the symptomatology and configuration of the aneurysm as well as on the access anatomy. For patients presenting with progressive visual loss caused by mass effect, surgical aneurysm clipping with decompression or parent vessel occlusion results in an increased likelihood of improved visual function when compared with coil embolization [18]. For patients presenting with a progressive increase in aneurysm size or SAH and for some asymptomatic patients, treatment patterns are trending toward endovascular coiling because of the less invasive nature of that approach compared with craniotomy [19]. Paraclinoid aneurysms may require stent or balloon assistance for coil embolization, and this is a common site for use of these devices. Craniotomy can involve drilling of the clinoid process and surgical exposure of the cervical ICA.

Aneurysms located on the posterior communicating artery are lesions for which surgical and endovascular treatment approaches are considered to have clinical equipoise. Features like a fetal configuration of the posterior cerebral artery or complex access anatomy tend to favor surgical exploration in these cases. From an endovascular perspective, these are often straightforward aneurysms to treat if the configuration of the carotid siphon is amenable to catheterization [20].

The configuration of an ICA bifurcation aneurysm is similar to that of a basilar apex aneurysm with respect to the orientation of the artery and the aneurysm, but surgical approaches are safer in this region than in the basilar apex region. The decision between coiling and clipping is often based on operator experience, aneurysm anatomy, and patient comorbidities.

Aneurysms of the anterior communicating artery territory can be difficult lesions to treat by surgical or endovascular approaches because of the complexity of the regional anatomy. More than 50% of the aneurysms in patients enrolled in the International Subarachnoid Aneurysm Trial (ISAT) were located in the anterior communicating artery territory, and patients in the endovascular arm had better short-term outcomes than those in the surgical arm [3]. These results may have been a result of the degree of brain retraction or resection that is necessary for an operative approach. For those anterior communicating artery aneurysms in which the neck is undefined and stent-assisted coiling might be appropriate, surgical clipping may be preferable, however, because the A1 segment is usually too small to allow for the intravascular placement of a stent [21].

Pericallosal artery aneurysms and other aneurysms located on distal segments of the anterior cerebral artery are less technically complex to treat surgically than are aneurysms in the territory of the anterior communicating artery. The ability to perform endovascular coil embolization of these aneurysms is heavily influenced by intracranial vessel tortuosity and the aneurysm configuration and cause (traumatic versus infectious) [22].

Aneurysms of the middle cerebral artery (MCA) tend to possess a complex anatomy at the neck region, with the aneurysm typically occurring at a bifurcation or trifurcation of the M1 segment. The aneurysm neck often involves the origin of one or more vessels, making the treatment of such lesions challenging for endovascular approaches. In most cases, the neck anatomy precludes complete coil embolization of the inflow zone, which may lead to aneurysm regrowth [23,24]. Because of the proximity of the artery to the cortical surface, these aneurysms are often best treated with craniotomy and clipping. Some patients with more proximal M1 segment aneurysms may benefit from endovascular embolization.

Dome-to-neck ratio

The anatomy of aneurysms with an aspect ratio of greater than 2 is favorable for conventional endovascular coiling; moreover, such aneurysms seem to present a greater risk for rupture [25]. For aneurysms with an aspect ratio of less than 2 or with a neck size greater than 4 mm, primary coiling may result in herniation of coils into the parent artery or inability to pack the neck region tightly [4,26,27]. This leads to a higher incidence of partially treated aneurysms and a higher risk for recanalization or growth of the aneurysm. For aneurysms with unfavorable aspect ratios or neck size, adjunctive balloon or stent assistance may be necessary. Preprocedural management with antiplatelet medication is necessary if stent- or balloon-assisted coiling is planned. This is not ideal for nonsecured ruptured aneurysms, given the potential risk of rebleeding when administrating such agents.

Fusiform aneurysms

A comprehensive description of the selection of appropriate therapy for fusiform aneurysms is beyond the scope of this article. In general, these lesions have a poor natural history, and the treatment is high risk. Patients with fusiform aneurysms can manifest with a variety of symptoms as the result of SAH, aneurysmal growth with direct compression of neural structures, distal embolization of intraluminal thrombus, or progressive occlusion of the ostia of small perforating arteries along the length of the aneurysm.

Therapy must address the symptomatology, because the risk of treating these aneurysms can approach or exceed the natural history of the disease. As opposed to saccular aneurysms, in which the goal is to exclude the aneurysm from the circulation, complete exclusion is often not possible with fusiform aneurysms, despite adequate collateralization, because of the presence of vital perforating end arteries. For patients presenting with thromboembolic events, anticoagulation can be considered, but this therapy must be weighed against the likelihood of fatal SAH in the event of aneurysm rupture. Compression-related symptoms can be treated by occlusion of one or more feeding arteries, which may lead to hemodynamic changes within the aneurysm and may result in the alleviation of symptoms caused by mass effect and, in some cases, complete aneurysm thrombosis. Surgical bypass procedures may or may not be necessary in these cases. If permanent vessel occlusion is required, it is performed only after BTO. An appealing option for the treatment of such lesions is the placement of intravascular stents (one or more) to reconstruct the parent vessel. The use of stents in this situation can change the hemodynamic environment within the aneurysm, potentially leading to thrombosis. The deployment of two or more stents in the same location can provide a lower porosity mesh, favoring the flow changes within the lesion.

Covered and partially covered stents should soon be available and surely have a place in the treatment of fusiform aneurysms. The issue of perforators and branch patency remains to be studied and defined.

Summary

Although attempts at treatment of most aneurysms by endovascular methods may be possible, a wise practitioner recognizes the limitations that apply in each particular case. As with any specialty, sound judgment is as important as operative skills to avoid procedural complications and provide good patient care. All practitioners, whether cerebrovascular neurosurgeons or neurointerventionists, need to possess an understanding of the available treatment options for their patients. The continued evolution of endovascular technology and techniques will undoubtedly expand the application of this approach to a broader patient population.

Devices and agents for endovascular treatment of aneurysms

Detachable balloons and alternatives to permanent vessel occlusion

Permanent vessel occlusion may be a viable endovascular therapeutic option for patients tolerating BTO in whom treatment of the aneurysm with preservation of the parent vessel cannot be safely achieved. The goals of endovascular treatment by parent artery occlusion are to induce intra-aneurysmal thrombosis through alterations in the local hemodynamics and subsequent shrinkage of the aneurysm and to maintain collateral blood flow. Clot organization and fibrosis as well as elimination of hemodynamic factors responsible for aneurysm growth can lead to a reduction in the size of the aneurysm, thereby relieving the symptoms caused by neural compression. Aneurysm involution can take a long time, especially if the walls are thick and calcified [28]. Pressure-related signs and symptoms usually improve soon after parent artery occlusion or flow reversal within the parent artery, because the pulsation of the sac is diminished and small reductions in aneurysm size occur. Transient swelling can occur acutely after thrombosis of the aneurysm, however, and can exacerbate symptoms like cranial nerve palsies [29] or hydrocephalus.

The traditional endovascular approach to parent vessel sacrifice involves the use of detachable silicone balloons. In this technique, the balloon is prepared and advanced through a guide catheter to the appropriate location. Balloon placement for permanent occlusion is dependent on aneurysm location and test occlusion findings relative to the presence or absence of aneurysm reperfusion from collateral flow. Ideally, the aneurysm should be excluded from the circulation, with a first balloon being placed distal to the aneurysm neck and a second balloon placed proximal to it. This approach can be used in the treatment of cavernous carotid aneurysms.

For the more common anatomic configuration in which the perforating arteries originate distal to the aneurysm, two balloons are placed in a tandem fashion proximal to the aneurysm to occlude the parent vessel. The second balloon is added to prevent migration of the first balloon. Both detachable balloons are delivered through a single guide catheter. After the more distal of the two balloons has been positioned and inflated, the other balloon is partially inflated to arrest the flow in the proximal portion of the vessel. Before detachment of the balloons, additional angiograms should be obtained and may indicate the risk of aneurysm reperfusion via collaterals. In the event of massive aneurysm reperfusion, balloon repositioning or reassessment of the effectiveness of this treatment may be necessary. If the position of the balloons is judged to be optimal, the distal balloon is detached; the proximal balloon is then fully inflated and detached as well. Changes in hemodynamics within the aneurysm induce thrombosis of the sac.

In cases of carotid ophthalmic aneurysms, the balloons can be positioned (1) over the aneurysm neck, between the aneurysm and the ophthalmic artery, if there is more than a 5-mm segment in which to deposit the balloon; (2) in front of the orifice of the ophthalmic artery if there is a functional anastomosis with the external carotid artery; or (3) below the ophthalmic artery if there is no reperfusion of the aneurysm by collateral circulation [7]. The recent withdrawal of the only US Food and Drug Administration (FDA)–approved detachable silicone balloon from the United States market has led to the development of other strategies for permanent parent vessel occlusion. One such strategy involves the combination of temporary proximal flow arrest with a nondetachable balloon with permanent parent vessel occlusion with coils [30].

In cases of vertebrobasilar system aneurysms, striving to attain the dual goals of inducing thrombosis of the aneurysm lumen and maintaining collateral blood presents somewhat of a dilemma. Although thrombosis is best achieved by placing the occluding balloon as close as possible to the aneurysm, the presence of vital perforators just proximal to the aneurysm precludes the placement of the balloon in this position. Placement of the balloon in a more proximal position leads to preservation of adequate collateral flow through or past the aneurysm orifice. In most cases, unilateral occlusion of the dominant vertebral artery is sufficient to induce thrombosis within the aneurysm. Otherwise, occlusion of the contralateral vertebral artery can be performed 3 or 4 weeks later, after repeat test occlusion of this artery to verify adequate retrograde flow from the posterior communicating artery [7]. When bilateral vertebral artery occlusion is indicated for the treatment of a basilar aneurysm, the authors perform occlusion distal to the origin of the PICA on one side and proximal to the PICA origin contralaterally.

The indications for endovascular permanent vessel occlusion are becoming rarer with the advent of newer techniques, such as stent-assisted coiling, and the development of new technology, such as specifically designed devices for the intracranial circulation.

Results of permanent vessel occlusion

The likelihood of aneurysm thrombosis after proximal endovascular parent artery occlusion is related to the magnitude of persistent flow from collaterals [29]. Higashida et al [31] reported stable complete thrombosis in 68 (100%) cavernous aneurysms in their series after endovascular parent artery sacrifice. Symptoms of local compression caused by giant aneurysms improved, despite the lack of evidence of a reduction in aneurysm size on follow-up CT scans. The effectiveness of this procedure decreases in the anterior circulation when it is performed for aneurysms distal to the ophthalmic artery. Fox et al [29] reported that although all cavernous-carotid aneurysms in their series were completely thrombosed after proximal parent vessel occlusion, only 10 (48%) of 21 aneurysms located above the ophthalmic artery origin became thrombosed without an additional aneurysm trapping procedure. Similarly, vertebral artery occlusion for proximal aneurysms, such as those arising from the intracranial vertebral artery, is quite effective, with results being progressively less successful for aneurysms of the vertebrobasilar junction, basilar artery, superior cerebellar artery, and basilar bifurcation [32].

Despite a negative preoperative test occlusion, neurologic deficits can occur after parent artery sacrifice. The rate of permanent postprocedural neurologic deficits in patients with a negative BTO after endovascular sacrifice of the ICA varies from 0% to 10% [29,31,32]. When the neurologic deterioration is related to hemodynamic factors, the collateral flow can be augmented with aggressive hyperdynamic therapy, which may lead to reversal of the deficit. An emergency arterial bypass procedure might also be considered in this setting.

The long-term changes in intracranial circulation hemodynamics occurring after elective parent artery sacrifice are not completely understood. The major concern is that by increasing blood flow in collateral vessels, parent artery sacrifice may lead to the formation of de novo aneurysms [33]. In a review of the literature, Dyste and Beck [34] reported the presence of symptomatic aneurysm formation or enlargement after carotid occlusion in 4% to 10% of cases after therapeutic carotid occlusion. In their series, Timperman et al [35] found de novo aneurysms in 2 (3%) of 58 cases of therapeutic carotid occlusion. Both patients in these cases presented with ruptured anterior communicating artery aneurysms. Whether these de novo aneurysms are related to the same pathologic process that caused the original aneurysm or result from increased blood flow in the intact carotid artery remains to be proved.

Era of aneurysm coiling

The major paradigm shift in intracranial aneurysm treatment was initiated by the introduction of electrolytically detachable coils by Guido Guglielmi. The persistence and creativity of this Italian neurosurgeon led to the major advancement represented by the invention of the GDC system, thus beginning a new era in the endovascular treatment of aneurysms. In the early 1980s, while applying current to a stainless steel electrode introduced into an experimental aneurysm to promote electrothrombosis, Guglielmi observed accidental electrolytic detachment of the electrode tip. Several years later, Guglielmi and engineer Ivan Sepetka worked to combine the processes of endovascular electrolysis and electrothrombosis, an undertaking that eventually led to the development of the GDC system [1,36]. Theoretically, with the GDC system, an aneurysm could be excluded from the intracranial circulation while the patency of the parent vessel was preserved. Different types of coils have been used successfully for endovascular occlusion of intracranial aneurysms. At present, FDA-approved coils are available from the following six device manufacturing companies: Boston Scientific Target, Micrus, Cordis (Miami Lakes, Florida), MicroVention (Aliso Viejo, California), MicroTherapeutics (Irvine, California), and Cook (Bloomington, Indiana). Undeniably, the evolution of detachable coil technology has revolutionized the overall approach to the management of intracranial aneurysms. The recent development of bioactive coils has strengthened the role of coils even more in the treatment of intracranial aneurysms.

Aneurysm coiling technology: basic treatment concepts

The concept of aneurysm coiling is based on the ability to fill the sac with a soft compliant platinum agent that can be retrieved in the event of an improper fit. Controlled delivery is the primary advantage of the detachable systems, with the coil being detached only when the correct position is documented by angiography. A further advantage is the flexibility and softness of the coils, which varies from one system to another; this enables filling of the aneurysm sac and minimizes the risk of rupture during deployment.

Most coil systems consist of a thin, spiral-woven, platinum wire formed in the shape of a helix and soldered to a stainless steel delivery wire. When positioned within a microcatheter, the coil assumes a straight shape and can easily be advanced into the aneurysm. The coils have a circular memory that is expressed when the coil is pushed out of the microcatheter and deployed within the aneurysm. Coil softness refers to the ease with which a coil can compress and expand and is influenced primarily by the diameter of the platinum wire. Soft coils are made of a thinner platinum wire than are standard ones. Soft and standard coils are available in a range of sizes and lengths so that aneurysms can be packed piecemeal with appropriately sized coils. Changes in coil design have made the coils resistant to stretching. More elaborate designs have become available, including two-diameter coils in which the helix of the initial coil segment defines a smaller diameter than the remaining helices. With two-diameter coils, the leading coil loop tends to remain inside the aneurysm sac while avoiding contact between the advancing coil tip and the aneurysm wall because of the smaller loop diameter. This design also reduces the predisposition of the first coil to herniate from the aneurysm during deployment. In an attempt to decrease the incidence and degree of coil compaction [37], 3D coils were developed. These coils spontaneously form a complex 3D configuration during delivery and have been used successfully to occlude aneurysms with an unfavorable geometry for conventional coil embolization. In fibered coils, the thrombogenicity of the platinum coil is enhanced by the attachment of Dacron fibers.

The GDC detachment system is described here because it was the first aneurysm coiling system developed and served as the basis for the development of other coil systems. The stainless steel delivery wire is insulated, except for the most distal part, the detachment zone. A radiopaque marker is incorporated in the delivery wire 3 cm proximal to the detachment zone. During detachment, this marker aligns with the proximal marker on the microcatheter (the microcatheter contains two markers; the distal one goes inside the aneurysm and the proximal one gives the operator the ability to check the advancement and alignment of the coil before detachment). By checking the position of the proximal markers on the delivery wire and microcatheter, the operator can ensure that the coil has advanced outside the microcatheter tip (even though the distal marker on the catheter tip may be obscured by overlying previously placed coils) and avoid advancing the stiff delivery wire into aneurysm sac. When the coil has been placed in a satisfactory position, a positive, low-voltage, direct current is applied to the delivery wire. The current induces electrolysis at the solder junction between the coil and delivery wire, and the coil is gradually detached. This technique allows delivery of the coil without displacement from its location. Ideally, the aneurysm is progressively filled with coils until angiographic obliteration of the sac and preservation of the parent artery are achieved.

The coil systems have general characteristics in common but vary in their size, shape, and detachment system. Methods of detachment currently available include electricity-based (Boston Scientific Target, Micrus, MicroTherapeutics) and hydraulic (Cordis, MicroVention, Cook) approaches. Nuances for each system exist, but the details are not within the scope of this article.

The most recent innovation in the coil systems is the addition of bioactive agents to the classic platinum coil. The theoretic advantage is to promote the organization of thrombus within the aneurysm and thus to reduce the incidence of aneurysm recanalization. The Matrix coil (Boston Scientific Target) was the first bioactive coil introduced in the United States. These coils are made of platinum covered with a bioabsorbable polymeric material (polyglycolic acid [PGA]/lactide) [38]. The advantage of the Matrix system over conventional platinum coil systems has been shown in animal studies [38,39], but its effectiveness in preventing aneurysm recanalization in human beings remains to be seen. The Cerecyte coil (Micrus) is another example of a PGA-modified platinum coil.

Another bioactive coil, the Hydrogel coil (MicroVention), uses a different concept. Rather than facilitating thrombus organization, this device has been designed to improve filling within the aneurysm sac, with complete or near-complete exclusion of thrombus. The device consists of a carrier platinum coil coupled to an expandable hydrogel material, which undergoes a three- to nine-fold increase in volume when placed in a physiologic environment (acid pH–induced swelling occurs within 20 minutes). The presence of the hydrogel within the coil mass leads to a greater filling of the aneurysm sac, potentially serving as a base for a more elaborate healing response. Unlike thrombus, the hydrogel material is stable and unaffected by natural thrombolytic processes and thus may diminish observed rates of aneurysm recanalization [40]. This benefit has been shown in animals [40]; again, the long-term benefits and limitations of clinical application remain to be seen.

Basic technique of coil embolization

The basic technique described here assumes that intensive medical decision making has been performed with consideration of the indications for the procedure, individual characteristics of the patient and his or her aneurysm, and goals for the coiling procedure (complete occlusion whenever safe and feasible or partial coiling when protecting the dome of a ruptured aneurysm unsuitable for primary coiling or clipping).

Anesthesia

At most centers, aneurysm coil embolization is performed with the patient in a state of general anesthesia. This approach does not allow direct intraprocedural assessment of the patient's neurologic status. Although some advocate that intraprocedural monitoring can be performed using motor or somatosensory evoked potentials and electroencephalography, the risks associated with general anesthesia and mechanical ventilation would still be present. As reported by Henkes et al [41] in cases performed under general anesthesia, most ischemic complications cause symptoms immediately after the procedure. At the authors' institutions, GDC embolization of intracranial aneurysms is performed in awake patients after the administration of sedative and analgesic agents (midazolam, fentanyl, morphine, or hydromorphone) [42]. The potential advantages of this approach, including decreased cardiopulmonary morbidity rates, a shorter hospital stay, and lower hospital costs, still require confirmation by a direct comparison with other anesthetic procedures [42]. Qureshi et al [42] pointed out that thromboembolic complications can be promptly recognized and treated in awake patients.

Preprocedural medications

For patients with unruptured and nonacutely ruptured aneurysms scheduled for primary coiling, we routinely administer aspirin (81–325 mg daily) for at least 4 days before the procedure. If balloon- or stent-assisted coiling is anticipated, clopidogrel (75 mg daily for 4 days before the procedure or a loading dose of 450 mg 4 hours before the procedure) is added to the regimen. Intravenous heparin (50–70 U/kg) is given just after placement of the introducer sheath, with the aim of obtaining an activated coagulation time in the range of 250 to 300 seconds. For patients with ruptured aneurysms, we routinely proceed without administering heparin and antiplatelet agents. If balloon or stent assistance is necessary, we may opt for partially coiling the aneurysm, completing the treatment during the same admission but after the acute phase of rupture has passed (ie, when the patient has recovered neurologically).

Procedure

After a femoral sheath has been placed (6 or 7 French) in the right groin, a diagnostic angiogram is obtained. Appreciation of the aneurysm neck and its relation to adjacent perforating and major arteries is a prerequisite to the embolization procedure. It is particularly important to isolate the aneurysm neck from the parent vessel angiographically so that any coil prolapse into the parent vessel can easily be detected. This often requires the acquisition of multiple oblique views. Once a "working projection" is identified, it is recorded for use during the embolization procedure. In some cases, the complex 3D geometry of the aneurysm and surrounding vessels or the overlapping of different structures prevents the acquisition of an adequate view for safe embolization of the aneurysm.

Once the diagnostic angiogram has been obtained, a guide catheter is placed in the target vessel as distal as is safely possible. Such positioning of the guide catheter provides a stable platform to carry out the steps of the coiling procedure.

A coaxial system consisting of a microcatheter and microwire is used to catheterize the aneurysm. The coaxial system and guide catheter are flushed continuously with a solution of saline and heparin (1000 IU of heparin per 1000 mL of saline) to prevent thrombus formation between the two catheters or while the coils are being advanced through the microcatheter.

Access to the aneurysm is obtained via the micro-guide wire, followed by microcatheter placement. Road mapping is helpful during this part of the procedure. Care is taken to avoid touching the aneurysm wall with the tip of the wire or microcatheter. An appropriately sized coil is chosen by matching the helix radius of the coil to the estimated diameter of the aneurysm. The best choice for the first coil is one that bridges the aneurysm neck and allows dense homogeneous packing of the aneurysm. In principle, the longest coil available to fill as much of the aneurysm sac as possible should be used. The first and second coils are critical for achieving complete occlusion. The first coil should be placed in a basket-like configuration within the aneurysm. The placement of a second basket coil within the first may provide a more stable configuration for the deposition of subsequent coils.

After placement and before detachment of each coil, a control angiogram is obtained with injection of contrast material through the guide catheter to confirm proper placement of the coil as well as to demonstrate patency of the adjacent arteries. After placement of the initial basket coil or coils, the remaining cavity is filled with smaller diameter coils, which are placed within the loops of the basket to prevent bulging into the parent artery. Coils are deposited until dense packing is achieved or when the aneurysm accepts no more coils (resistance is encountered with risk of herniation into the parent vessel). Although some authors suggest packing the aneurysm as much as possible and stopping the procedure only when the last coil cannot be introduced inside the sac (thus, the last coil is always wasted), we prefer to individualize the degree of packing to the aneurysm morphology and the procedural goals.

Balloon remodeling technique

The balloon remodeling technique was the initial alternative to surmount the problem presented by coil embolization of wide-necked aneurysms [43]. In this technique, a soft semicompliant or conformable balloon is positioned across the neck of an aneurysm and inflated during coiling. The balloon works as a mechanical barrier that allows tighter packing of the aneurysm while preventing coil herniation into the parent artery during coil delivery. Also, the balloon stabilizes the microcatheter during coil delivery and forces the coils to conform to the 3D shape of the aneurysm. This technique is most suitable and less technically challenging for proximal aneurysms of the ICA or the vertebrobasilar system. To avoid undesired movements of the microcatheter within the aneurysm when the remodeling technique is used, the balloon must be placed first in the parent vessel in front of the aneurysm neck. Selective microcatheterization of the aneurysm is then performed. Inflation of the balloon in front of the aneurysm neck temporarily occludes the neck and the parent vessel. Under balloon protection, coils are then deposited into the aneurysm. After placement of each coil into the aneurysm but before detachment, the balloon is deflated to test the stability of the coil. If no displacement of the coil is observed, the coil is detached. If movement is detected after balloon deflation, the coil is considered unstable and repositioned or removed.

In experienced hands, application of the remodeling technique has been associated with complete angiographic occlusion in 77% to 83% of aneurysms immediately after treatment [43,44]. The technique has several drawbacks, however. The procedure is technically demanding, and the operator is required to use two microcatheters simultaneously. The dangers of local thrombus formation and distal embolization are increased by temporary interruption of blood flow in the parent vessel, and thromboembolic complications have been observed in 5% to 8% of patients treated [43,44]. The need to inflate and deflate the balloon repeatedly risks intimal damage. There is also concern that an increase in intra-aneurysmal pressure during balloon inflation across the aneurysm neck [45], coupled with forceful placement of coils in a closed space [44], may increase the risk of bleeding, especially during treatment of acutely ruptured aneurysms. The incidence of intraprocedural rupture with the remodeling technique can be as high as 5%, which is a rate twice that encountered with conventional coil embolization [44]. In the event of rupture, however, the balloon can be inflated immediately to stop the hemorrhage and allow placement of additional coils to occlude the aneurysm. In this way, bleeding is rapidly managed, and clinical consequences can be minimized. Despite these limitations, this technique is a valid part of the armamentarium of endovascular surgeons and has been used by experienced teams to treat between 1.4% and 20% of the aneurysms embolized at their centers [41,43,44]. Although the long-term effectiveness of this technique in promoting stable occlusion of wide-necked aneurysms is unknown, short-term outcomes are promising. In their series of 56 patients, Moret et al [43] reported that 20 of 21 completely occluded aneurysms remained completely occluded at follow-up angiography 3 to 6 months later.

Stent-assisted coiling technique

Although the balloon remodeling technique constitutes an important method for the endovascular treatment of intracranial aneurysms, the adjunctive use of stents seems to offer an appealing alternative. Incentive for the use of a stent in conjunction with coils includes the potential for a lower risk of dissection or vessel rupture [41]. In the authors' experience, the implantation of a stent across the neck area serves as a buttress to the coil mass and contributes to changing the hemodynamic parameters locally by redirecting the flow and providing a substrate for endothelialization in that area [46,47].

Several concerns have been raised about the safety of stents in the treatment of intracranial aneurysms [48]; however, preliminary clinical experience suggests that some of these concerns are unjustified. For example, stents are known to induce intimal hyperplasia, and it has been argued that excessive neointimal proliferation after stent placement can result in hemodynamically significant stenosis, especially of the smaller intracranial branches. The occurrence of neointimal hyperplasia is usually evident in the first few months after treatment as a consequence of the vessel reacting to the presence of a foreign body. In the authors' series of stent-assisted coiling (with coronary stents) for the treatment of 12 ophthalmic segment aneurysms in 11 patients, no case of in-stent stenosis was found over the course of angiographic follow-up (mean of 26.5 months; range: 5–55 months) [49].

Concerns also exist that occlusion of the ostia of small side branches and perforating arteries by stent placement may result in ischemia or infarction in the territory of these vessels. The authors' experience with stenting in the basilar artery in a canine model did not reveal any effect of the stents struts on the perforators, however [50]. These experimental results were mirrored by our clinical observations. Lopes et al [51] examined the postprocedural cerebral angiograms of 10 patients (7 had aneurysms and 3 had intracranial stenosis) in which the stent was placed across a normal major branch artery. Over the course of a mean follow-up interval of 10 months, all major branches remained patent, no infarctions were associated with the territory of the major branch arteries crossed by the stents, and no patient experienced a related episode of clinical ischemia. It is also possible that in patients with fusiform aneurysms of the basilar trunk and other critical segments, the involved perforating vessels have become "nonfunctional," thus explaining the absence of permanent neurologic sequelae after stent placement with or without secondary coil placement. Because of the high porosity of the stents used, lateral branches, such as the ophthalmic artery and the anterior inferior cerebellar artery, remain patent after a stent is placed across their origins.

Self-expandable intracranial stents

Some potential pitfalls associated with the use of balloon-mounted stents in the intracranial circulation have prevented widespread application of stent implantation. Intended for use in the coronary circulation, balloon-mounted stents lack the suppleness necessary to navigate the tortuousities inherent to the intracranial circulation to reach lesions beyond the carotid siphon. They are ideal for side wall aneurysms on straight vessels, but because most intracranial aneurysms arise at branch points, the efficacy of coronary stents in the treatment of these lesions is greatly reduced. Also, the balloon inflation needed to deploy the stent can be associated with a small risk of vessel dissection or rupture [52,53] and theoretically could lead to delayed stenosis [54,55]. In an attempt to minimize these risks, a push was made to develop a self-expanding stent pliable enough to navigate the turns of intracranial vessels and effectively span the neck of a branch point aneurysm yet with enough radial force to contain an intra-aneurysmal coil mass. The first available such stent was the Neuroform stent (Boston Scientific Target).

The Neuroform stent is constructed of nitinol (a nickel-titanium alloy), which possesses a high degree of elasticity and deformability. This self-expanding stent has an ultrathin open-cell mesh design and exerts a lower amount of radial force than stents used in the treatment of atherosclerotic disease. Instead of being mounted on a balloon, the stent comes preloaded in a coaxial, over-the-wire, 3-French microcatheter delivery system. The delivery catheter has a braided shaft with a hydrophilic coating to facilitate vascular access. Because the stent is fully enclosed within the microcatheter, it can be passed through vessels without abrading the vessel wall. The ultrathin property of the stent struts makes the stent essentially radiolucent, and this feature is offset by four radiopaque platinum marker bands at each end. The entire system consists of the 3-French micro-delivery catheter with the stent preloaded and a second 2-French stabilizer catheter. Usually, the delivery system for the stent is advanced over the exchange wire to the point that it spans the neck of the aneurysm. At this point, the stent is deployed by holding the stabilizer in position and pulling back the delivery catheter.

Use of the Neuroform stent was associated with the pitfalls common to a first-generation device. Howington et al [56] described difficulties with navigation and delivery of this stent in tortuous vessels and thromboembolic complications, especially in acutely ruptured aneurysms. As is the case with any stent implantation, patients receiving this self-expanding stent require dual antiplatelet therapy (aspirin plus clopidogrel or ticlopidine). Unfortunately, the aspirin-clopidogrel regimen is contraindicated in patients with an acutely ruptured aneurysm who might benefit from stent-assisted coiling. Although it is possible to administer the loading dose of clopidogrel in these patients and then deploy the stent, such an approach could be complicated by recurrent hemorrhage. Moreover, if thrombus forms during the procedure, the use of intra-arterial thrombolysis would increase the risk of repeat hemorrhage significantly. Howington et al [56] suggested that the ideal aneurysm for the Neuroform stent is one that has not ruptured and is treated in an elective fashion after appropriate antiplatelet therapy has been initiated.

Reports of the experience with the first-generation Neuroform stent at two centers are available. Fiorella et al [20] reported the results obtained with attempted implantation of this device in 19 patients with 22 aneurysms during a 5-month period. A total of 25 stents were deployed, with 5 patients having multiple stents placed. Fourteen patients had unruptured aneurysms at the time of treatment. The indications for use of the device in their series were broad-necked aneurysms in 13 patients, fusiform or dissecting aneurysms in 3, salvage or bailout in 1, and giant aneurysms in 2. Technical problems included difficulty in deploying the stent in six cases; stent displacement in two cases; and inability to deploy the stent, inadvertent stent deployment, and coil stretching, respectively, in one case each. Twenty-one of the 22 aneurysms were treated with the Neuroform stent: 4 with the stent alone and 17 with stent-assisted coiling. Among the coiled aneurysms, complete or nearly complete (more than 95%) occlusion was achieved in 6 aneurysms and partial occlusion was achieved in 11. Clinically significant adverse events included two periprocedural thromboembolic complications. One of the patients died after thrombolysis was attempted. The other patient made an excellent functional recovery after undergoing successful thrombolysis of a thrombosed basilar artery stent. In the series reported by Benitez et al [57], 56 patients were identified as having wide-necked intracranial aneurysms suitable for stent-assisted coiling. A total of 49 aneurysms in 48 patients were treated with the Neuroform stent associated or not associated with coils. Stent deployment failed in eight cases (14%). Six aneurysms were stented only; 1 aneurysm was initially coiled, followed by stent placement; and 41 aneurysms were initially stented, followed by coil placement. There were five (8.9%) deaths, one (1.8%) of which occurred secondary to a stroke after the procedure. Four (7%) patients experienced thromboembolic events, of which three (5.3%) events were related to the procedure. In addition, there were two femoral pseudoaneurysms. The overall complication rate was 10.7%.The combination of two Neuroform stents implanted in a "Y-shaped" configuration to treat wide-necked basilar apex aneurysms has been suggested [58]. The overall impact of this technique application remains to be seen.

Unquestionably, the introduction of the Neuroform stent represented an important advance in the endovascular treatment of aneurysms with a low dome-to-neck ratio, which otherwise would be difficult to treat with coils. Second and third-generation Neuroform stents are now available, and in our personal experience, their performance is improved in comparison with the original device.

Many other specifically designed intracranial stents are being developed and should become available in the near future. Design modifications are expected to include asymmetric and covered stents and should enhance the results of endovascular approaches for the treatment of intracranial aneurysms.

Liquid embolic agents

Given the significant number of recurrences after coiling, especially in large and giant aneurysms with wide necks [26,59,60], other avenues of endovascular treatment were sought. The use of a liquid agent that would be able to obliterate the aneurysm sac completely and seal the neck has significant attractions and has been examined for several years [61–63]. The liquid nonadhesive embolic agent proposed for this purpose is Onyx (MicroTherapeutics). Specifically designed for endovascular use, Onyx is an ethylene vinyl alcohol copolymer dissolved in an organic solvent, dimethyl sulfoxide (DMSO). When this liquid embolic agent comes into contact with an aqueous solution, it precipitates and initially forms an outer soft and spongy polymer cast, with a semi-liquid center. As further material is injected into the cast, it fills the space into which it is injected, and additional material then breaks out through the outer layer of the existing cast [64]. Experimental studies in different animal models have demonstrated the feasibility and safety of endovascular treatment of aneurysms by the use of this method [65,66].

The technique of Onyx embolization begins with the placement of a highly compliant DMSO-compatible occlusion balloon (Equinox or Hyperglide; MicroTherapeutics) within the parent vessel over the aneurysm neck. The balloon is left deflated while a DMSO-compatible microcatheter (Rebar; MicroTherapeutics) is placed within the aneurysm. A slow test injection of contrast material through the microcatheter is made with the balloon inflated to ensure that the neck is "controlled," and a satisfactory seal is achieved with stasis of contrast material within the aneurysm. The microcatheter is then purged with saline to clear any contrast residue and primed with DMSO with a volume to match the dead space within the catheter. Onyx (HD 500) is then introduced into the microcatheter. After a volume of approximately 0.2 mL has been injected, the Onyx approaches the end of the microcatheter and the balloon is inflated to the predetermined volume (measured when creating the seal between the aneurysm neck and parent vessel, as mentioned previously). The balloon maintains the patency of the parent vessel during the procedure while the aneurysm is filled with the Onyx, which forms a cast that seals the aneurysm off from the circulation and, in effect, reconstructs the parent vessel wall (Fig. 1).

The disadvantage of Onyx embolization is that it increases the technical complexity of the procedure [64]. The agent is injected at a rate of approximately 0.1 mL/min by using the specifically designed Cadence Precision Injector syringe (MicroTherapeutics), which operates by means of a screw thread. Because Onyx is a viscous material, it accumulates around the microcatheter tip and gradually enlarges to form a kernel that remains attached to the end of the microcatheter. After each injection, the balloon is left inflated for another 3 minutes and is then deflated to allow cerebral reperfusion for at least 2 minutes, and the cycle is repeated. With each injection, new portions of the aneurysm fill; eventually, the material flows down to the margins of the balloon and occludes the aneurysm neck. When the material comes into contact with the balloon, the injection is slowed or stopped with brief 15- to 30-second pauses to minimize the risk of leakage into the parent artery and beyond the balloon. It is important to ensure that material covers the aneurysm neck to achieve complete and durable occlusion and reduce the risk of aneurysm regrowth. The microcatheter position is not adjusted once the injection has begun. After angiographic confirmation of complete or satisfactory occlusion of the aneurysm, the catheter syringe is decompressed by aspiration of 0.2 mL of the material and a 10-minute pause is taken to allow complete solidification of the polymer with the balloon deflated. The balloon is then reinflated, and the microcatheter is removed by gentle traction [64].

Mawad et al [67] described their experience with stent-assisted Onyx embolization for the treatment of giant aneurysms in 11 patients. In their series, all aneurysms were excluded from the circulation, with preservation of the parent artery. Six-month follow-up angiographic images documented no recanalization of the aneurysm in 9 patients and minimal recanalization in 1 patient. The complications in this series included one death (vessel dissection, resulting in fatal intracranial hemorrhage) and one case of transient hemiparesis caused by watershed ischemia (prolonged balloon inflation occluding the ICA). Some concerns regarding the safety of the clinical use of DMSO are mentioned in the literature, especially with respect to the risks of parent vessel occlusion and DMSO-induced angionecrosis [64–67].

Two clinical trials, one European and one American, were designed to investigate the safety and efficacy of the Onyx embolic system in selected patients with intracranial aneurysms. The American trial, comparing Onyx versus coil embolization, was recently halted, and the results are not yet available. The results of the Cerebral Aneurysm Multicenter European Onyx trial were recently published [64]. This prospective single-arm observational study was conducted at 20 European centers, enrolling a consecutive series of 119 patients with 123 aneurysms judged suitable for Onyx treatment. The definition of a suitable aneurysm was one that was likely to be difficult to treat or presented a high risk for conventional coil techniques or neurosurgical clip placement, had recurred after coil embolization, or had failed to respond to surgical or endovascular treatment. Their results comprised data obtained for 97 of 119 patients with 100 of 123 aneurysms; 87% of patients harbored unruptured aneurysms, and 81% of aneurysms were large or giant. Angiographic images obtained at the 12-month follow-up examination were available for 71 of 97 patients. Of these, aneurysm

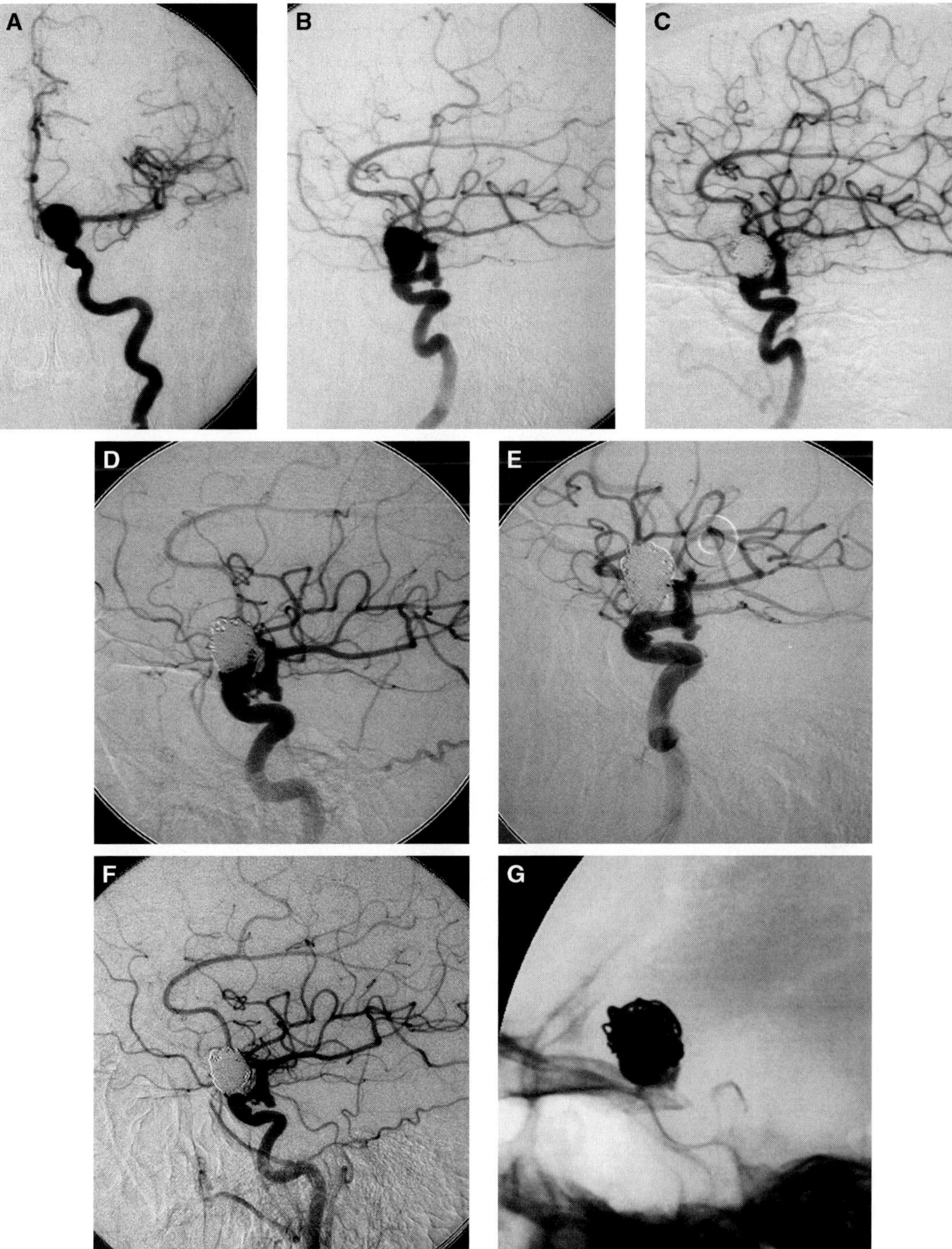

Fig. 1. Case illustration. This 64-year-old woman presented with an unruptured left internal carotid artery aneurysm (*A*, anteroposterior view; *B*, lateral view). (*C*) The patient initially underwent primary coiling of her aneurysm with partial occlusion of the sac. Three months after the procedure, the aneurysm remnant was found to be larger. (*D*) A further increase in size was noticed at 9 months. (*E*) At this point, the patient received retreatment with Onyx, which resulted in complete occlusion of the aneurysm. (*F*) No aneurysm regrowth was observed on the follow-up angiogram obtained 28 months after the second treatment. (*G*) Note that the Onyx conforms to the coil mass.

occlusion was complete in 79% of patients, subtotal in 13%, and incomplete in 8%. Permanent neurologic morbidity related to the procedure was present in 8.2% of patients, including monocular blindness caused by leakage of the agent into the ophthalmic artery (two cases), ipsilateral infarctions (two cases), SAH caused by dissection (two cases), and worsening of cranial nerve palsy (one case). An additional 8.2% of patients had transient neurologic complications. During the study period, 7.2% of the patients died: two deaths were related to the procedure, one was related to SAH (pulmonary complications), and four were of unrelated causes. The two procedure-related deaths were associated with femoral access site complications. The functional status of 75 of the 82 patients alive and with follow-up at 12 months was Rankin Scale grade 2 or better. Delayed occlusion of the parent vessel occurred in 9 patients; delayed occlusion was asymptomatic in 5 patients and resulted in permanent neurologic deficit in 2. Retreatment was required for recurrence of 10 (10%) aneurysms between 3 and 12 months after initial treatment, which seemed to be dependent on the aneurysm size (5%, 13%, and 5% of small, large, and giant aneurysms, respectively) [64].

Outcomes of coiling for intracranial aneurysm treatment

The immediate clinical and angiographic results after GDC embolization of ruptured intracranial aneurysms were assessed by Vinuela et al [60]. These authors reported 403 patients treated at eight United States centers participating in the FDA study between December 1990 and July 1995, which led to device approval in September 1995. All aneurysms were treated within 15 days of rupture. The most common reasons for selecting endovascular treatment in this series included high surgical risk because of aneurysm size and location (69%), failed surgical exploration (12.7%), and poor neurologic (12.2%) or medical (4.7%) status. Because of this preselection, most (57%) aneurysms were in the posterior circulation. Immediate angiographic results varied, primarily according to the size of the aneurysm neck and sac. Complete aneurysm occlusion at the conclusion of the embolization procedure was observed in 70.8% of small aneurysms (4 to 10 mm in largest diameter) with small necks (<4 mm). In this subgroup, technical failures (inability to place coils because of technical difficulties, such as vessel tortuosity or wide neck) were uncommon (occurring in only 3.6% of cases). In contrast, complete occlusion was achieved in only 31% of small aneurysms with wide necks and technical failure occurred in 16.9%. Despite the high-risk preselected population, overall rates of morbidity (8.9%) and mortality (6.2%) were low and were not significantly influenced by aneurysm location when anterior and posterior circulation aneurysms were compared (morbidity: 8.1% versus 9.6%, mortality: 6.4% versus 6.1%, respectively). In critically assessing these results, it must be remembered that the aneurysms treated represented the early experience at the participating centers. As more experience has been accumulated, several centers have reported their results after coiling of intracranial aneurysms [68–71]. Current success rates can be expected to be higher because of improved selection criteria and treatment strategies, along with the availability of a greater range of coil sizes and types.

Murayama et al [26] reported their 11-year experience (beginning in December 1990) with GDC embolization at the University of California at Los Angeles Medical Center. For comparative purposes, the patients were divided into two groups: group A included their initial 5 years' experience with 230 patients harboring 251 aneurysms, and group B included the later 6 years' experience with 588 patients harboring 665 aneurysms. Overall, angiographically demonstrated complete occlusion was achieved in 55% of aneurysms and a neck remnant was displayed in 35.4% of lesions. Coil occlusion was incomplete in 3.5% of aneurysms and attempted unsuccessfully in 5%. A comparison between the two groups revealed a higher rate of complete embolization in group B than in group A (56.8 versus 50.2%, respectively). The overall morbidity/mortality rate was 9.4%. Follow-up angiograms were obtained in 53.4% of cases of aneurysms, and recanalization was exhibited in 26.1% of aneurysms in group A and 17.2% of those in group B. The overall recanalization rate was 20.9%. Aneurysm recanalization was related primarily to neck remnants and larger size. The overall incidence of delayed aneurysm rupture was 1.6%, a rate that improved in the more recent 5 years to 0.5%. Ten of 12 delayed ruptures occurred in large or giant aneurysms.

The addition of improved 3D coils and softer stretch-resistant coils to allow more complete packing at the region of the aneurysm neck seems to have resulted in an improvement in the overall results of treatment. Niemann et al [72] reported a series of 133 patients with 141 aneurysms treated by a single neurointerventionist with ACT microcoils (Micrus), a new generation of spherically shaped 3D coils. Of the aneurysms treated, 110 were ruptured and 31 were unruptured. Complete angiographic occlusion was achieved in 74% of aneurysms, 24% had subtotal (≥95%) occlusion, and 2% had incomplete (<95%) occlusion.

As mentioned, the long-term stability (efficacy) of aneurysm occlusion with coils is still unknown, because some aneurysms recanalize [73] and even rupture [74,75] despite initial satisfactory treatment (complete angiographic occlusion). Raftopoulos et al [76] analyzed a prospective series of 103 patients with 132 aneurysms treated with coiling considered the first therapeutic option. In this study, clipping was performed only for cases in which endovascular embolization was deemed unlikely because of aneurysm characteristics or for those cases in which embolization had failed. Three groups were defined: group A comprised 64 aneurysms treated by endovascular embolization (these aneurysms had a neck-to-sac ratio of <1:3), group B comprised 63 aneurysms that were not considered suitable for endovascular treatment and were surgically clipped, and group C comprised 12 aneurysms that were not satisfactorily (>95%) embolized and were subsequently clipped. The frequency of residual aneurysms was 31.2% in group A, 1.6% in group B, and 0% in group C. Poor outcomes (defined as Glasgow Outcome Scale score of 1–3) at 2 to 6 months after treatment in patients with good clinical status before treatment occurred in 10.7% of the patients in group A, 0% in group B, and 8.3% in group C.

More recent reports have concentrated on the results and importance of follow-up angiography. Cognard et al [77] reported their observations in 169 aneurysms (ruptured and unruptured) in which at least one follow-up angiogram was obtained a minimum of 3 months after treatment. At the end of the initial procedure, occlusion was judged to be total in 95 (56%) cases, subtotal in 66 (39%), and incomplete in 8 (5%). Because of initial subtotal or incomplete occlusion, a second procedure was performed in 18 patients, with subsequent total occlusion achieved in 14. The first follow-up angiogram confirmed total occlusion in an additional 39 aneurysms that initially had been considered subtotally occluded. Overall, total occlusion was obtained in 148 (88%) aneurysms. This study underscores the importance of long-term follow-up angiographic studies. Recurrence was observed in 5% of the totally occluded aneurysms at 3 months of follow-up and in 9% of 99 aneurysms that were totally occluded on the first follow-up angiogram and were assessed with a second follow-up study a mean of 18 months later. Of 39 aneurysms totally occluded on the second follow-up angiogram, 3 (8%) had recurred when a third angiogram was obtained an average of 38 months later. Recurrence was more frequent in ruptured aneurysms than in unruptured aneurysms (17% versus 7%) as well as in large aneurysms compared with small aneurysms, but there was no difference in the frequency of recurrence relative to aneurysm location.

Byrne and colleagues [78] reviewed the 5-year experience at Oxford University with GDC treatment of ruptured intracranial aneurysms. Surviving patients were followed up for a median of 22 months. Angiographic occlusion was assessed in 259 aneurysms in 250 patients. After treatment, 64% of the aneurysms were completely occluded. At angiographic follow-up, usually obtained between 6 and 12 months later, the degree of occlusion observed at the conclusion of the embolization procedure remained stable in 86.4% of small aneurysms and in 85.2% of large aneurysms. In 38 aneurysms (14.7%), a remnant had enlarged to some degree. In 8.5% of cases, improvement of the initial degree of occlusion was observed at follow-up angiography as a result of thrombosis that occurred subsequent to the completion of packing.

Raymond et al [59] retrospectively reviewed the angiograms of 466 patients with 501 aneurysms, of which 54.1% were ruptured and 45.9% were unruptured. The mean size of the aneurysms was 9.67 mm, with a mean neck size of 4.31 mm. The most frequent aneurysm sites were the basilar bifurcation (27.7%) and the carotid ophthalmic artery (18.0%). Recurrences were subjectively divided into minor and major (suitable for retreatment) categories. In their series, short-term (≤1 year) follow-up angiograms were available in 70.5% of cases and long-term (>1 year) follow-up angiograms were available in 55%, for a total of 76.5% cases followed up. Recurrences were found in 33.6% of treated aneurysms that were followed up for a mean duration of 12.31 months after treatment. Major recurrence was present in 20.7% at a mean of 16.49 months. Aneurysm hemorrhage occurred in 3 (0.8%) patients during a mean clinical follow-up period of 31 months. Predictors of aneurysm recurrence included an aneurysm size of 10 mm or greater, treatment during the acute phase of rupture, incomplete initial occlusion, and longer duration of follow-up. Aneurysms completely occluded in the initial treatment were found to have recurred even after 37 months of follow-up. The aforementioned series have confirmed the overall safety of this technique; however, concerns remain because of the lack of long-term follow-up data regarding efficacy (procedural durability).

No agreement exists as to the timing and duration of angiographic follow-up after coil embolization of intracranial aneurysms. In general, we obtain an initial follow-up angiogram at 3 to 6 months in patients with aneurysms that are totally occluded or those having a minimal residual neck. In patients with residual aneurysm filling that extends beyond the neck, an earlier study (usually at 1–3 months after coiling) is indicated to assess the stability and size of the remnant and the possible need for additional treatment. The necessity and timing of additional follow-up studies are determined on an individual basis; however, all patients, even those with stable occlusion on the first follow-up angiogram, should undergo a 1-year follow-up study. The need for repeat angiographic follow-up, which exposes patients to the low but definite risk of an invasive procedure, is one of the current limitations of endovascular treatment of aneurysms. The results obtained with magnetic resonance angiography suggest that this imaging technology has the potential to replace angiography for assessing aneurysm occlusion after coiling [79]. Transcranial color Doppler imaging has been described as a useful tool to assess aneurysm occlusion after coiling [80].

Several factors are directly related to the possibility of achieving complete and stable angiographic occlusion of aneurysms, especially aneurysm and neck size and dome-to-neck ratio. Fernandez Zubillaga et al [81] reported complete aneurysm occlusion in 85% of small-necked (4 mm or smaller) aneurysms and in only 15% of aneurysms with necks exceeding 4 mm. The importance of the ratio between maximal sac diameter and neck diameter (dome-to-neck ratio) has been debated [77,82]. It has been suggested that when this ratio is less than 2, the aneurysm has a so-called "wide neck" and that optimal results are obtained when this ratio is at least 2 [82]. When aneurysms are selected for endovascular treatment on the basis of this favorable anatomic-geometric consideration, complete angiographic occlusion can be achieved in 72% of acutely ruptured aneurysms and in 80% of unruptured ones [82]. Small-sized aneurysms with wide necks present the greatest technical challenge [60].

The recent addition of bioactive coils is expected to improve the overall results obtained with bare platinum coils. Vinuela et al [83] reported a 19% recanalization rate for aneurysms with a neck remnant treated with Matrix coils compared with 50% for those treated with GDCs after 18 months of follow-up. Chaloupka et al [84] reported a 15.3% rate of retreatment with Matrix coils compared with a rate of 29.6% with GDCs. Alexander et al [85] reported a 3.9% rate of retreatment in 51 of 101 patients treated with Matrix coils who had a 6-month follow-up, with no information available about the remaining 50 patients.

The preliminary results for the Acceleration of Connective Tissue Formation in Endovascular Aneurysm Repair study, a company-sponsored (Boston Scientific Target) registry evaluating patients treated with Matrix coils, were recently presented [86]. The primary end point for the study was the rate of angiographic recanalization at 3 months; secondary end points were angiographic recanalization rates at 12 months and the occurrence of adverse events and clinical outcomes. Patients with de novo aneurysms of less than 25 mm in diameter and Hunt and Hess (HH) grade 0 to 3 at admission were included in the study. Ninety-nine aneurysms were treated in 96 patients at 11 centers in the United States and Europe. The median age of these patients was 53 years (range: 20–82 years), and 72% were women. Median aneurysm size was 8 mm (range: 1.3–19.6 mm); 27% of the aneurysms were considered large and the remaining 73% were considered small. Regarding neck size, 79% of the aneurysms were considered to have wide necks (neck >4 mm or <2:1 dome-to-neck ratio). Seventy-seven percent of the aneurysms were in the anterior circulation. Forty-five percent of patients presented with SAH with the following HH grade distribution: I, 46%; II, 27%; and III, 27%. Angiographic images analyzed at 3 months for 74 (75%) of the 99 aneurysms treated demonstrated a 12% recanalization rate, with 5% considered minor (no treatment required) and 7% major, and there was a 15% total recanalization rate at 12 months (results available for 62% of aneurysms treated).

A company-sponsored (MicroVention) multicenter prospective study to evaluate the results of aneurysm treatment with a bioactive coil

(HydroCoil Embolic System; MicroVention), HydroCoil for Aneurysm Occlusion, is being conducted [87]. This hybrid hydrogel-platinum coil was used for the endovascular treatment of 186 patients with 191 aneurysms enrolled between October 2002 and February 2004 at 15 sites worldwide. The primary end points for the study are adverse events at the time of the treatment and at 3 to 6 months and 12 to 18 months thereafter plus angiographic recurrence of the aneurysm at 3 to 6 months and 12 to 18 months after treatment. Among the study patients, 71 (37%) of 191 aneurysms had ruptured. The mean aneurysm size was 8 mm, the mean neck size was 4.4 mm, and the mean dome-to-neck ratio was 1.7. The immediate angiographic results demonstrated rates of complete occlusion, near-complete occlusion, and incomplete occlusion of 49.4%, 42.4%, and 8.2%, respectively. These rates are equivalent to those obtained with bare platinum coils. Angiographic images analyzed at 3 months for 101 of the 186 treated patients demonstrated a 15.9% recanalization rate for aneurysms smaller than 10 mm and a 36.4% recanalization rate for those equal to or larger than 10 mm. The major criticism of this study was that any combination of HydroCoil and bare platinum coils could be used, and the percentage of HydroCoils used relative to all coils used varied from 5% to 100% [87].

The need for improvement in the long-term durability of coiling is still an open issue. The addition of bioactive coils, intracranial stents, and the upcoming new technology is likely to lead to a dramatic improvement in technical achievement of complete aneurysm obliteration, but the effect of the addition of new technology on the durability of the results remains to be proved.

Randomized trials of coiling versus clipping

Vanninen et al [88] reported the results of a single center, prospective, randomized study of GDC embolization versus surgery for the treatment of recently (<72 hours) ruptured intracranial aneurysms suitable for either treatment approach. Fifty-two patients were assigned to the endovascular treatment group and 57 to the surgical treatment group. The two groups were demographically well matched. Despite the relatively broad inclusion criteria, 70 other patients treated during the same period were not randomized because of the following reasons: endovascular treatment was not anatomically feasible (33 patients), presence of a large hematoma requiring evacuation (35 patients), or presence of cranial nerve compression (2 patients). There were no differences in 3-month clinical outcomes, as determined by the Glasgow Outcome Scale [9], in the two treatment groups: 81% of the patients initially assigned to endovascular treatment and 79% of the patients assigned to surgery had a good or moderate recovery. No differences were observed between the two groups when neuropsychologic outcome was assessed at 12 months, and the scores were significantly improved in both groups 3 to 12 months after treatment. According to the study protocol, MRI of the brain was performed at 12 months. Patients in the surgical group had more ischemic lesions in the parent artery territory of the ruptured aneurysm, in addition to signs of brain retraction injury. Although this trial showed equivalent outcomes with current endovascular embolization techniques and with surgery, it did not answer questions about long-term durability of the treatment.

The ISAT [3] was designed as a randomized multicenter trial to compare the safety and efficacy of endovascular coiling with that of standard neurosurgical clipping of aneurysms judged suitable for both treatments. During the study period, 9559 patients with SAH were identified: 2737 had primary coil embolization (coiling was preferred in elderly patients, patients with poor clinical grades, and patients with posterior circulation aneurysms), 3615 had clipping (chosen in young patients, patients with MCA aneurysms, and patients with larger aneurysms), and 1064 had unknown treatment. Of those 9559 patients, 2143 with ruptured intracranial aneurysms were randomly assigned to receive neurosurgical clipping (n = 1070) or endovascular treatment by detachable platinum coils (n = 1073). Among the randomized cases, 88% of patients were World Federation of Neurosurgical Societies (WFNS) grade 1 to 3, 93% of the aneurysms were 10 mm or smaller, and 97% of the aneurysms were located in the anterior circulation (50.5% anterior communicating and 27% posterior communicating or anterior choroidal).

Clinical outcomes were assessed at 2 months and at 1 year with planned interim ascertainment of recurrent hemorrhages and death. The primary objective was to determine whether endovascular coiling, compared with neurosurgical clipping, reduced the proportion of patients with a modified Rankin Scale score of 3 to 6 (dependency or death) at 1 year by 25%. Trial recruitment was stopped by the steering committee after the interim analysis on the basis of the following results: 190 (23.7%) of 801 patients allocated endovascular treatment were dependent or dead at 1 year compared with 243 (30.6%) of 793 patients allocated neurosurgical treatment. The relative and absolute risk reductions in dependency or death after allocation to endovascular versus neurosurgical treatment were 22.6% (95% confidence interval [CI], 8.9–34.2) and 6.9% (95% CI, 2.5–11.3), respectively. The risk of rebleeding from the ruptured aneurysm after 1 year was 2 per 1276 patient-years and 0 per 1081 patient-years for the groups allocated endovascular and neurosurgical treatment, respectively. The study conclusion was that in patients with ruptured intracranial aneurysms for which endovascular coiling and neurosurgical clipping are therapeutic options, the outcome in terms of survival free of disability at 1 year was significantly better with endovascular coiling. Furthermore, the most recent data available from this study suggested that the long-term risks of further bleeding from the treated aneurysm were low with either therapy, although somewhat more frequent with endovascular coiling. The cumulative risk of rebleeding at 1 year was 0.15% for coiling versus 0.07% for clipping [89].

As with any study of this magnitude, the ISAT evoked criticisms regarding the design, number of patients randomized, definition of an aneurysm suitable for both approaches, whether state-of-the-art aneurysm surgery was well represented, and other issues. Unquestionably, the ISAT has provided the only level I evidence available so far comparing endovascular coiling and surgical clipping of intracranial aneurysms. Moreover, in the hands of the ISAT investigators, endovascular coiling was a safer treatment option for patients with good WFNS grades and small anterior circulation aneurysms. The looming question regarding durability of aneurysm coiling is still open and much longer follow-ups are needed to assess this issue.

Complications: avoidance and management

Ischemic complications

The frequency of ischemic complications occurring during endovascular aneurysm embolization is reported to range from 2.5% to 24% [90,91]. The incidence of asymptomatic embolic events may be even greater [92]. Rordorf et al [92] used diffusion-weighted MRI performed within 48 hours in 14 consecutive elective GDC procedures to evaluate the incidence of silent ischemic events during aneurysm treatment. All embolizations were performed under systemic heparinization, and all flush solutions were heparinized; in addition, the guiding catheters and microcatheters were placed for continuous heparinized infusions. Small areas of restricted diffusion, presumed to represent procedure-related embolic infarctions, were found on the images of 8 of 14 patients. All except one of the areas were located ipsilateral to the catheterization. Six patients had evidence of multiple infarctions. Most lesions were small (<2 mm); 1 patient with coil stretch and herniation into the parent vessel had numerous infarctions, with a dominant posterior frontal infarction. Pre- and postprocedure National Institutes of Health Stroke Scale scores were unchanged for 13 of 14 patients. Overall, the rate of asymptomatic emboli was 61% (8 of 13 treatments) in uncomplicated procedures. These investigators concluded that silent thromboembolic events related to the use of the GDC system are a common occurrence, despite meticulous technique and systemic anticoagulation. Although clinical consequences are rare, the high occurrence rate suggests that alterations in technique, such as the addition of antiplatelet agents, should be considered [92].

Prevention of thromboembolic complications is fundamental. The authors routinely administer antiplatelet agents (eg, aspirin) before performing coiling procedures for nonacutely ruptured or unruptured aneurysms. This practice seems to be safe not only in the event of intraprocedural rupture but in terms of lowering the risk of thromboembolic complications in these patients. In the authors' opinion, antiplatelet agent therapy is even more important when bioactive coils are used. The rate of thromboembolic events when using such devices seems to be higher and justifies the use of such agents [86,87]. The addition of clopidogrel to the antiplatelet regimen is recommended for those patients in whom stent-assisted coiling is anticipated. Heparin is administered intravenously to achieve an activated coagulation time in the range of 250 to 300 seconds for nonacutely ruptured or unruptured aneurysms, because subtherapeutic levels of anticoagulation during the procedure may also lead to thromboembolic phenomena. The fact that heparin actually stimulates platelet aggregation should be kept in mind, especially with the advent of new direct thrombin inhibitors, such as bivalirudin [93].

Different stages of the procedure can trigger thrombus formation with or without consequent distal embolization. Meticulous attention to detail and extreme caution are recommended when trying to manipulate the guide catheter into a stable position. This portion of the procedure can be the most challenging and time-consuming, especially in elderly patients with tortuous atherosclerotic proximal vessels. During coil placement, thromboembolic complications can be a consequence of thrombus dislodged from within the aneurysm (particularly in partially thrombosed aneurysms) or thrombus formation around the coil mass during or even after the procedure. This risk is especially high in cases of coil herniation through the neck into the parent vessel or into distal branches arising near the aneurysm neck.

When coils herniate, several options are available, depending on the situation. The herniation of one or even several coils into the parent vessel is not necessarily associated with thromboembolic complications. As long as the herniation is well tolerated clinically, observation alone is a valid option. That is usually the case when a single loop of the coil herniates into the parent vessel. In this situation, the authors prefer to start or keep patients on a dual antiplatelet regimen (usually aspirin and clopidogrel) for 6 to 8 weeks. If the errant coil is noticed to be moving within the parent vessel, however, it should be considered a potential cause of secondary thromboembolism. In these cases, coil removal or trapping is a viable option, depending on the situation. Many devices are available for coil removal. For coil trapping or fixation, a stent can be deployed to force the herniated coil against the parent vessel wall, which may promote secondary endothelialization. As a maneuver of last resort in the setting of ischemia caused by the occluding effects of the migrated coil or coils, an emergency craniotomy with coil and thrombus extraction can be performed to re-establish flow and attempt to reverse the ongoing ischemia [94].

When distal embolism is suspected or documented, superselective thrombolytic therapy can restore patency and potentially reverse disabling neurologic deficits. Many agents have been reported for this application, including hyperheparinization, urokinase [95], alteplase [91], abciximab [96], eptifibatide [91], or a combination of these drugs [96]. Fiorella et al [96] reported their experience with the treatment of intraprocedural thromboembolic complications in 13 patients (10 aneurysm cases) with abciximab, alone or in combination with tissue plasminogen activator. After identification of the complication, patients received intra-arterial (n = 5) or intravenous (n = 8) abciximab. Complete (n = 7) or partial (n = 6) resolution of thrombus was observed in all cases. Five patients had small infarctions in the distribution of the thromboembolic complication. In the authors' experience, the results obtained with intra-arterial or intravenous injection of glycoprotein IIb or IIIa inhibitors, such as eptifibatide and abciximab, have been satisfactory, with a high rate of recanalization or thrombus degradation and a low rate of hemorrhagic complications.

To prevent or minimize the risk of aneurysm rerupture and catastrophic consequences, Cronqvist et al [95] suggest that fibrinolysis for thromboemboli that occur during coiling should be considered only if the aneurysm has been sufficiently embolized. In such cases, rapid completion of coiling should be performed, followed by thrombolysis. Prompt fibrinolysis is not always successful [95], and its success depends on clot composition. An embolus consisting of fresh thrombus that develops during the procedure is much more likely to be dissolved by thrombolysis than is an embolus consisting of an atherosclerotic plaque fragment dislodged during catheterization of the proximal vessels.

Intraprocedural rupture

Intraprocedural aneurysm rupture is reported to occur in 2% to 8% of patients during aneurysm coiling (Fig. 2) [60,68,97]. Rupture seems to be more common in the treatment of small aneurysms, especially in the acute phase immediately after SAH [60,68]. Operator experience is also an important factor, with intraoperative rupture being most common in the early phase of the learning curve. In 75 patients treated during the acute phase after SAH, Raymond and Roy [68] experienced five ruptures in the first 25 patients, one in the next 25 patients, and none in the last 25 patients treated.

Aneurysm rupture can occur during several phases of the embolization procedure, ranging from diagnostic angiography injection to coil insertion. Doerfler et al [98] reported five patients with intraprocedural aneurysmal rupture. In one patient, rupture was caused by guide wire perforation of the aneurysm wall. In two patients, the microcatheter itself perforated the aneurysm. In another two patients, rupture occurred during placement of the first coil. In this series,

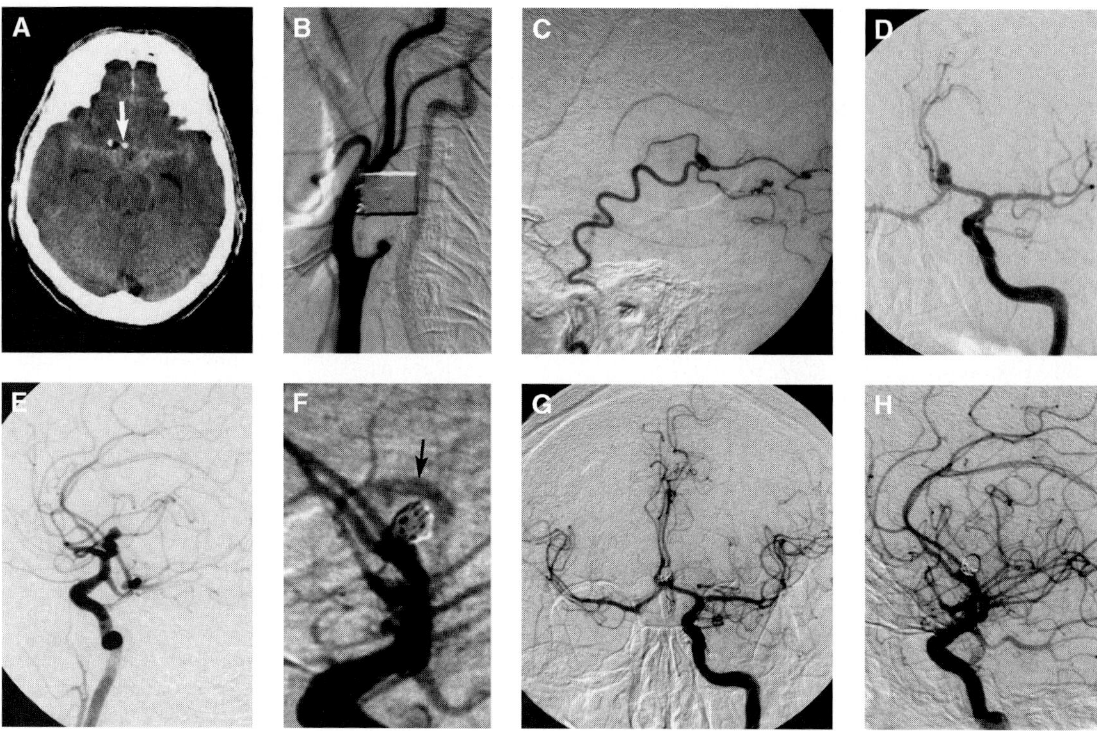

Fig. 2. Case illustration. This 59-year-old man presented with subarachnoid hemorrhage (*A*, CT scan), with Hunt and Hess grade 2 and Fisher grade 3. Twenty years previously, the patient underwent occlusion of the right internal carotid artery (ICA) (note the presence of calcification in the paraclinoid area on the right side [*white arrow*]) with a Selverstone clamp (*B*, angiogram) preceded by a superficial temporal artery–to–middle cerebral artery bypass (*C*, angiogram). A cerebral angiogram performed at the time of the present admission demonstrated an anterior communicating artery aneurysm filling from the left ICA (*D*, anteroposterior [AP] view; *E*, lateral view). The patient was brought to the angiography suite for aneurysm coiling. (*F*) After placement and detachment of the third coil within the aneurysm, contrast extravasation was noticed. Rapid completion of the coiling procedure with the placement of two additional coils resulted in cessation of contrast extravasation. The final angiographic result documents complete aneurysm occlusion with parent vessel preservation (*G*, AP view; *H*, lateral view). The patient had a good outcome (modified Rankin Scale score of 1 at 30 days).

intraprocedural rupture occurred in 3% of 164 patients with ruptured aneurysms and was associated with a mortality rate of 20%.

Levy et al [97] reported intraprocedural rupture in 6 (2%) of 274 patients with intracranial aneurysms treated with coil embolization. The rupture resulted from detachment of the last coil in 3 patients, detachment of the third coil (of four) in 1 patient, and insertion of the first coil in another patient.

Microwire-related perforations can be minimized by selecting the appropriate wire, with preference given to soft-tipped wires, particularly in the setting of acute rupture. Microcatheter-related ruptures occur while attempts are made to catheterize the aneurysm and obtain stable and optimal placement of the microcatheter within the aneurysm. During this maneuver, it is important to avoid excessive slack in the microcatheter, which can cause it to move forward suddenly and perforate the aneurysm [99]. When catheterizing the aneurysm, the guide wire precedes the entry of the microcatheter into the aneurysm. Using road mapping techniques, the microcatheter is slowly advanced and placed at the center of the aneurysm. Undesirable forward movements are avoided when positioning the microcatheter by relieving any forward tension that might remain within the microcatheter guide wire system before withdrawing the guide wire. Slack from the microcatheter is removed by making several passes with the guide wire. After ensuring that no residual forward tension is present, the guide wire is slowly withdrawn under direct fluoroscopic control. While the first coil is delivered, excessive stress against the aneurysm wall is avoided. This maneuver is greatly enhanced by the availability of 3D coils with a small inner loop. In acutely ruptured aneurysms, the hemorrhage site can be identified sometimes as a daughter sac on the aneurysm fundus. When possible, the first coil should be delivered away from these sites. Rupture occurs less often during delivery or after detachment of subsequent coils [100].

The clinical manifestations of intraprocedural rupture are variable. Although minimal extravasation of blood may not produce symptoms in some cases, awake patients tend to have headaches of varying severity. Neurologic focal deficits and impairment of the level of consciousness may follow, depending on the severity of the hemorrhage [42]. When an intraprocedural rupture occurs in anesthetized patients, hemodynamic monitoring reveals an otherwise unexplained increase in systemic blood pressure and heart rate [100]. Prompt management of the rupture is of utmost importance to minimize its consequences. Intraprocedural heparinization is promptly reversed by the administration of intravenous protamine. The authors routinely keep protamine (30 mg) on the back table in the angiography suite ready for infusion. This practice can save precious minutes in the case of an unexpected intraprocedural rupture. It is critical to avoid withdrawing the device responsible for the rupture (micro-guide wire, microcatheter, or coil). The device may tamponade the rupture site and limit the size of hemorrhage. When the microcatheter is responsible for the rupture, a coil can be delivered within the subarachnoid space as the microcatheter is slowly brought back to the sac in an attempt to seal the leak. Similarly, if a coil is responsible for the rupture, it is important to continue to deliver the coil. In general, once a rupture has occurred, the remaining aneurysm sac is packed with coils as quickly as possible. In refractory situations, temporary or permanent balloon occlusion of the parent artery can be performed [100]. The outcome of an intraprocedural rupture can be variable and is related primarily to the severity of the bleed. In the event of a severe rupture, monitoring and treating increased intracranial pressure are mandatory. Immediate placement of an external ventricular drain in the angiography suite can be a life-saving maneuver; thus, the operator should be familiar with this procedure.

Infection

Although infection is a concern after the placement of any endovascular implant, it is extremely rare after aneurysm coiling. Al-Okaili and Patel [101] reported a single case of peri-aneurysmal brain abscess formation after coil embolization of a giant unruptured right posterior communicating artery aneurysm. The possibility of infection should be considered especially when coils are placed in an aneurysm extending into or adjacent to a potentially contaminated space, such as the sphenoid sinus, or when they are used in the treatment of mycotic aneurysms. Periprocedural administration of antibiotic therapy for prophylaxis has been suggested in such cases [101]. Some authors recommend that all patients with endovascular implants receive appropriate prophylactic coverage during any invasive procedure in case of bacteremia, but no consensus exists regarding this practice [101].

Shunt-dependent hydrocephalus and vasospasm

Preliminary clinical evidence suggests that shunt-dependent hydrocephalus occurs less frequently in patients undergoing endovascular coiling than in those treated with surgical clipping. In the previously mentioned Finnish randomized trial reported by Vanninen et al [88], shunt insertion was required significantly more often in the surgical group. Similarly, in a retrospective series, Gruber et al [102] observed that shunt-dependent hydrocephalus developed in 23.2% of patients undergoing surgery and in 17.7% of patients undergoing early endovascular treatment. The reasons for these differences are unknown.

One potential limitation of the endovascular approach in patients treated acutely after aneurysm rupture is the inability to remove cisternal clot, with a theoretic risk of increasing the likelihood of vasospasm. Early series, however, suggested that the risk of delayed cerebral ischemia after endovascular treatment of acutely ruptured intracranial aneurysms is no higher than that encountered after surgical clipping [88,103]. Some authors maintain that the incidence of spasm after coiling may be even lower, because mechanical injury is decreased by endovascular treatment [104,105]. Murayama et al [103] reported that symptomatic vasospasm occurred in 23% of 69 HH grade I, II, or III patients who underwent GDC occlusion of intracranial aneurysms within 72 hours of rupture, resulting in an overall combined morbidity and mortality rate of

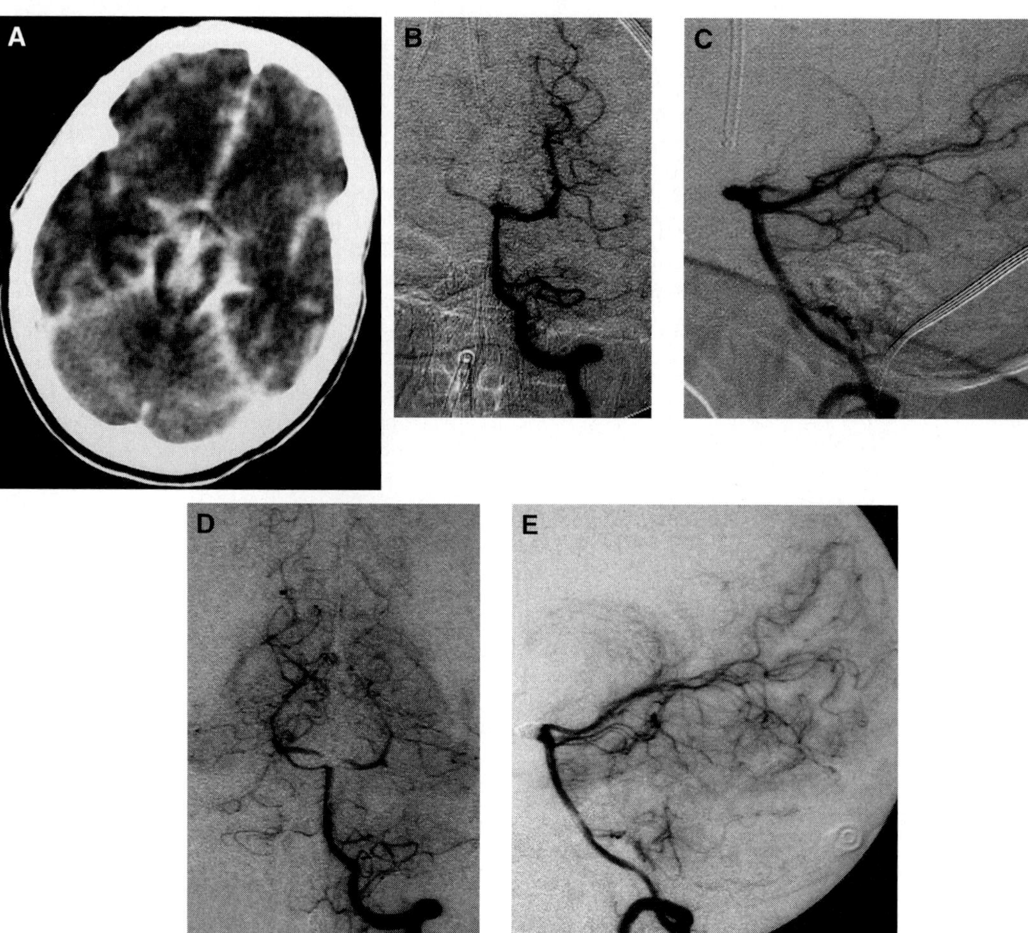

Fig. 3. Case illustration. This 59-year-old woman presented with severe headache. (*A*) An axial CT scan revealed diffuse subarachnoid hemorrhage. By digital subtraction angiography (DSA), anteroposterior (AP) (*B*) and lateral (*C*) views demonstrated a basilar tip aneurysm projecting anteriorly. (*D*, *E*) Aneurysm coiling was successfully performed with near-complete occlusion of the aneurysm after treatment. Daily serial transcranial Doppler (TCD) imaging demonstrated diffuse increased velocities 4 days after the initial aneurysm rupture. By DSA, AP (*F*) and lateral (*G*) projections revealed severe vasospasm of the basilar artery and its branches. (*H*) It also demonstrated severe vasospasm of the M1 segment of the right middle cerebral artery (MCA). (*I*) Note the resolution of vasospasm after the performance of balloon angioplasty. The same study also demonstrated severe diffuse vasospasm in the distribution of left MCA and anterior cerebral artery (*J*), which showed improvement after intra-arterial papaverine infusion (*K*). Two days later, increased left internal carotid artery (ICA) territory velocities were recorded. (*L*) DSA obtained at this time demonstrated severe vasospasm, which was more marked in the supraclinoid segment of the ICA. (*M*) Note the position of the angioplasty balloon over the wire on this unsubtracted image. (*N*) The vasospasm resolved after angioplasty. (*O*, *P*) Forty-eight hours later, TCD velocities were increased once again and DSA demonstrated severe diffuse vasospasm bilaterally in the distribution of the MCA and anterior cerebral artery. (*Q*, *R*) Note the improvement after intra-arterial papaverine infusion. After a 25-day admission, the patient was transferred to a rehabilitation unit (with a modified Rankin Scale score of 1). Six-month follow-up angiographic AP (*S*) and lateral (*T*) views show near-complete occlusion of the aneurysm, with some residual filling at the neck area.

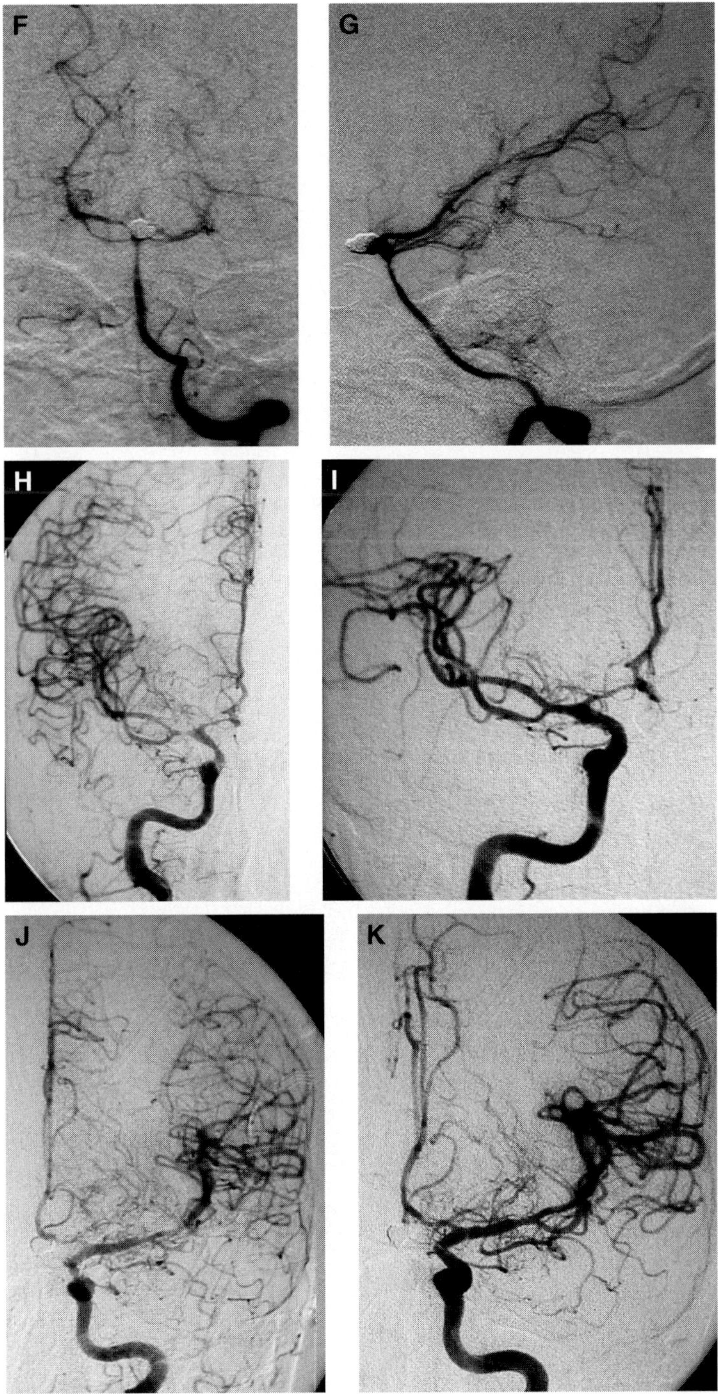

Fig. 3 (*continued*)

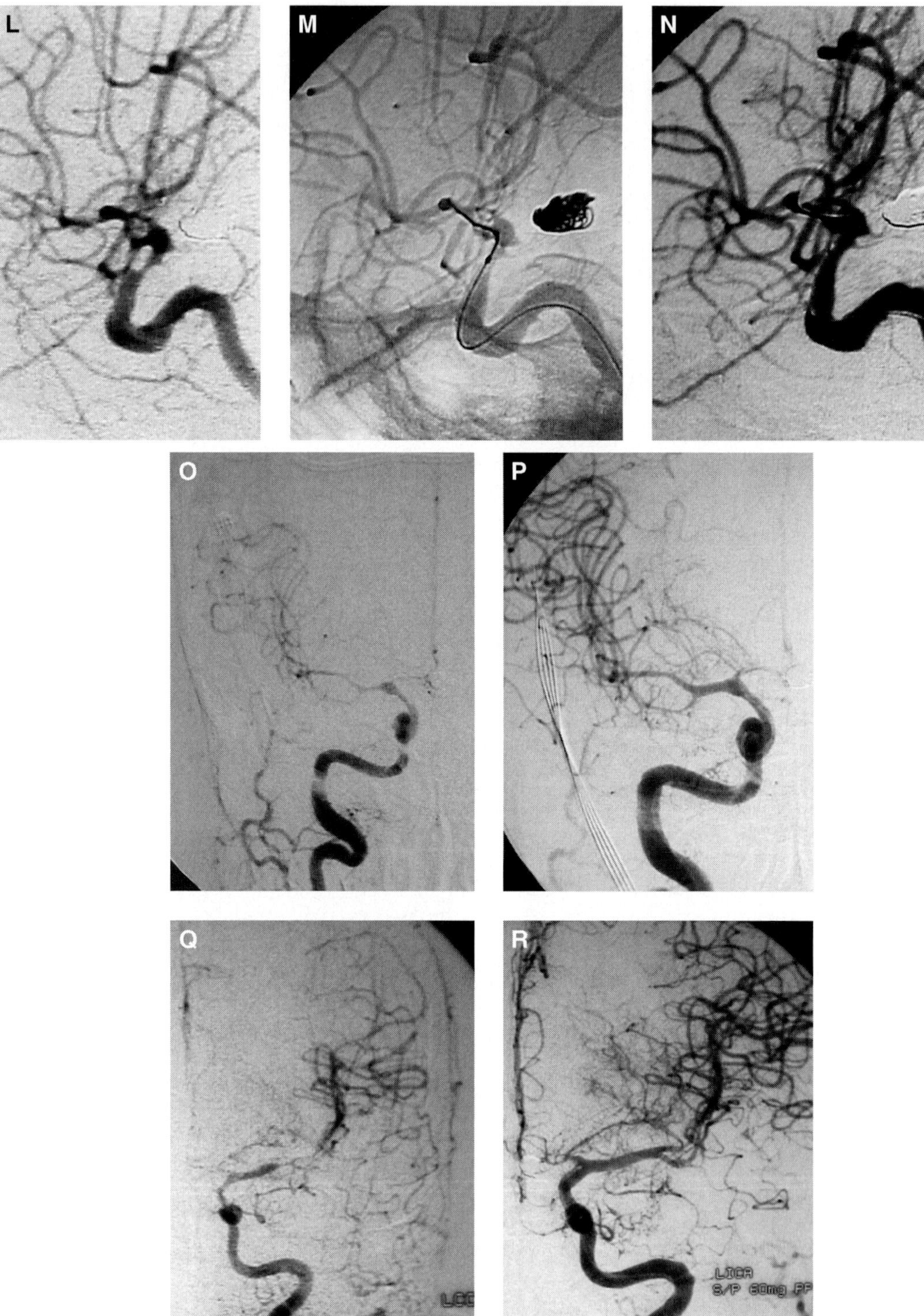

Fig. 3 (*continued*)

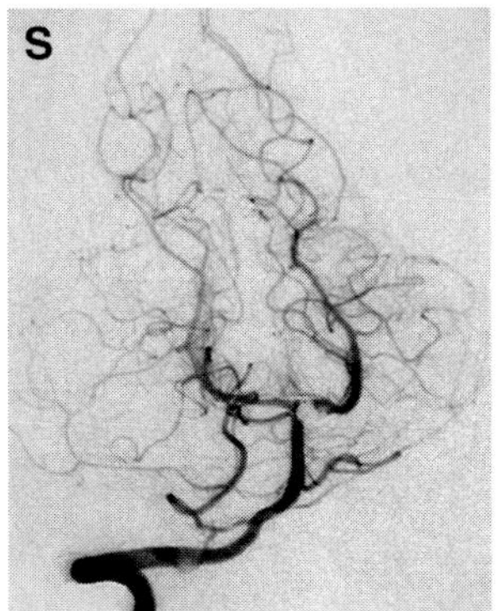

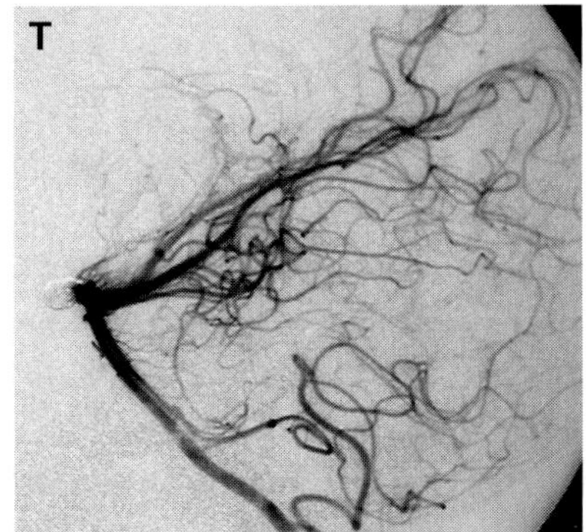

Fig. 3 (*continued*)

5.6% at 6 months. A negligible difference in the occurrence rate of clinically symptomatic vasospasm was observed in the Finnish randomized trial that compared surgery with GDC embolization for the treatment of acutely ruptured intracranial aneurysms [88]. No difference was found in the incidence of vasospasm in clipped and coiled aneurysms in two more recent studies [106,107].

Prevention and treatment of cerebral vasospasm

Given the importance of adequate management of vasospasm treatment in the overall outcome of patients with ruptured intracranial aneurysms and SAH, a discussion of the prevention and treatment of cerebral vasospasm is provided below.

Cerebral vasospasm is the delayed narrowing of the luminal diameter of the arteries at the base of the brain that occurs after SAH; it is often associated with radiographic or clinical evidence of diminished cerebral perfusion in the distal territory of the affected artery. Ischemic injury caused by vasospasm continues to be the leading cause of morbidity and mortality in patients with aneurysmal SAH [108]. In 1987, the Cooperative Aneurysm Study investigators reported an incidence of angiographic vasospasm exceeding 50%, with ischemic symptoms in 32% of these cases [109]. Despite extensive research regarding the prevention and treatment of this condition, these rates remain valid today [110–113]. Angiographic vasospasm is usually observed 3 to 5 days after the hemorrhage, with a peak at 5 to 14 days and resolution over the course of 2 to 4 weeks [114]. Approximately 50% of patients present with a clinical manifestation of delayed ischemic neurologic deficit (DIND). Among those with DIND, 15% to 20% experience permanent neurologic deficits or die from vasospasm, despite maximal medical therapy [115,116]. The DIND associated with symptomatic vasospasm usually appears shortly after the onset of angiographic vasospasm, with the acute or subacute development of focal or generalized symptoms and signs [114,117]. Cerebral angiography remains the "gold standard" for the evaluation and radiographic diagnosis of cerebral vasospasm. Transcranial Doppler ultrasound and newer modalities, such as CT perfusion [118], brain tissue oxygen content monitoring [119], microdialysis [120,121], and diffusion or perfusion magnetic resonance techniques [122,123], are helpful adjuncts in the early diagnosis and follow-up of this entity, however.

Awareness of the risk factors that predispose patients to developing vasospasm (location and volume of subarachnoid blood, younger age, and positive smoking history) [124–126] and early recognition of symptoms and clinical signs are essential for the optimal management of this condition. After early aneurysm clipping or embolization, the maintenance of a normovolemic state, as demonstrated by Lennihan et al [127], should be the aim (central venous pressure [CVP] >5 mm Hg, pulmonary artery diastolic pressure [PADP] >7 mm Hg) considering that prophylactic hypervolemic therapy (CVP >8 mm Hg, PADP >14 mm Hg) has failed to prove effectiveness in preventing vasospasm. Hypervolemic therapy should remain the initial treatment of choice when vasospasm exists, however. Pharmacologic treatment with calcium channel blockers, with nimodipine being the mainstay agent, has been

Table 1
Case series of balloon angioplasty in the treatment of cerebral vasospasm

Authors	No. patients and characteristics	Timing of angioplasty	Angiographic improvement (%)	Clinical improvement (%)	Recurrence (%)	Complications
Zubkov et al [145]	89 All grades with vasospasm	51 patients before surgery 16 patients after surgery	100	72	0 (at 5–7 days)	3 arterial ruptures, 1 TIA, 1 patient in worse condition
Eskridge et al [146]	48 No response to HV and HTN	<18 h of DIND	100	66	0	2 arterial ruptures, 2 rebleeds from unclipped aneurysms, 1 thrombosis (6 weeks after angioplasty)
Higashida et al [116]	13 No response to HV and HTN	No evidence of infarction on CT	100	69	0	1 hemorrhagic infarction
Coyne et al [137]	13 No response to HV and HTN	<48 h of DIND	100	31	—	None
Takahashi et al [162]	20 No response to HV and HTN	No evidence of infarction on CT	100	70	0	1 aneurysm rupture
Firlik et al [155]	14 No response to HV and HTN	Days 6–12	100	92 (12 of 13 patients) improved, 58% complete resolution	0	—
Nemoto [163]	10 No response to HV and HTN	—	60	40	—	—

Elliot et al [164]	Comparison between angioplasty and IA papaverine: 39 patients angioplasty, 13 patients papaverine No response to HV and HTN	—	(results measured by TCD imaging)	GOS score favorable in 67% of angioplasty cases	1	—
Polin and Kassell [165]	Comparison between 38 patients treated by balloon angioplasty and matched controls (North American Tirilazad Trial)	—	(angiogram)	Logistic regression: no difference in outcome between groups	—	—

Abbreviations: DIND, delayed ischemic neurologic deficit; GOS, Glasgow Outcome Scale; HTN, hypertension; HV, hypervolemia; IA, intra-arterial; TCD, transcranial Doppler; TIA, transient ischemic attack; —, not mentioned.

Modified from Newell DW, Eskridge J, Mayberg M, et al. Endovascular treatment of intracranial aneurysms and cerebral vasospasm. Clin Neurosurg 1992;39:348–60.

shown to improve the final outcome [128]. Nimodipine has been shown to improve the overall outcome in SAH cases in spite of not changing the absolute incidence of radiographic vasospasm [129]. The mechanisms by which nimodipine exerts its beneficial effect after aneurysmal SAH remain uncertain. There is no evidence that nicardipine and AT877 improve overall outcome. Mixed results have been associated with U74006F (tirilazad mesylate) [130,131].

Therapy with intravenous magnesium sulfate infusion has been suggested [132,133]. By acting as a calcium antagonist (calcium and magnesium have opposing effects on vascular tone), this agent might exert a neuroprotective effect, leading to a reduction in the incidence of clinical vasospasm as well as to an improvement in outcome for patients with symptomatic vasospasm [134]. Also, magnesium sulfate may compete with calcium for intracellular sites or limit the influx of calcium from damaged cellular membranes [134], producing beneficial effects by antagonizing the damaging actions of increased intracellular calcium concentration induced by cerebral ischemia [133].

Recently, lumbar drainage has been proposed as an effective way to reduce the risk of developing clinical vasospasm through removal of spasmogenic factors in the cerebrospinal fluid (CSF). In a retrospective study, Klimo et al [135] showed that CSF lumbar drainage performed after SAH was associated with a marked reduction in the risk of clinically evident vasospasm and its sequelae, shortened hospital stay, and improved outcome.

Endovascular treatment of cerebral vasospasm

Endovascular treatment with angioplasty and intra-arterially delivered drugs is often reserved for patients who fail to improve with the use of maximal medical therapy. In these cases, early endovascular intervention could play an important role (Fig. 3).

First described by Zubkov in 1984 [136], endovascular treatment of vasospasm using balloon angioplasty has been performed with increasing frequency in selected patients by mechanical dilation of the stenotic arteries through a microballoon catheter under fluoroscopic guidance. The results from initial clinical trials of angioplasty showed no recurrence of vasospasm within 7 days of treatment, with some rare cases of vessel dissection or rupture [116,137–140].

Angioplasty is effective in reversing vessel constriction and may lead to significant and sustained neurologic improvement, which is seen in many cases. Recurrent vasospasm at the angioplasty site is rare, although it may occur in vessel segments just proximal and distal to the site. After balloon dilation of arteries, transient alteration in myocyte structure [141], resulting in a degree of functional impairment of vascular smooth muscle cells persisting for at least 7 days, has been noticed. The long-lasting effect of balloon dilation is caused by disruption of the normal architecture of the collagen matrix in the arterial wall [142]. Hypothesizing that normal smooth muscle function is required for the development of vasospasm, preventive balloon angioplasty has been suggested by some authors [143]. In animal models of SAH, early angioplasty was shown to prevent the development of vasospasm [143]. On the basis of these findings, Muizelaar et al [144] conducted a phase I study in which 13 patients with Fisher grade 3 SAH underwent multivessel angioplasty within 3 days of SAH. None of these patients developed clinical vasospasm, but 1 of them had a vessel rupture during the procedure.

Table 1 [166] summarizes several case series in which balloon angioplasty was evaluated for the treatment of cerebral vasospasm. Despite successful dilation of vasospastic arteries, clinical outcome may not improve in one third of patients, however. Maximum benefits with angioplasty may be seen in patients with good clinical status at admission who experience subsequent acute deterioration because of vasospasm unresponsive to intensive medical therapy. Zubkov et al [145] found that improvement was most prominent in patients who presented with HH grade I or II and subsequently deteriorated; all such 13 patients in their series experienced neurologic improvement after angioplasty. Among the SAH patients with HH grade III at presentation, 85% improved with angioplasty compared with a 40% improvement in patients with HH grades IV and V. Angioplasty for patients with cerebral infarction does not seem to cause hemorrhagic transformation. Nevertheless, the clinical benefit seems to be limited [137]. Eskridge et al [146] found that angioplasty was most successful if performed within 12 hours of symptom onset. Other studies indicate that a shorter 2-hour window may exist to improve patient outcome before irreversible ischemic damage occurs [147]. Comparing two groups of patients undergoing endovascular treatment for symptomatic cerebral vasospasm (one group within 2 hours of symptom onset and the other 2 hours or more thereafter), Rosenwasser et al [147] found

Table 2
Case series involving intra-arterial injection of papaverine in the treatment of cerebral vasospasm

Authors	No. and characteristics of patients	Dosage and timing of papaverine	Angiogram improvement (%)	Clinical improvement (%)/results	Recurrence (%)	Comments
Kassell et al [157]	12	100–300-mg infusion	66	33	17	1 patient transient deterioration of mental status and hemiparesis
Kaku et al [156]	14 No response to HV and HTN, no evidence of infarction on CT	6–20 mg in repeated doses with angioplasty and IA nicardipine	92	80	0	Tachycardia
Clouston et al [153]	10 No response to HV and HTN	150–600-mg manual injection <48 hours after DIND	93	50	21	1 patient permanent monocular blindness, 1 patient arterial rupture without neurologic decline
Numaguchi et al [159]	Analysis of repeat IA papaverine in 24 patients (12 with no improvement)		100	50 after second infusion, 33 after third infusion	100	
Milburn et al [158]	34 patients, 81 arterial territories	300-mg infusion over 15 to 60 minutes, day 3 to day 19 after SAH	100	Not mentioned	100	
Fandino et al [154]	10 patients/23 vascular territories, no response to HV and HTN	360 mg/120 ml, infusion rate of 0.1 mL/s, days 4 to 16 after SAH	100	Good recovery 70%, moderate disability 30%	Not mentioned	Improvement of cerebral oxygenation
Firlik et al [155]	15 patients, 32 arteries		78	26	40% (6 of 15 patients)	4 complications: 1 brain stem depression, 1 systemic hypotension, 1 seizure, 1 symptom aggravation
Polin et al [167]	Comparison between 31 patients treated by balloon angioplasty and matched controls (North American Tirilazad Trial)	Not mentioned	13 (immediate)	Logistic regression: no difference in outcome between groups	Not mentioned	Not mentioned

Abbreviations: DIND, delayed ischemic neurologic deficit; HTN, hypertension; HV, hypervolemia; IA, intra-arterial; SAH, subarachnoid hemorrhage; TIA, transient ischemic attack.

Modified from Qureshi AI, Dawson R, Frankel MR, et al. Recent advances in the management of vasospasm in patients with subarachnoid hemorrhage. The Neurologist 1996;2:53–65.

Table 3
Advantages and disadvantages of balloon angioplasty and intra-arterial injection of papaverine for the treatment of cerebral vasospasm

Modality	Advantages	Disadvantages
Papaverine injection	Low risk of vessel injury Possibility of treating branches distal to A1, M2, and P1	High incidence of spasm recurrence Can cause an increase in intracranial pressure Can cause seizures
Balloon angioplasty	Low incidence of spasm recurrence Re-establishes vessel lumen diameter May be useful as prophylactic maneuver	Risky to treat branches distal to A1, M2, and P1 Risk of vessel dissection by microwires Risk of vessel rupture during balloon inflation May be limited by tortuous anatomy and severe spasm distal to the target vessel

similar good angiographic resolution of spasm in both groups (approximately 90% in each group) but distinct differences in sustained clinical improvement (70% in the early treatment group versus 40% in the delayed treatment group).

Despite continuous advances in catheter technology, vessel rupture and dissection remain the primary complications of angioplasty [138, 146,148]. The performance of an angioplasty at a site proximal to an unclipped aneurysm may present a risk for rupture of the aneurysm [146]. Therefore, treatment of the aneurysm before angioplasty has been recommended for patients with unsecured ruptured aneurysms [138,149]. Murayama et al [150] reported their experience with combined endovascular treatment for cerebral aneurysm occlusion and vasospasm in a single session. They concluded that this combination is safe and feasible. In some cases, this is not possible and the severity of spasm precludes aneurysm catheterization. In such cases, dilation of the vessel with intra-arterial infusion of papaverine (30-mg dose) can facilitate microcatheter navigation.

Papaverine is an opium alkaloid that causes vasodilation of cerebral vessels through direct action on smooth muscle cells. It also prevents the constriction of smooth muscle secondary to a wide variety of stimuli [151]. It is essential that papaverine be infused just proximal to the spastic arterial segments to maximize the therapeutic effect of the drug [152].

Intra-arterial injection of papaverine for the treatment of cerebral vasospasm has been reported in several series (Table 2) [153–159]. The results of these studies suggest that the vasodilating effect of intra-arterial papaverine may be long lasting and even more apparent more than 10 days after the onset of SAH. The benefit was most prominent in patients who underwent angioplasty along with intra-arterial papaverine administration for symptomatic vasospasm in vascular territories not accessible to angioplasty [156]. Evaluation of various dosages indicated that using papaverine at a rate of 300 mg in 100-mL saline was adequate and safe in most cases [157]. Delayed responses (up to 30 minutes) have been described in some patients. Recurrence rates of up to 20% were seen in patients who received only intra-arterial papaverine. Vasospasm recurrence, probably caused by the short duration of action of the drug [152], has been described after papaverine administration [157] but seems to respond to a second infusion. Notable adverse effects of papaverine administration include increased intracranial pressure, seizures, and hemodynamic compromise [160,161]. A summary of the advantages and disadvantages of intra-arterial papaverine injection and balloon angioplasty for the treatment of cerebral vasospasm is provided in Table 3.

New horizons

Forthcoming additions to the current armamentarium of aneurysm treatment are likely to influence this field in the near future. A better understanding of aneurysm population genetics is likely to enhance the selection of candidates for treatment. The development of new devices, such as asymmetric stents, covered stents, coiling adjuncts, and improved bioactive agents, should allow for improvements in the effectiveness and durability of intracranial aneurysm treatment. Controlled studies to assess the impact of each addition to the endovascular armamentarium should be performed in an attempt to quantify the impact of any given new device or therapy on the outcomes of this condition. A better understanding of intra-aneurysm hemodynamics and the possibility of simulating aneurysm flow before treatment might make it possible to assess the magnitude of different therapeutic options on the specific aneurysm harbored by a particular patient. In the future, it might be possible to use computer modeling of a patient's radiographic data to predict the changes caused by the placement of a coil or a stent.

Technologic advances are likely to continue to affect the treatment of intracranial aneurysms. The swing of the pendulum toward less invasive modalities seems to be irreversible, for the betterment of the patients.

References

[1] Guglielmi G, Vinuela F, Dion J, et al. Electrothrombosis of saccular aneurysms via endovascular approach. Part 2: preliminary clinical experience. J Neurosurg 1991;75(1):8–14.

[2] Wiebers DO, Whisnant JP, Huston J III, et al. Unruptured intracranial aneurysms: natural history, clinical outcome, and risks of surgical and endovascular treatment. Lancet 2003;362(9378):103–10.

[3] Molyneux A, Kerr R, Stratton I, et al. International Subarachnoid Aneurysm Trial (ISAT) of neurosurgical clipping versus endovascular coiling in 2143 patients with ruptured intracranial aneurysms: a randomised trial. Lancet 2002;360(9342):1267–74.

[4] Lozier AP, Connolly ES Jr, Lavine SD, et al. Guglielmi detachable coil embolization of posterior circulation aneurysms: a systematic review of the literature. Stroke 2002;33(10):2509–18.

[5] Lusseveld E, Brilstra EH, Nijssen PC, et al. Endovascular coiling versus neurosurgical clipping in patients with a ruptured basilar tip aneurysm. J Neurol Neurosurg Psychiatry 2002;73(5):591–3.

[6] Uda K, Murayama Y, Gobin YP, et al. Endovascular treatment of basilar artery trunk aneurysms with Guglielmi detachable coils: clinical experience with 41 aneurysms in 39 patients. J Neurosurg 2001;95(4):624–32.

[7] Valee JN, Aymard A, Casasco AE. Endovascular test and permanent occlusion of extracranial and intracranial cerebral vessels: indications, techniques and management. In: Connons JJ, Wojak JC, editors. Interventional neuroradiology, strategies and practical techniques. Philadelphia: WB Saunders; 1999. p. 394–408.

[8] Vallee JN, Aymard A, Vicaut E, et al. Endovascular treatment of basilar tip aneurysms with Guglielmi detachable coils: predictors of immediate and long-term results with multivariate analysis 6-year experience. Radiology 2003;226(3):867–79.

[9] Lawton MT. Basilar apex aneurysms: surgical results and perspectives from an initial experience. Neurosurgery 2002;50(1):1–10.

[10] Nagashima H, Kobayashi S, Tanaka Y, et al. Endovascular therapy versus surgical clipping for basilar artery bifurcation aneurysm: retrospective analysis of 117 cases. J Clin Neurosci 2004;11(5):475–9.

[11] Osawa M, Hongo K, Tanaka Y, et al. Results of direct surgery for aneurysmal subarachnoid haemorrhage: outcome of 2055 patients who underwent direct aneurysm surgery and profile of ruptured intracranial aneurysms. Acta Neurochir (Wien) 2001;143(7):655–64.

[12] Gruber DP, Zimmerman GA, Tomsick TA, et al. A comparison between endovascular and surgical management of basilar artery apex aneurysms. J Neurosurg 1999;90(5):868–74.

[13] Lozier AP, Kim GH, Sciacca RR, et al. Microsurgical treatment of basilar apex aneurysms: perioperative and long-term clinical outcome. Neurosurgery 2004;54(2):286–99.

[14] Haw C, Willinsky R, Agid R, et al. The endovascular management of superior cerebellar artery aneurysms. Can J Neurol Sci 2004;31(1):53–7.

[15] Mukonoweshuro W, Laitt RD, Hughes DG. Endovascular treatment of PICA aneurysms. Neuroradiology 2003;45(3):188–92.

[16] Lewis SB, Chang DJ, Peace DA, et al. Distal posterior inferior cerebellar artery aneurysms: clinical features and management. J Neurosurg 2002;97(4):756–66.

[17] Beyerl BD, Heros RC. Multiple peripheral aneurysms of the posterior inferior cerebellar artery. Neurosurgery 1986;19(2):285–9.

[18] Hoh BL, Carter BS, Budzik RF, et al. Results after surgical and endovascular treatment of paraclinoid aneurysms by a combined neurovascular team. Neurosurgery 2001;48(1):78–90.

[19] Park HK, Horowitz M, Jungreis C, et al. Endovascular treatment of paraclinoid aneurysms: experience with 73 patients. Neurosurgery 2003;53(1):14–24.

[20] Fiorella D, Albuquerque FC, Han P, et al. Preliminary experience using the Neuroform stent for the treatment of cerebral aneurysms. Neurosurgery 2004;54(1):6–17.

[21] Proust F, Debono B, Hannequin D, et al. Treatment of anterior communicating artery aneurysms: complementary aspects of microsurgical and endovascular procedures. J Neurosurg 2003;99(1):3–14.

[22] Pierot L, Boulin A, Castaings L, et al. Endovascular treatment of pericallosal artery aneurysms. Neurol Res 1996;18(1):49–53.

[23] Regli L, Dehdashti AR, Uske A, et al. Endovascular coiling compared with surgical clipping for the treatment of unruptured middle cerebral artery aneurysms: an update. Acta Neurochir Suppl (Wien) 2002;82:41–6.

[24] Szajner M, Szczepanek D, Trojanowski T, et al. Comparison of effectiveness of percutaneous embolization and microsurgery in the treatment of

60 patients with MCA berry aneurysms. Neurol Neurochir Pol 2003;37(1):133–49.

[25] Weir B, Amidei C, Kongable G, et al. The aspect ratio (dome/neck) of ruptured and unruptured aneurysms. J Neurosurg 2003;99(3):447–51.

[26] Murayama Y, Nien YL, Duckwiler G, et al. Guglielmi detachable coil embolization of cerebral aneurysms: 11 years' experience. J Neurosurg 2003; 98(5):959–66.

[27] Vallee JN, Pierot L, Bonafe A, et al. Endovascular treatment of intracranial wide-necked aneurysms using three-dimensional coils: predictors of immediate anatomic and clinical results. AJNR Am J Neuroradiol 2004;25(2):298–306.

[28] Vazquez Anon V, Aymard A, Gobin YP, et al. Balloon occlusion of the internal carotid artery in 40 cases of giant intracavernous aneurysm: technical aspects, cerebral monitoring, and results. Neuroradiology 1992;34(3):245–51.

[29] Fox AJ, Vinuela F, Pelz DM, et al. Use of detachable balloons for proximal artery occlusion in the treatment of unclippable cerebral aneurysms. J Neurosurg 1987;66(1):40–6.

[30] Graves VB, Perl J II, Strother CM, et al. Endovascular occlusion of the carotid or vertebral artery with temporary proximal flow arrest and microcoils: clinical results. AJNR Am J Neuroradiol 1997;18(7):1201–6.

[31] Higashida RT, Halbach VV, Dowd C, et al. Endovascular detachable balloon embolization therapy of cavernous carotid artery aneurysms: results in 87 cases. J Neurosurg 1990;72(6):857–63.

[32] Aymard A, Gobin YP, Hodes JE, et al. Endovascular occlusion of vertebral arteries in the treatment of unclippable vertebrobasilar aneurysms. J Neurosurg 1991;74(3):393–8.

[33] Hodes JE, Fox AJ, Pelz DM, et al. Rupture of aneurysms following balloon embolization. J Neurosurg 1990;72(4):567–71.

[34] Dyste GN, Beck DW. De novo aneurysm formation following carotid ligation: case report and review of the literature. Neurosurgery 1989;24(1): 88–92.

[35] Timperman PE, Tomsick TA, Tew JM Jr, et al. Aneurysm formation after carotid occlusion. AJNR Am J Neuroradiol 1995;16(2):329–31.

[36] Guglielmi G, Vinuela F, Sepetka I, et al. Electrothrombosis of saccular aneurysms via endovascular approach. Part 1: electrochemical basis, technique, and experimental results. J Neurosurg 1991;75(1): 1–7.

[37] Guglielmi G. Treatment of an intracranial aneurysm using a new three-dimensional-shape Guglielmi detachable coil: technical case report. Neurosurgery 1999;45(4):959–61.

[38] Murayama Y, Tateshima S, Gonzalez NR, et al. Matrix and bioabsorbable polymeric coils accelerate healing of intracranial aneurysms: long-term experimental study. Stroke 2003;34(8):2031–7.

[39] Murayama Y, Vinuela F, Tateshima S, et al. Bioabsorbable polymeric material coils for embolization of intracranial aneurysms: a preliminary experimental study. J Neurosurg 2001;94(3):454–63.

[40] Kallmes DF, Schweickert PA, Marx WF, et al. Vertebroplasty in the mid- and upper thoracic spine. AJNR Am J Neuroradiol 2002;23(7): 1117–20.

[41] Henkes H, Fischer S, Weber W, et al. Endovascular coil occlusion of 1811 intracranial aneurysms: early angiographic and clinical results. Neurosurgery 2004;54(2):268–85.

[42] Qureshi AI, Suri MF, Khan J, et al. Endovascular treatment of intracranial aneurysms by using Guglielmi detachable coils in awake patients: safety and feasibility. J Neurosurg 2001;94(6):880–5.

[43] Moret J, Cognard C, Weill A, et al. Reconstruction technic in the treatment of wide-neck intracranial aneurysms. Long-term angiographic and clinical results. Apropos of 56 cases. J Neuroradiol 1997; 24(1):30–44.

[44] Lefkowitz MA, Gobin YP, Akiba Y, et al. Balloon-assisted Guglielmi detachable coiling of wide-necked aneurysms: Part II—clinical results Neurosurgery 1999;45(3):531–8.

[45] Akiba Y, Murayama Y, Vinuela F, et al. Balloon-assisted Guglielmi detachable coiling of wide-necked aneurysms: Part I—experimental evaluation. Neurosurgery 1999;45(3):519–30.

[46] Lanzino G, Wakhloo AK, Fessler RD, et al. Efficacy and current limitations of intravascular stents for intracranial internal carotid, vertebral, and basilar artery aneurysms. J Neurosurg 1999;91(4): 538–46.

[47] Wakhloo AK, Tio FO, Lieber BB, et al. Self-expanding nitinol stents in canine vertebral arteries: hemodynamics and tissue response. AJNR Am J Neuroradiol 1995;16(5):1043–51.

[48] Wakhloo AK, Lanzino G, Lieber BB, et al. Stents for intracranial aneurysms: the beginning of a new endovascular era? Neurosurgery 1998; 43(2):377–9.

[49] Bendok BR, Hanel RA, Boulos AS, et al. Stent-assisted coiling of intracranial internal carotid artery aneurysms: clinical and angiographic follow up [abstract]. Am J Cardiol 2002;90(Suppl 6A): 190H.

[50] Levy EI, Boulos AS, Hanel RA, et al. In vivo model of intracranial stent implantation: a pilot study to examine the histological response of cerebral vessels after randomized implantation of heparin-coated and uncoated endoluminal stents in a blinded fashion. J Neurosurg 2003;98(3): 544–53.

[51] Lopes DK, Ringer AJ, Boulos AS, et al. Fate of branch arteries after intracranial stenting. Neurosurgery 2003;52(6):1275–9.

[52] Lylyk P, Cohen JE, Ceratto R, et al. Endovascular reconstruction of intracranial arteries by stent

placement and combined techniques. J Neurosurg 2002;97(6):1306–13.

[53] Wada H, Piotin M, Boissonnet H, et al. Carotid rupture during stent-assisted aneurysm treatment. AJNR Am J Neuroradiol 2004;25(5):827–9.

[54] Wainwright CL, Miller AM, Wadsworth RM. Inflammation as a key event in the development of neointima following vascular balloon injury. Clin Exp Pharmacol Physiol 2001;28(11):891–5.

[55] Anderson PG, Boerth NJ, Liu M, et al. Cyclic GMP-dependent protein kinase expression in coronary arterial smooth muscle in response to balloon catheter injury. Arterioscler Thromb Vasc Biol 2000;20(10):2192–7.

[56] Howington JU, Hanel RA, Harrigan MR, et al. The Neuroform stent, the first microcatheter-delivered stent for use in the intracranial circulation. Neurosurgery 2004;54(1):2–5.

[57] Benitez RP, Silva MT, Klem J, et al. Endovascular occlusion of wide-necked aneurysms with a new intracranial microstent (Neuroform) and detachable coils. Neurosurgery 2004;54(6):1359–68.

[58] Perez-Arjona E, Fessler RD. Basilar artery to bilateral posterior cerebral artery 'Y stenting' for endovascular reconstruction of wide-necked basilar apex aneurysms: report of three cases. Neurol Res 2004;26(3):276–81.

[59] Raymond J, Guilbert F, Weill A, et al. Long-term angiographic recurrences after selective endovascular treatment of aneurysms with detachable coils. Stroke 2003;34(6):1398–403.

[60] Vinuela F, Duckwiler G, Mawad M. Guglielmi detachable coil embolization of acute intracranial aneurysm: perioperative anatomical and clinical outcome in 403 patients. J Neurosurg 1997;86(3): 475–82.

[61] Kinugasa K, Mandai S, Terai Y, et al. Direct thrombosis of aneurysms with cellulose acetate polymer. Part II: preliminary clinical experience. J Neurosurg 1992;77(4):501–7.

[62] Kinugasa K, Mandai S, Tsuchida S, et al. Cellulose acetate polymer thrombosis for the emergency treatment of aneurysms: angiographic findings, clinical experience, and histopathological study. Neurosurgery 1994;34(4):694–701.

[63] Mandai S, Kinugasa K, Ohmoto T. Direct thrombosis of aneurysms with cellulose acetate polymer. Part I: results of thrombosis in experimental aneurysms. J Neurosurg 1992;77(4):497–500.

[64] Molyneux AJ, Cekirge S, Saatci I, et al. Cerebral Aneurysm Multicenter European Onyx (CAMEO) trial: results of a prospective observational study in 20 European centers. AJNR Am J Neuroradiol 2004;25(1):39–51.

[65] Murayama Y, Vinuela F, Tateshima S, et al. Endovascular treatment of experimental aneurysms by use of a combination of liquid embolic agents and protective devices. AJNR Am J Neuroradiol 2000;21(9):1726–35.

[66] Yang X, Wu Z, Li Y, et al. Comparison of cellulose acetate polymer and electrolytic detachable coils for treatment of canine aneurysmal models. Chin Med Sci J 2002;17(1):47–51.

[67] Mawad ME, Cekirge S, Ciceri E, et al. Endovascular treatment of giant and large intracranial aneurysms by using a combination of stent placement and liquid polymer injection. J Neurosurg 2002; 96(3):474–82.

[68] Raymond J, Roy D. Safety and efficacy of endovascular treatment of acutely ruptured aneurysms. Neurosurgery 1997;41(6):1235–46.

[69] Kuether TA, Nesbit GM, Barnwell SL. Clinical and angiographic outcomes, with treatment data, for patients with cerebral aneurysms treated with Guglielmi detachable coils: a single-center experience. Neurosurgery 1998;43(5):1016–25.

[70] Byrne JV, Adams CB, Kerr RS, et al. Endosaccular treatment of inoperable intracranial aneurysms with platinum coils. Br J Neurosurg 1995;9(5): 585–92.

[71] Byrne JV, Molyneux AJ, Brennan RP, et al. Embolisation of recently ruptured intracranial aneurysms. J Neurol Neurosurg Psychiatry 1995;59(6): 616–20.

[72] Niemann D, Aviv R, Cowsill C, et al. Anatomically conformable, three-dimensional, detachable platinum microcoil system for the treatment of intracranial aneurysms. AJNR Am J Neuroradiol 2004; 25(5):813–8.

[73] Mericle RA, Wakhloo AK, Lopes DK, et al. Delayed aneurysm regrowth and recanalization after Guglielmi detachable coil treatment. Case report. J Neurosurg 1998;89(1):142–5.

[74] Hodgson TJ, Carroll T, Jellinek DA. Subarachnoid hemorrhage due to late recurrence of a previously unruptured aneurysm after complete endovascular occlusion. AJNR Am J Neuroradiol 1998;19(10): 1939–41.

[75] Manabe H, Fujita S, Hatayama T, et al. Rerupture of coil-embolized aneurysm during long-term observation. Case report. J Neurosurg 1998;88(6): 1096–8.

[76] Raftopoulos C, Mathurin P, Boscherini D, et al. Prospective analysis of aneurysm treatment in a series of 103 consecutive patients when endovascular embolization is considered the first option. J Neurosurg 2000;93(2):175–82.

[77] Cognard C, Weill A, Spelle L, et al. Long-term angiographic follow-up of 169 intracranial berry aneurysms occluded with detachable coils. Radiology 1999;212(2):348–56.

[78] Byrne JV, Sohn MJ, Molyneux AJ, et al. Five-year experience in using coil embolization for ruptured intracranial aneurysms: outcomes and incidence of late rebleeding. J Neurosurg 1999;90(4):656–63.

[79] Derdeyn CP, Graves VB, Turski PA, et al. MR angiography of saccular aneurysms after treatment with Guglielmi detachable coils: preliminary

experience. AJNR Am J Neuroradiol 1997;18(2): 279–86.
[80] Turner CL, Higgins JN, Kirkpatrick PJ. Assessment of transcranial color-coded duplex sonography for the surveillance of intracranial aneurysms treated with Guglielmi detachable coils. Neurosurgery 2003;53(4):866–72.
[81] Fernandez Zubillaga A, Guglielmi G, Vinuela F, et al. Endovascular occlusion of intracranial aneurysms with electrically detachable coils: correlation of aneurysm neck size and treatment results. AJNR Am J Neuroradiol 1994;15(5): 815–20.
[82] Debrun GM, Aletich VA, Kehrli P, et al. Selection of cerebral aneurysms for treatment using Guglielmi detachable coils: the preliminary University of Illinois at Chicago experience. Neurosurgery 1998;43(6):1281–97.
[83] Vinuela F, Marayama Y, Duckwiler G, et al. The UCLA experience with Matrix bioactive coil. Presented at the Japanese Society of Intravascular Neurology Meeting, November 2003.
[84] Chaloupka J. Single-center experience with Matrix detachable coils in more than 100 aneurysms with Matrix coils. Presented at the American Society of Interventional and Therapeutic Neuroradiology Meeting, San Diego, February 1–4, 2004.
[85] Alexander M. The Duke experience with treatment of the first 100 aneurysms with Matrix coils. Presented at the American Society of Interventional and Therapeutic Neuroradiology Meeting, February 1–4, 2004.
[86] Vinuela F. The ACTIVE study. For the investigators of the ACTIVE study. Presented at the American Society of Neuroradiology Annual Meeting, Seattle, June 5–11, 2004.
[87] Cloft H. HydroCoil for Endovascular Aneurysm Occlusion (HEAL). For the HEAL investigators. Presented at the American Society of Neuroradiology Annual Meeting, Seattle, June 5–11, 2004.
[88] Vanninen R, Koivisto T, Saari T, et al. Ruptured intracranial aneurysms: acute endovascular treatment with electrolytically detachable coils—a prospective randomized study. Radiology 1999; 211(2):325–36.
[89] Kerr R. Data from the ISAT. The influence of the ISAT on neurosurgery training. Presented at the Brazilian Meeting of Neurosurgery, Goiania, Brazil, September 7, 2004.
[90] Alexander MJ, Duckwiler GR, Gobin YP, et al. Management of intraprocedural arterial thrombus in cerebral aneurysm embolization with abciximab: technical case report. Neurosurgery 2002;50(4): 899–902.
[91] Qureshi AI, Luft AR, Sharma M, et al. Prevention and treatment of thromboembolic and ischemic complications associated with endovascular procedures: Part II—clinical aspects and recommendations. Neurosurgery 2000;46(6):1360–76.
[92] Rordorf G, Bellon RJ, Budzik RE Jr, et al. Silent thromboembolic events associated with the treatment of unruptured cerebral aneurysms by use of Guglielmi detachable coils: prospective study applying diffusion-weighted imaging. AJNR Am J Neuroradiol 2001;22(1):5–10.
[93] Harrigan MR, Levy EI, Bendok BR, et al. Bivalirudin for endovascular intervention in acute ischemic stroke: case report. Neurosurgery 2004;54(1): 218–23.
[94] Gurian JH, Martin NA, King WA, et al. Neurosurgical management of cerebral aneurysms following unsuccessful or incomplete endovascular embolization. J Neurosurg 1995;83(5):843–53.
[95] Cronqvist M, Pierot L, Boulin A, et al. Local intraarterial fibrinolysis of thromboemboli occurring during endovascular treatment of intracerebral aneurysm: a comparison of anatomic results and clinical outcome. AJNR Am J Neuroradiol 1998;19(1): 157–65.
[96] Fiorella D, Albuquerque FC, Han P, et al. Strategies for the management of intraprocedural thromboembolic complications with abciximab (ReoPro). Neurosurgery 2004;54(5):1089–98.
[97] Levy E, Koebbe CJ, Horowitz MB, et al. Rupture of intracranial aneurysms during endovascular coiling: management and outcomes. Neurosurgery 2001;49(4):807–13.
[98] Doerfler A, Wanke I, Egelhof T, et al. Aneurysmal rupture during embolization with Guglielmi detachable coils: causes, management, and outcome. AJNR Am J Neuroradiol 2001;22(10):1825–32.
[99] McDougall CG, Halbach VV, Dowd CF, et al. Causes and management of aneurysmal hemorrhage occurring during embolization with Guglielmi detachable coils. J Neurosurg 1998; 89(1):87–92.
[100] Ricolfi F, Le Guerinel C, Blustajn J, et al. Rupture during treatment of recently ruptured aneurysms with Guglielmi electrodetachable coils. AJNR Am J Neuroradiol 1998;19(9):1653–8.
[101] Al-Okaili R, Patel SJ. Brain abscess after endovascular coiling of a saccular aneurysm: case report. AJNR Am J Neuroradiol 2002;23(4):697–9.
[102] Gruber A, Reinprecht A, Bavinzski G, et al. Chronic shunt-dependent hydrocephalus after early surgical and early endovascular treatment of ruptured intracranial aneurysms. Neurosurgery 1999;44(3):503–12.
[103] Murayama Y, Malisch T, Guglielmi G, et al. Incidence of cerebral vasospasm after endovascular treatment of acutely ruptured aneurysms: report on 69 cases. J Neurosurg 1997;87(6):830–5.
[104] Strother CM. Does reduction in vascular trauma during treatment of acutely ruptured saccular aneurysms reduce the incidence of vasospasm? AJNR Am J Neuroradiol 1998;19(3):190.
[105] Yalamanchili K, Rosenwasser RH, Thomas JE, et al. Frequency of cerebral vasospasm in patients

treated with endovascular occlusion of intracranial aneurysms. AJNR Am J Neuroradiol 1998;19(3): 553–8.

[106] Dehdashti AR, Mermillod B, Rufenacht DA, et al. Does treatment modality of intracranial ruptured aneurysms influence the incidence of cerebral vasospasm and clinical outcome? Cerebrovasc Dis 2004; 17(1):53–60.

[107] Goddard AJ, Raju PP, Gholkar A. Does the method of treatment of acutely ruptured intracranial aneurysms influence the incidence and duration of cerebral vasospasm and clinical outcome? J Neurol Neurosurg Psychiatry 2004;75(6):868–72.

[108] Qureshi AI, Dawson R, Frankel MR, et al. Recent advances in the management of vasospasm in patients with subarachnoid hemorrhage. The Neurologist 1996;2:53–65.

[109] Adams HP Jr, Kassell NF, Torner JC, et al. Predicting cerebral ischemia after aneurysmal subarachnoid hemorrhage: influences of clinical condition, CT results, and antifibrinolytic therapy. A report of the Cooperative Aneurysm Study. Neurology 1987;37(10):1586–91.

[110] Auer LM. Acute operation and preventive nimodipine improve outcome in patients with ruptured cerebral aneurysms. Neurosurgery 1984; 15(1):57–66.

[111] Awad IA, Carter LP, Spetzler RF, et al. Clinical vasospasm after subarachnoid hemorrhage: response to hypervolemic hemodilution and arterial hypertension. Stroke 1987;18(2):365–72.

[112] Megyesi JF, Vollrath B, Cook DA, et al. In vivo animal models of cerebral vasospasm: a review. Neurosurgery 2000;46(2):448–60.

[113] Treggiari-Venzi MM, Suter PM, Romand JA. Review of medical prevention of vasospasm after aneurysmal subarachnoid hemorrhage: a problem of neurointensive care. Neurosurgery 2001;48(2): 249–61.

[114] Sundt TM Jr, Kobayashi S, Fode NC, et al. Results and complications of surgical management of 809 intracranial aneurysms in 722 cases. Related and unrelated to grade of patient, type of aneurysm, and timing of surgery. J Neurosurg 1982;56(6): 753–65.

[115] Heros RC, Zervas NT, Varsos V. Cerebral vasospasm after subarachnoid hemorrhage: an update. Ann Neurol 1983;14(6):599–608.

[116] Higashida RT, Halbach VV, Cahan LD, et al. Transluminal angioplasty for treatment of intracranial arterial vasospasm. J Neurosurg 1989;71(5 Part 1):648–53.

[117] Longstreth WT Jr, Nelson LM, Koepsell TD, et al. Clinical course of spontaneous subarachnoid hemorrhage: a population-based study in King County. Neurology 1993;43(4):712–8.

[118] Nabavi DG, LeBlanc LM, Baxter B, et al. Monitoring cerebral perfusion after subarachnoid hemorrhage using CT. Neuroradiology 2001;43(1):7–16.

[119] Vath A, Kunze E, Roosen K, et al. Therapeutic aspects of brain tissue pO2 monitoring after subarachnoid hemorrhage. Acta Neurochir Suppl (Wien) 2002;81:307–9.

[120] Sarrafzadeh AS, Sakowitz OW, Kiening KL, et al. Bedside microdialysis: a tool to monitor cerebral metabolism in subarachnoid hemorrhage patients? Crit Care Med 2002;30(5):1062–70.

[121] Unterberg AW, Sakowitz OW, Sarrafzadeh AS, et al. Role of bedside microdialysis in the diagnosis of cerebral vasospasm following aneurysmal subarachnoid hemorrhage. J Neurosurg 2001;94(5): 740–9.

[122] Condette-Auliac S, Bracard S, Anxionnat R, et al. Vasospasm after subarachnoid hemorrhage: interest in diffusion-weighted MR imaging. Stroke 2001;32(8):1818–24.

[123] Phan T, Houston J III, Campeau N, et al. Value of diffusion-weighted imaging in patients with a nonlocalizing examination and vasospasm from subarachnoid hemorrhage. Cerebrovasc Dis 2003; 15(3):177–81.

[124] Fisher CM, Kistler JP, Davis JM. Relation of cerebral vasospasm to subarachnoid hemorrhage visualized by computerized tomographic scanning. Neurosurgery 1980;6(1):1–9.

[125] Macdonald RL, Wallace MC, Coyne TJ. The effect of surgery on the severity of vasospasm. J Neurosurg 1994;80(3):433–9.

[126] Weir BK, Kongable GL, Kassell NF, et al. Cigarette smoking as a cause of aneurysmal subarachnoid hemorrhage and risk for vasospasm: a report of the Cooperative Aneurysm Study. J Neurosurg 1998;89(3):405–11.

[127] Lennihan L, Mayer SA, Fink ME, et al. Effect of hypervolemic therapy on cerebral blood flow after subarachnoid hemorrhage: a randomized controlled trial. Stroke 2000;31(2):383–91.

[128] Allen GS, Ahn HS, Preziosi TJ, et al. Cerebral arterial spasm—a controlled trial of nimodipine in patients with subarachnoid hemorrhage. N Engl J Med 1983;308(11):619–24.

[129] Feigin VL, Rinkel GJ, Algra A, et al. Calcium antagonists in patients with aneurysmal subarachnoid hemorrhage: a systematic review. Neurology 1998;50(4):876–83.

[130] Lanzino G, Kassell NF. Double-blind, randomized, vehicle-controlled study of high-dose tirilazad mesylate in women with aneurysmal subarachnoid hemorrhage. Part II. A cooperative study in North America. J Neurosurg 1999;90(6):1018–24.

[131] Lanzino G, Kassell NF, Dorsch NW, et al. Double-blind, randomized, vehicle-controlled study of high-dose tirilazad mesylate in women with aneurysmal subarachnoid hemorrhage. Part I. A cooperative study in Europe, Australia, New Zealand, and South Africa. J Neurosurg 1999;90(6):1011–7.

[132] Boet R, Mee E. Magnesium sulfate in the management of patients with Fisher Grade 3 subarachnoid

hemorrhage: a pilot study. Neurosurgery 2000; 47(3):602–6.

[133] Veyna RS, Seyfried D, Burke DG, et al. Magnesium sulfate therapy after aneurysmal subarachnoid hemorrhage. J Neurosurg 2002;96(3): 510–4.

[134] Ram Z, Sadeh M, Shacked I, et al. Magnesium sulfate reverses experimental delayed cerebral vasospasm after subarachnoid hemorrhage in rats. Stroke 1991;22(7):922–7.

[135] Klimo P Jr, Kestle JR, MacDonald JD, et al. Marked reduction of cerebral vasospasm with lumbar drainage of cerebrospinal fluid after subarachnoid hemorrhage. J Neurosurg 2004;100(2): 215–24.

[136] Zubkov YN, Nikiforov BM, Shustin VA. Balloon catheter technique for dilatation of constricted cerebral arteries after aneurysmal SAH. Acta Neurochir (Wien) 1984;70(1–2):65–79.

[137] Coyne TJ, Montanera WJ, Macdonald RL, et al. Percutaneous transluminal angioplasty for cerebral vasospasm after subarachnoid hemorrhage. Can J Surg 1994;37(5):391–6.

[138] Eskridge JM, McAuliffe W, Song JK, et al. Balloon angioplasty for the treatment of vasospasm: results of first 50 cases. Neurosurgery 1998;42(3):510–7.

[139] Eskridge JM, Song JK, Elliott JP, et al. Balloon angioplasty of the A1 segment of the anterior cerebral artery narrowed by vasospasm. Technical note. J Neurosurg 1999;91(1):153–6.

[140] Zubkov AY, Lewis AI, Scalzo D, et al. Morphological changes after percutaneous transluminal angioplasty. Surg Neurol 1999;51(4):399–403.

[141] Chavez L, Takahashi A, Yoshimoto T, et al. Morphological changes in normal canine basilar arteries after transluminal angioplasty. Neurol Res 1990;12(1):12–6.

[142] Yamamoto Y, Smith RR, Bernanke DH. Mechanism of action of balloon angioplasty in cerebral vasospasm. Neurosurgery 1992;30(1):1–5.

[143] Megyesi JF, Findlay JM, Vollrath B, et al. In vivo angioplasty prevents the development of vasospasm in canine carotid arteries. Pharmacological and morphological analyses. Stroke 1997;28(6): 1216–24.

[144] Muizelaar JP, Zwienenberg M, Rudisill NA, et al. The prophylactic use of transluminal balloon angioplasty in patients with Fisher Grade 3 subarachnoid hemorrhage: a pilot study. J Neurosurg 1999; 91(1):51–8.

[145] Zubkov YN, Alexander LF, Smith RR, et al. Angioplasty of vasospasm: is it reasonable? Neurol Res 1994;16(1):9–11.

[146] Eskridge JM, Newell DW, Pendleton GA. Transluminal angioplasty for treatment of vasospasm. Neurosurg Clin N Am 1990;1(2):387–99.

[147] Rosenwasser RH, Armonda RA, Thomas JE, et al. Therapeutic modalities for the management of cerebral vasospasm: timing of endovascular options. Neurosurgery 1999;44(5):975–80.

[148] Linskey ME, Horton JA, Rao GR, et al. Fatal rupture of the intracranial carotid artery during transluminal angioplasty for vasospasm induced by subarachnoid hemorrhage. Case report. J Neurosurg 1991;74(6):985–90.

[149] Le Roux PD, Newell DW, Eskridge J, et al. Severe symptomatic vasospasm: the role of immediate postoperative angioplasty. J Neurosurg 1994; 80(2):224–9.

[150] Murayama Y, Song JK, Uda K, et al. Combined endovascular treatment for both intracranial aneurysm and symptomatic vasospasm. AJNR Am J Neuroradiol 2003;24(1):133–9.

[151] Bolton TB. Mechanisms of action of transmitters and other substances on smooth muscle. Physiol Rev 1979;59(3):606–718.

[152] Vorkapic P, Bevan RD, Bevan JA. Longitudinal time course of reversible and irreversible components of chronic cerebrovasospasm of the rabbit basilar artery. J Neurosurg 1991;74(6):951–5.

[153] Clouston JE, Numaguchi Y, Zoarski GH, et al. Intraarterial papaverine infusion for cerebral vasospasm after subarachnoid hemorrhage. AJNR Am J Neuroradiol 1995;16(1):27–38.

[154] Fandino J, Kaku Y, Schuknecht B, et al. Improvement of cerebral oxygenation patterns and metabolic validation of superselective intraarterial infusion of papaverine for the treatment of cerebral vasospasm. J Neurosurg 1998;89(1): 93–100.

[155] Firlik KS, Kaufmann AM, Firlik AD, et al. Intraarterial papaverine for the treatment of cerebral vasospasm following aneurysmal subarachnoid hemorrhage. Surg Neurol 1999;51(1):66–74.

[156] Kaku Y, Yonekawa Y, Tsukahara T, et al. Superselective intra-arterial infusion of papaverine for the treatment of cerebral vasospasm after subarachnoid hemorrhage. J Neurosurg 1992;77(6): 842–7.

[157] Kassell NF, Helm G, Simmons N, et al. Treatment of cerebral vasospasm with intra-arterial papaverine. J Neurosurg 1992;77(6):848–52.

[158] Milburn JM, Moran CJ, Cross DT, et al. Increase in diameters of vasospastic intracranial arteries by intraarterial papaverine administration. J Neurosurg 1998;88(1):38–42.

[159] Numaguchi Y, Zoarski GH, Clouston JE, et al. Repeat intra-arterial papaverine for recurrent cerebral vasospasm after subarachnoid haemorrhage. Neuroradiology 1997;39(10):751–9.

[160] Cross DT, Moran CJ, Angtuaco EE, et al. Intracranial pressure monitoring during intraarterial papaverine infusion for cerebral vasospasm. AJNR Am J Neuroradiol 1998;19(7):1319–23.

[161] Carhuapoma JR, Qureshi AI, Tamargo RJ, et al. Intra-arterial papaverine-induced seizures: case

report and review of the literature. Surg Neurol 2001;56:159–63.

[162] Takahashi A, Yoshimoto T, Mizoi K, et al. Transluminal balloon angioplasty for vasospasm after subarachnoid hemorrhage. In: Sano K, Takakura K, Kassell NF, et al, editors. Cerebral vasospasm. Tokyo: University of Tokyo Press; 1990. p. 429–32.

[163] Nemoto S. Percutaneous transluminal angioplasty. No To Shinkei 2000;52(7):571–9.

[164] Elliott JP, Newell DW, Lam DJ, et al. Comparison of balloon angioplasty and papaverine infusion for the treatment of vasospasm following aneurysmal subarachnoid hemorrhage. J Neurosurg 1998; 88(2):277–84.

[165] Polin RS, Kassell NF. Treatment of vasospasm. J Neurosurg 1998;88(5):933.

[166] Newell DW, Eskridge J, Mayberg M, et al. Endovascular treatment of intracranial aneurysms and cerebral vasospasm. Clin Neurosurg 1992;39:348–60.

[167] Polin RS, Hansen CA, German P, et al. Intra-arterially administered papaverine for the treatment of symptomatic cerebral vasospasm. Neurosurgery 1998;42(6):1256–7.

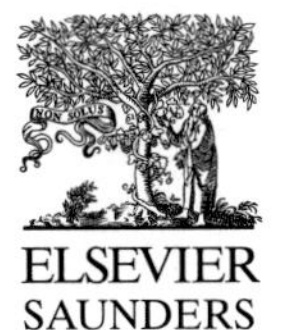
ELSEVIER
SAUNDERS

Neurosurg Clin N Am 16 (2005) 355–363

NEUROSURGERY
CLINICS
OF NORTH AMERICA

Liquid Embolic Agents in the Treatment of Intracranial Arteriovenous Malformations

Jay U. Howington, MD[a], Charles W. Kerber, MD[b], L. Nelson Hopkins, MD, FACS[a,*]

[a]*Department of Neurosurgery and Toshiba Stroke Research Center, School of Medicine and Biomedical Sciences, State University of New York at Buffalo, 3 Gates Circle, Buffalo, NY 14209, USA*

[b]*Departments of Radiology and Neurosurgery, University of California at San Diego, 200 West Arbor Drive, San Diego, CA 92103, USA*

The morbidity and mortality associated with the surgical treatment of intracranial arteriovenous malformations (AVMs) has decreased over the past two decades, mainly because of advances in endovascular therapy and the increased use of stereotactic radiosurgery. Those AVMs traditionally associated with high surgical risk are now often treated with radiosurgery instead. Several studies have demonstrated the direct relation between AVM size and surgical difficulty and operative morbidity [1–8]. When considering endovascular therapy for AVMs, the aim is to obliterate the malformation or to reduce its size to enhance the patient's outcome through surgery or radiosurgery. The first embolization of an AVM was performed by Luessenhop and Spence [9] in 1960 by injecting silastic spheres through a surgical exposure of the cervical carotid artery. Although this method was technically simple to perform, it was nonselective and often resulted in inadvertent occlusion of normal vessels and neurologic injury [10,11]. In 1973, Djindjian et al [12] developed a technique of selective catheterization involving the external carotid artery, but it was Serbinenko [13] who, in 1974, succeeded in accessing the cerebral arteries using a detachable balloon mounted on a floating catheter. Unfortunately, this technique was not vessel specific, because the balloon was carried distally within the vessel with the most flow. Also, the balloon was too large to occlude anything distal to the arterial feeder and thus left the nidus of the malformation unpenetrated.

Polyvinyl alcohol (PVA) particles have also been used as embolic agents in the treatment of AVMs. Porstmann et al [14] first reported the use of PVA particles, but this agent proved to be problematic in the treatment of AVMs for several reasons [15,16]. First, the particles needed to be large enough to embolize the lesion effectively but small enough to be injected through the catheter without blocking the lumen. This problem was solved by later catheter innovations, but other problems with this agent have persisted and include the lack of radiopacity and inability to effect a permanent occlusion of the feeding artery or nidus.

Zanetti et al [17] first described the use of the monomer isobutyl-2-cyanoacrylate for endovascular embolization using canine renal arteries in 1972, but it was not until 1976 that Kerber [18] reported the use of a calibrated-leak balloon mounted on a microcatheter to navigate the intracranial circulation and deliver this novel adhesive agent to the small feeding vessels of an AVM. This technique required the repeated inflation and deflation of the balloon to flow-direct the microcatheter, which was technically difficult and linked with numerous complications [19–22]. In addition, although the initial acrylates were excellent embolic agents, they were associated with toxic reactions and reported to have carcinogenic properties [23,24]. The basic cyanoacrylate monomer was therefore modified, and the resulting embolic agent, N-butyl cyanoacrylate (NBCA; Trufill,

* Corresponding author.

1042-3680/05/$ - see front matter
doi:10.1016/j.nec.2004.08.013

Cordis Neurovascular, Miami Lakes, Florida), has become the standard liquid acrylic adhesive agent in endovascular neurosurgery. Recently, a nonadhesive liquid embolic agent known as Onyx (Onyx Liquid Embolic System, Micro Therapeutics, Irvine, California) has undergone evaluation for embolization at several centers [25–27]. Onyx and NBCA have in common the ability to be injected in liquid form through a microcatheter, although they differ significantly in their various properties and chemical composition. This article focuses on these two agents and the techniques used with each for the embolization of intracranial AVMs.

Provocative testing

The goal of therapeutic embolization is occlusion of the AVM without hindering flow to normal brain parenchyma; however, endovascular cerebral AVM procedures are reported to produce permanent neurologic deficits in approximately 10% of cases [28]. Once a microcatheter is in position, discerning whether embolization will result in a neurologic deficit can be difficult. Some neurointerventionists choose to place patients under general anesthesia and rely on the lack of normal cerebral vessel filling observed on superselective angiography to make this decision. The authors prefer to perform pharmacologic provocative testing while the patient is awake to predict the safety of embolization. The lack of normal cerebral vessels on superselective angiography does not guarantee a risk-free embolization [28]. Pharmacologic provocative testing has been shown to be extremely helpful in discerning whether embolization will result in a neurologic deficit [29–34]. The three main agents used for pre-embolic provocative testing are amobarbital, methohexital, and lidocaine. Traditionally, the short-acting barbiturates have been used to evaluate the potential for injury in the cerebral gray matter because of their action on the gamma-amino butyric acid A ($GABA_A$) receptor. Barbiturates may have little to no effect on cerebral white matter, however, because of a lack of $GABA_A$-ergic synapses. Lidocaine, through its blockage of voltage-gated sodium channels present on all nerve cell membranes, inhibits gray and white matter structures and has been used as an adjunct to barbiturate testing by some [29,35]. Fitzsimmons et al [35] have reported the use of amobarbital and lidocaine in pre-embolization assessment and argue that the addition of lidocaine may increase the sensitivity and predictive value of pre-embolization provocative testing. Although a negative provocative test result predicts the safety of permanent vessel occlusion, it does not eliminate the risk of neurologic injury. Any transient neurologic deficit produced by pharmacologic testing, however, should be expected to produce a permanent deficit with arterial embolization [29–35].

N-butyl cyanoacrylate

Particulate agents, such as PVA, were the mainstay of preoperative embolic therapy for AVMs before advances were made in microcatheter technology. The particles cause a temporary occlusion, which results in vessel thrombosis. This thrombus is subsequently broken down so that there is a relatively high recanalization rate when using PVA [36]. Histopathologic studies of NBCA demonstrate that cyanoacrylate provokes a more intense inflammatory reaction than that caused by PVA and involves the wall of the vessel and the adjacent interstitial areas [37–41]. This inflammatory reaction ultimately leads to vessel necrosis, fibrous ingrowth, and a fairly permanent occlusion [39,42]. The US Food and Drug Administration approved the use of NBCA for the endovascular treatment of AVMs in 2000. The results of the N-BCA Trial, which demonstrated that NBCA was equivalent to PVA as a preoperative embolic agent for the treatment of cerebral AVMs, have been published [14].

Liquid monomeric NBCA is converted to a solid long-chain polymer by anionic initiators (nucleophiles), which are found in excess in blood and on endothelium. Once the polymerization reaction begins, it proceeds at a rapid rate to completion and generates heat in the process. The reaction proceeds so rapidly that the NBCA solidifies in a catheter without the addition of a medium that permits adjustments to be made in the polymerization time. Cromwell and Kerber [19] published their experience with iophendylate oil as an additive, and subsequent investigations have defined the optimal ratio of cyanoacrylate to oil to range from 1:5 to 2:5 [43,44]. Mixing the glue and oil at these ratios extends the polymerization time to allow for adequate penetration of the nidus. Iophendylate oil has been replaced by other oil-based mediums (eg, ethiodized oil, lipiodol) because of greater ease of use with these latter agents. The mixture of glue and oil enables a delay in polymerization; unfortunately, it changes the character of the adhesive so that it comes out of the tip of the catheter in droplets, which can then pass uncontrolled through the AVM and to the lung. Powdered tantalum is also used to increase radiopacity during injection. The kit supplied by Cordis Neurovascular comes with NBCA, ethiodized oil, and tantalum powder. These are then combined at the operator's discretion, depending on the hemodynamics of the lesion. The authors often add glacial acetic acid to the mixture to prolong the polymerization time further, allowing for better control of the injection and fuller casting of the nidus.

Proponents of embolization with cyanoacrylate glue argue that it causes permanent occlusion and can even cure small AVMs if adequate nidal penetration is accomplished [22,42,45–48]. Lesions that can potentially be cured with NBCA embolization are small AVMs with a single feeding pedicle (Fig. 1). The multiplicity of arterial feeders usually seen in larger complex AVMs makes angiographic obliteration of the nidus difficult to obtain. The patent areas of the nidus retain flow and have the potential to recruit secondary feeders. These secondary feeders are often too small to catheterize; therefore, achieving a cure requires surgery or radiosurgery [49,50]. Advocates of NBCA embolization claim that the well-cast portion of the nidus is permanently occluded and that this effectively transforms an inoperable AVM into an operable one by reducing the size of the lesion as well as the number of its arterial feeders [42,45,51–57]. The permanence of the occlusion appeals to proponents of stereotactic radiosurgery because it reduces the risk of hemorrhage during the interval between radiation and vessel sclerosis. (If quadrants of the nidus are embolized, higher doses at the time of radiosurgery can be given, but if the perimeter of the nidus is unchanged, the radiation dosimetry would be the same as if the AVM had not been embolized). NBCA embolization also appeals to the neurosurgeon resecting the AVM because it softens the vessels and makes them retractable, thereby decreasing the amount of blood loss and serving to establish a boundary zone between the AVM vessels and those of normal brain parenchyma. Giant AVMs that are too large to be embolized completely or resected without incurring significant neurologic deficit can be treated in a palliative fashion with NBCA embolization. These lesions often cause symptoms because of the steal phenomenon generated by the blood volume shunted through the AVM. Partial embolization decreases the shunt volume and potentially reduces seizure activity and focal hypoxia.

The following is a general description of the technique used at the authors' institution for NBCA embolization. The tip of the microcatheter

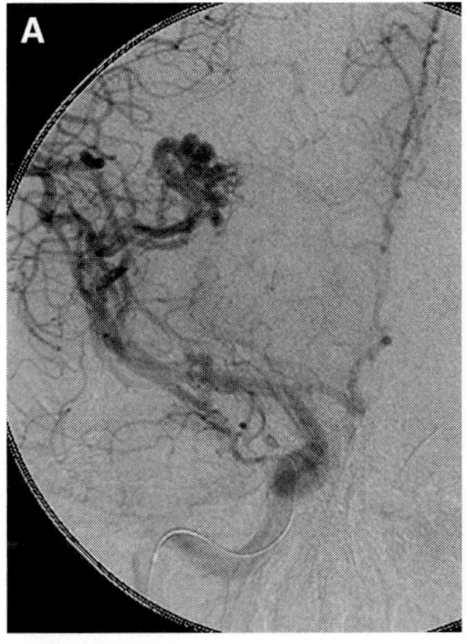

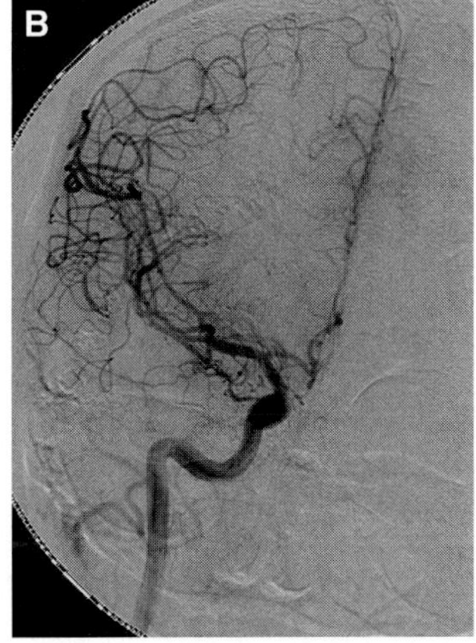

Fig. 1. (*A*) Anteroposterior intracranial angiogram of the right internal carotid artery in a 26-year-old woman obtained 2 months after she presented with an intracerebral hemorrhage. This small arteriovenous malformation is supplied by only one feeder. (*B*) Right common carotid artery angiogram obtained after embolization with N-butyl cyanoacrylate (Trufill; Cordis Neurovascular, Miami Lakes, Florida) demonstrating complete obliteration of the malformation. (*From* Howington JU, Kerber CW, Guterman LR, Hopkins LN. Liquid embolic agents in the treatment of intracranial arteriovenous malformations. In: Horowitz MB, Levy EI, editors. Neuroendovascular surgery series. Basel: Karger 2004;17:138.)

is advanced as close to the nidus as possible, and superselective angiography is performed. If normal vessels are not appreciated, provocative testing is performed. While this is being done, a second physician mixes the NBCA, ethiodized oil, and tantalum powder (and possibly glacial acetic acid) on a separate table, which must be uncontaminated by any ionizing material. The authors prefer to use a standard concentration of 30% (NBCA [0.9 mL] and oil [2.1 mL]) mixed with the standard vial of tantalum supplied by the manufacturer. The cyanoacrylate is modified with glacial acetic acid on the basis of the hemodynamic properties observed during the superselective angiogram. The glacial acetic acid is added to the mixture using a 3-mL syringe with a 30-gauge needle. It is critical that the preparation takes place in an ion-free environment to prevent premature polymerization. Each physician changes gown and gloves before handling the adhesive. Although the standard concentration of NBCA is 30%, this concentration can be adjusted to the hemodynamics of the AVM so as to provide adequate penetration of the nidus without occlusion of the venous drainage system. Before the embolization is performed, the microcatheter is manually flushed continuously with nonionic 5% dextrose in water (D5W). The operator who is to inject the NBCA should also be the one flushing the catheter so as to avoid an injection that is too weak or too strong. In a rapid exchange, the D5W syringe is removed (allowing no air entry) and replaced with the syringe containing the adhesive. With steady force, the NBCA is pushed through the catheter until the first drops appear at the tip of the catheter. The rate of injection is then adjusted to establish a good nidal cast by keeping the drops from coming out too fast or too slow. Reflux around the microcatheter must be avoided. When the embolization is complete, negative pressure is applied to the syringe containing the adhesive, and the microcatheter is quickly withdrawn. This final maneuver usually requires the cooperation of two physicians. Whether more pedicles are to be embolized is a decision made by the endovascular surgeon based on the amount of nidus occluded. As a general rule, the authors think that no more than 50% of the nidus should be embolized in the first attempt. The authors give credence to the theory of normal perfusion pressure breakthrough and think that a greater percentage of occlusion without complete nidal obliteration increases the risk of postprocedure hemorrhage [58]. Also, incomplete nidal obliteration in conjunction with significant occlusion of the venous drainage system increases the risk of postprocedural hemorrhage. Smaller AVMs with only one feeder can often be cured during a single embolization procedure, whereas larger more complex lesions usually require multiple sessions spaced over several months.

A long-known risk of using cyanoacrylates to embolize AVMs is that of rapid polymerization and reflux, which results in gluing the catheter in place [14,59]. Early polymerization can also result in the undesired effect of feeding vessel occlusion without nidal penetration. If the polymerization time is too long, the cyanoacrylate can pass into the venous circulation, resulting in pulmonary emboli. With a thorough understanding of the flow dynamics of the AVM, along with the ability to titrate the polymerization time with additive media, these risks can be largely minimized.

Onyx

Taki and colleagues [60] were the first to describe the use of ethylene-vinyl alcohol copolymer (EVOH) in combination with dimethyl sulfoxide (DMSO) for the embolization of cerebral AVMs. They combined the solid copolymer (5 g) with metrizamide powder (35 g, for opacification) dissolved in DMSO (60 g). DMSO is an organic solvent, and when the polymer-powder-solvent mixture comes in contact with an aqueous medium, such as blood, the DMSO diffuses away and the EVOH precipitates and solidifies. The resultant embolic material is cohesive without being adhesive, which means that it does not adhere to the wall of the vessel or the catheter but is thick enough to become lodged in the vessel. Subsequent studies led to a premixed solution of EVOH, tantalum, and DMSO known as Onyx, which comes in three different concentrations of EVOH (6.0%, 6.5%, and 8.0%) [26,61,62]. The varied concentrations of EVOH are used to vary the precipitation rate. The lower the concentration of EVOH, the less viscous the solution will be and the longer it will take to precipitate in the AVM.

Nonadhesive nature of Onyx enhances controllability during delivery

DMSO was chosen as the solvent for two main reasons: it readily diffuses in water, and its physiologic properties in human beings have been well studied [60,63]. This compound is extremely angiotoxic, however, and its adverse effects range from vasospasm to angionecrosis and arterial rupture. The damage to the vessel wall can be so great that an occlusion occurs, which then alters the flow dynamics. As in cases of premature NBCA polymerization, an inadvertent reflux of Onyx can lead to inadequate nidal penetration or parent artery embolization. The angiotoxicity of DMSO is directly related to the volume infused and the length of time the compound is in contact with the vessel wall. In fact, Murayama et al [61] demonstrated that these factors were the two most important determinants of the angiotoxicity of DMSO. Some investigators have argued that the toxicity of DMSO actually benefits the embolization process, however, by speeding up the intravascular thrombosis, endothelial injury, and eventual inflammatory foreign body reaction that is seen with embolization [64]. The effectiveness of DMSO as a solvent is so great that it has been shown to damage some of the catheters used for its delivery [26,61,65]. For this reason, specially designed DMSO-compatible catheters must be employed when Onyx is used for AVM embolization. Currently, only three catheters are able to tolerate the infusion of DMSO without being destroyed, and they are the Radifocus GT III catheter (Terumo, Tokyo, Japan) and the Flow Rider Plus and Rebar catheters (Micro Therapeutics). Another potential drawback to the use of Onyx as an adjunctive modality for the treatment of cerebral AVMs is the discomfort that many awake patients report as it is injected. At times, this discomfort can be so severe that the induction of general anesthesia may be necessary. Therefore, institutions that routinely use provocative testing as part of their embolization protocol may have difficulty in using Onyx. Finally, the ready-made vials of the EVOH-DMSO-tantalum (Onyx) mixture settle out of suspension if not shaken. The operator must be aware of this fact and remember to agitate the vial constantly until the time of the injection. If the mixture is injected without the tantalum being adequately suspended in the EVOH-DMSO, the radiopacity might be lessened. In their report of 23 patients treated using Onyx, Jahan et al [26] advocate the use of the Vortex-Genie shaker (Micro Therapeutics) for keeping the tantalum evenly dispersed so as to maximize radiopacity.

The nonadhesive nature of Onyx as a liquid embolic agent gives it several advantages over NBCA. Inadvertent gluing of the catheter to the arterial pedicle is not a concern. Because Onyx is nonadhesive, it can be injected in a slower and more controlled fashion; during this time, serial angiograms can be used to evaluate the progress of the embolization. Some preliminary experience indicates that because Onyx hardens slowly, extended injection times are possible, which means that there might be higher AVM cure rates with Onyx compared with NBCA [25]. After one pedicle is embolized, the same catheter can be repositioned in another pedicle for another embolization, which is something that is not possible with NBCA embolization. Fig. 2 demonstrates an AVM with multiple feeding vessels that was treated with Onyx during one setting. The presence of tantalum darkens the Onyx and also aids at the time of surgical resection by delineating AVM vessels from normal cerebral vessels (the same is true for NBCA). At the time of operation, the Onyx-filled nidus is reported to be spongy and easily retractable, which also benefits surgical resection [26,60,64,66]. In an effort to analyze the form that embolic agents take with the involved vessel, their pliability for resection, and the degree of blood loss during resection, Akin et al [64] performed a surgical handling study comparing NBCA and Onyx using a swine AVM resection model. They found that vessels embolized with Onyx were soft and easily manipulated, whereas vessels embolized with NBCA tended to be considerably tougher to manipulate and not as easy to cut. Also, during the surgical resection, the rete mirabile embolized with Onyx bled less than those treated with NBCA.

The basic technique of embolization with Onyx is similar to that of NBCA except that no preparation of the embolic material in an ion-free environment is necessary. The catheter must be primed with normal saline and then with DMSO (0.27 mL) to fill the dead space and prevent premature solidification of the Onyx. The operator chooses the particular concentration of EVOH on the basis of the flow dynamics of the AVM. Using a 1-mL syringe, the DMSO is slowly (over the course of 40 seconds) injected and then replaced by the Onyx. Under fluoroscopy, the Onyx is injected slowly enough to achieve adequate nidal penetration without reflux. The catheter is withdrawn or primed again with DMSO if further embolization is warranted.

Histopathologically, vascular structures embolized with EVOH show mild inflammatory changes in the acute setting and chronic inflammatory changes after only several days [26,

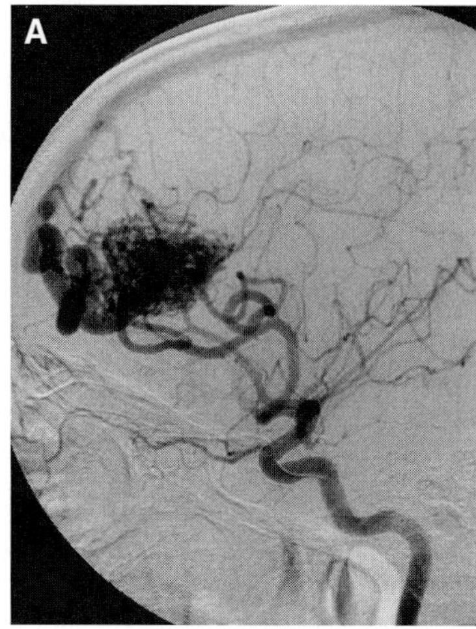

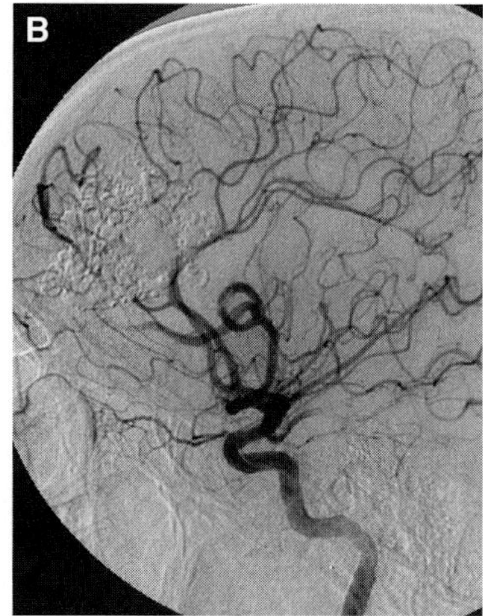

Fig. 2. (*A*) Lateral intracranial angiogram of the right internal carotid artery in a 37-year-old woman who presented with refractory epilepsy. The malformation is fed by branches from the anterior and middle cerebral arteries. (*B*) Lateral intracranial angiogram obtained after embolization with Onyx (Micro Therapeutics, Irvine, California) demonstrating no residual malformation. (*From* Howington JU, Kerber CW, Guterman LR, Hopkins LN. Liquid embolic agents in the treatment of intracranial arteriovenous malformations. In: Horowitz MB, Levy EI, editors. Neuroendovascular surgery series. Basel: Karger 2004;17:141.)

60–62,64–66]. These changes are usually found within the vessel lumen, with only focal areas of elastica disruption, and usually spare much of the vessel wall. This lack of necrosis allows the vessel to remain viable and makes future recanalization a possibility. Some authors have cautioned against the use of Onyx as an embolic agent for AVMs because of this recanalization risk [67,68]. Angionecrosis can occur, but this is thought to be caused by the improper injection of DMSO rather than by the presence of Onyx. Examination of resected AVMs treated with Onyx has revealed complete filling of some vessels, whereas others are only partially filled with the embolic material. The thrombus that fills the remainder of the vessel lumen can undergo recanalization over time. To date, there have been no long-term angiographic follow-up analyses of patients treated with Onyx. Late recanalization of AVMs treated with Onyx must be considered a possibility given the histopathologic findings published thus far and needs to be evaluated further.

Summary

The endovascular treatment of cerebral AVMs has advanced greatly in the four decades since Luessenhop and Spence [9] first described the use of silastic spheres to embolize an AVM. The innovations have been in the agents used to embolize as well as in the devices used to deliver the agent to the AVM. Endovascular therapies have helped to decrease operative morbidity by making it easier for the surgeon to resect the AVM and, in some cases, by eliminating the need for surgery altogether. The benefit of size reduction not only benefits the surgical treatment of AVMs but improves the efficacy of stereotactic radiosurgery. The authors expect that the future will bring continued advances; with such advances, the morbidity associated with AVM treatment should drop even lower.

References

[1] Heros RC, Tu YK. Unruptured arteriovenous malformations: a dilemma in surgical decision making. Clin Neurosurg 1986;33:187–236.

[2] Luessenhop AJ, Gennarelli TA. Anatomical grading of supratentorial arteriovenous malformations for determining operability. Neurosurgery 1977;1(1):30–5.

[3] Pasqualin A, Barone G, Cioffi F, Rosta L, Scienza R, Da Pian R. The relevance of anatomic and hemodynamic factors to a classification of cerebral arteriovenous malformations. Neurosurgery 1991;28(3):370–9.

[4] Spetzler RF, Martin NA. A proposed grading system for arteriovenous malformations. J Neurosurg 1986;65(4):476–83.

[5] Tamaki N, Ehara K, Lin TK, et al. Cerebral arteriovenous malformations: factors influencing the surgical difficulty and outcome. Neurosurgery 1991;29(6):856–63.

[6] Chang SD, Marcellus ML, Marks MP, Levy RP, Do HM, Steinberg GK. Multimodality treatment of giant intracranial arteriovenous malformations. Neurosurgery 2003;53(1):1–13.

[7] Morgan MK, Johnston IH, Hallinan JM, Weber NC. Complications of surgery for arteriovenous malformations of the brain. J Neurosurg 1993;78(2):176–82.

[8] Heros RC, Korosue K, Diebold PM. Surgical excision of cerebral arteriovenous malformations: late results. Neurosurgery 1990;26(4):570–8.

[9] Luessenhop AJ, Spence WT. Artificial embolization of cerebral arteries: report of use in a case of arteriovenous malformation. JAMA 1960;172:1153–5.

[10] Wolpert SM. Silastic sphere embolization of intracranial arteriovenous malformations. In: Wilson CB, Stein BM, editors. Intracranial arteriovenous malformations. Baltimore: Williams & Wilkins; 1988. p. 274–94.

[11] Wolpert SM, Stein BM. Catheter embolization of intracranial arteriovenous malformations as an aid to surgical excision. Neuroradiology 1975;10(2):73–85.

[12] Djindjian R, Cophignon J, Rey Theron J, Merland JJ, Houdart R. Superselective arteriographic embolization by the femoral route in neuroradiology. Study of 50 cases. 3. Embolization in craniocerebral pathology. Neuroradiology 1973;6(3):143–52.

[13] Serbinenko FA. Balloon catheterization and occlusion of major cerebral vessels. J Neurosurg 1974;41(2):125–45.

[14] Porstmann W, Wierny L, Warnke H, Gerstberger G, Romaniuk PA. Catheter closure of patent ductus arteriosus. 62 cases treated without thoracotomy. Radiol Clin N Am 1971;9(2):203–18.

[15] The N-BCA Trial Investigators. N-butyl cyanoacrylate embolization of cerebral arteriovenous malformations: results of a prospective, randomized, multi-center trial. AJNR Am J Neuroradiol 2002;23(5):748–55.

[16] Sorimachi T, Koike T, Takeuchi S, et al. Embolization of cerebral arteriovenous malformations achieved with polyvinyl alcohol particles: angiographic reappearance and complications. AJNR Am J Neuroradiol 1999;20(7):1323–8.

[17] Zanetti PH, Sherman FE. Experimental evaluation of a tissue adhesive as an agent for the treatment of aneurysms and arteriovenous anomalies. J Neurosurg 1972;36:72–9.

[18] Kerber C. Balloon catheter with a calibrated leak. A new system for superselective angiography and occlusive catheter therapy. Radiology 1976;120(3):547–50.

[19] Cromwell LD, Kerber CW. Modification of cyanoacrylate for therapeutic embolization: preliminary experience. AJR Am J Roentgenol 1979;132(5):799–801.

[20] Merland JJ, Rufenacht D, Laurent A, Guimaraens L. Endovascular treatment with isobutyl cyano acrylate in patients with arteriovenous malformation of the brain. Indications, results and complications. Acta Radiol Suppl 1986;369:621–2.

[21] Vinuela F, Fox AJ, Pelz D, Debrun G. Angiographic follow-up of large cerebral AVMs incompletely embolized with isobutyl-2-cyanoacrylate. AJNR Am J Neuroradiol 1986;7(5):919–25.

[22] Vinuela F, Duckwiler G, Guglielmi G. Intravascular embolization of brain arteriovenous malformations. In: Maciunas RJ, editor. Endovascular neurological intervention. Park Ridge, IL: American Association of Neurological Surgeons; 1995. p. 189–99.

[23] Samson D, Marshall D. Carcinogenic potential of isobutyl-2-cyanoacrylate. J Neurosurg 1986;65(4):571–2.

[24] Vinters HV, Galil KA, Lundie MJ, Kaufmann JC. The histotoxicity of cyanoacrylates. A selective review. Neuroradiology 1985;27(4):279–91.

[25] Cekirge S, Saatci I, Arat A. Long-term intranidal Onyx injections in the endovascular treatment of pial brain AVMs: description of a new technique and philosophy aimed at cure [abstract]. J Neurosurg 2002;96:173A.

[26] Jahan R, Murayama Y, Gobin YP, Duckwiler GR, Vinters HV, Vinuela F. Embolization of arteriovenous malformations with Onyx: clinicopathological experience in 23 patients. Neurosurgery 2001;48(5):984–97.

[27] Niemann DB, Molyneux AJ. Embolization of brain AVMs with ethylene-vinyl alcohol copolymer dissolved in DMSO (Onyx-liquid embolic system): evidence in a prospective series of 31 patients [abstract]. J Neurosurg 2002;96:171A.

[28] Arteriovenous malformations of the brain in adults. N Engl J Med 1999;340(23):1812–8.

[29] Sadato A, Taki W, Nakahara I, et al. Improved provocative test for the embolization of arteriovenous malformations—technical note. Neurol Med Chir (Tokyo) 1994;34(3):187–90.

[30] Peters KR, Quisling RG, Gilmore R, Mickle P, Kuperus JH. Intraarterial use of sodium methohexital for provocative testing during brain embolotherapy. AJNR Am J Neuroradiol 1993;14(1):171–4.

[31] Mathis JM, Barr JD. Pharmacologic testing as an adjunct to neuroendovascular procedures. Neurosurg Clin N Am 2000;11(1):21–6.

[32] Rauch RA, Vinuela F, Dion J, et al. Preembolization functional evaluation in brain arteriovenous malformations: the superselective Amytal test. AJNR Am J Neuroradiol 1992;13(1):303–8.

[33] Rauch RA, Vinuela F, Dion J, et al. Preembolization functional evaluation in brain arteriovenous malformations: the ability of superselective Amytal test to predict neurologic dysfunction before embolization. AJNR Am J Neuroradiol 1992;13(1):309–14.

[34] Moo LR, Murphy KJ, Gailloud P, Tesoro M, Hart J. Tailored cognitive testing with provocative amobarbital injection preceding AVM embolization. AJNR Am J Neuroradiol 2002;23(3):416–21.

[35] Fitzsimmons BF, Marshall RS, Pile-Spellman J, Lazar RM. Neurobehavioral differences in superselective Wada testing with amobarbital versus lidocaine. AJNR Am J Neuroradiol 2003;24(7): 1456–60.

[36] Standard SC, Guterman LR, Chavis TD, Hopkins LN. Delayed recanalization of a cerebral arteriovenous malformation following angiographic obliteration with polyvinyl alcohol embolization. Surg Neurol 1995;44(2):109–13.

[37] Brothers MF, Kaufmann JC, Fox AJ, Deveikis JP. n-Butyl 2-cyanoacrylate—substitute for IBCA in interventional neuroradiology: histopathologic and polymerization time studies. AJNR Am J Neuroradiol 1989;10(4):777–86.

[38] Duffner F, Ritz R, Bornemann A, Freudenstein D, Wiendl H, Siekmann R. Combined therapy of cerebral arteriovenous malformations: histological differences between a non-adhesive liquid embolic agent and n-butyl 2-cyanoacrylate (NBCA). Clin Neuropathol 2002;21(1):13–7.

[39] Kerber CW, Wong W. Liquid acrylic adhesive agents in interventional neuroradiology. Neurosurg Clin N Am 2000;11(1):85–99.

[40] Kish KK, Rapp SM, Wilner HI, Wolfe D, Thomas LM, Barr J. Histopathologic effects of transarterial bucrylate occlusion of intracerebral arteries in mongrel dogs. AJNR Am J Neuroradiol 1983;4(3): 385–7.

[41] Standard SC, Hopkins LN. Principles of neuroendovascular intervention. In: Maciunas RJ, editor. Endovascular neurological intervention. Park Ridge, IL: American Association of Neurological Surgeons; 1995. p. 1–34.

[42] Wikholm G. Occlusion of cerebral arteriovenous malformations with N-butyl cyano-acrylate is permanent. AJNR Am J Neuroradiol 1995;16(3): 479–82.

[43] Stoesslein F, Muenster W. A new technique for safe embolization using cyanoacrylate/contrast medium mixtures. Ann Radiol (Paris) 1984;27(4): 296–8.

[44] Stoesslein F, Ditscherlein G, Romaniuk PA. Experimental studies on new liquid embolization mixtures (histoacryl-lipiodol, histoacryl-panthopaque). Cardiovasc Intervent Radiol 1982;5(5):264–7.

[45] Fournier D, TerBrugge KG, Willinsky R, Lasjaunias P, Montanera W. Endovascular treatment of intracerebral arteriovenous malformations: experience in 49 cases. J Neurosurg 1991;75(2):228–33.

[46] Hurst RW, Berenstein A, Kupersmith MJ, Madrid M, Flamm ES. Deep central arteriovenous malformations of the brain: the role of endovascular treatment. J Neurosurg 1995;82(2):190–5.

[47] Mansmann U, Lasjaunias P, Meisel HJ. Treatment of patients with cerebral arteriovenous malformations. Radiology 2002;223(3):879–81.

[48] Wikholm G, Lundqvist C, Svendsen P. Embolization of cerebral arteriovenous malformations: part I—technique, morphology, and complications. Neurosurgery 1996;39(3):448–59.

[49] Fournier D, Terbrugge K, Rodesch G, Lasjaunias P. Revascularization of brain arteriovenous malformations after embolization with bucrylate. Neuroradiology 1990;32(6):497–501.

[50] Gobin YP, Laurent A, Merienne L, et al. Treatment of brain arteriovenous malformations by embolization and radiosurgery. J Neurosurg 1996;85(1): 19–28.

[51] Debrun GM, Aletich V, Ausman JI, Charbel F, Dujovny M. Embolization of the nidus of brain arteriovenous malformations with n-butyl cyanoacrylate. Neurosurgery 1997;40(1):112–21.

[52] DeMeritt JS, Pile-Spellman J, Mast H, et al. Outcome analysis of preoperative embolization with N-butyl cyanoacrylate in cerebral arteriovenous malformations. AJNR Am J Neuroradiol 1995; 16(9):1801–7.

[53] Frizzel RT, Fisher WS III. Cure, morbidity, and mortality associated with embolization of brain arteriovenous malformations: a review of 1246 patients in 32 series over a 35-year period. Neurosurgery 1995;37(6):1031–40.

[54] Jafar JJ, Davis AJ, Berenstein A, Choi IS, Kupersmith MJ. The effect of embolization with N-butyl cyanoacrylate prior to surgical resection of cerebral arteriovenous malformations. J Neurosurg 1993; 78(1):60–9.

[55] Pasqualin A, Scienza R, Cioffi F, et al. Treatment of cerebral arteriovenous malformations with a combination of preoperative embolization and surgery. Neurosurgery 1991;29(3):358–68.

[56] Richling B, Killer M. Endovascular management of patients with cerebral arteriovenous malformations. Neurosurg Clin N Am 2000;11(1):123–45.

[57] Vinuela F, Dion JE, Duckwiler G, et al. Combined endovascular embolization and surgery in the management of cerebral arteriovenous malformations: experience with 101 cases. J Neurosurg 1991;75(6): 856–64.

[58] Spetzler RF, Wilson CB, Weinstein P, Mehdorn M, Townsend J, Telles D. Normal perfusion pressure breakthrough theory. Clin Neurosurg 1978;25: 651–72.

[59] Bank WO, Kerber CW, Cromwell LD. Treatment of intracerebral arteriovenous malformations with isobutyl 2-cyanoacrylate: initial clinical experience. Radiology 1981;139(3):609–16.

[60] Taki W, Yonekawa Y, Iwata H, Uno A, Yamashita K, Amemiya H. A new liquid material for embolization of arteriovenous malformations. AJNR Am J Neuroradiol 1990;11(1):163–8.

[61] Murayama Y, Vinuela F, Ulhoa A, et al. Nonadhesive liquid embolic agent for cerebral arteriovenous malformations: preliminary histopathological studies in swine rete mirabile. Neurosurgery 1998;43(5):1164–75.

[62] Yamashita K, Taki W, Iwata H, et al. Characteristics of ethylene vinyl alcohol copolymer (EVAL) mixtures. AJNR Am J Neuroradiol 1994;15(6):1103–5.

[63] Marshall LF, Camp PE, Bowers SA. Dimethyl sulfoxide for the treatment of intracranial hypertension: a preliminary trial. Neurosurgery 1984;14(6):659–63.

[64] Akin ED, Perkins E, Ross IB. Surgical handling characteristics of an ethylene vinyl alcohol copolymer compared with N-butyl cyanoacrylate used for embolization of vessels in an arteriovenous malformation resection model in swine. J Neurosurg 2003;98(2):366–70.

[65] Chaloupka JC, Vinuela F, Vinters HV, Robert J. Technical feasibility and histopathologic studies of ethylene vinyl copolymer (EVAL) using a swine endovascular embolization model. AJNR Am J Neuroradiol 1994;15(6):1107–15.

[66] Terada T, Nakamura Y, Nakai K, et al. Embolization of arteriovenous malformations with peripheral aneurysms using ethylene vinyl alcohol copolymer. Report of three cases. J Neurosurg 1991;75(4):655–60.

[67] Higashida R. Embolization of arteriovenous malformations with Onyx: clinicopathological experience in 23 patients [comment]. Neurosurgery 2001;48:995.

[68] Lagares A, Lobato RD, Ricoy JR, Campollo J. Embolization of arteriovenous malformations with Onyx: clinicopathological experience in 23 patients. Neurosurgery 2002;51(6):1525–6.

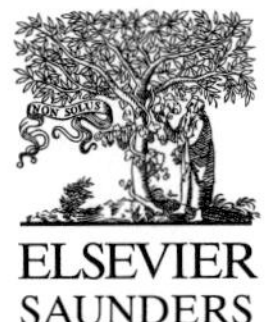

ELSEVIER
SAUNDERS

Neurosurg Clin N Am 16 (2005) 365–366

NEUROSURGERY
CLINICS
OF NORTH AMERICA

Indications for Surgical Treatment of Arteriovenous Malformations

Peter Nakaji, MD, Robert F. Spetzler, MD*

Division of Neurological Surgery, Barrow Neurological Institute, St. Joseph's Hospital and Medical Center, 350 West Thomas Road, Phoenix, AZ 85013, USA

The indications for surgical treatment of arteriovenous malformations (AVMs) of the brain are evolving. In general, any AVM whose natural history and anatomic characteristics make it more likely to cause morbidity or mortality than the treatment itself should be treated. Given the relatively high rate of hemorrhage associated with AVMs without treatment, their obliteration is usually desirable. Microsurgical removal remains the mainstay of definitive treatment, but the management of AVMs fundamentally requires a team approach. Advances in endovascular therapy and radiosurgery offer options that must be considered when formulating any treatment plan. Most patients' plans incorporate a combination of modalities. As we critically evaluate treatment outcomes, it has become clear that microsurgical removal is only one branch in a decision tree that may include the option of no treatment for some patients. This article reviews the indications for treatment of AVMs in general and then focuses on the selection of surgery as a treatment modality, alone and in combination with embolization and radiosurgery.

The decision about whether and how to treat an AVM depends on a number of factors, the most important elements of which are the patient's age, symptoms, and medical condition; the size of the AVM; its location; the type of venous drainage; the history of the AVM; and the natural history of AVMs in general. The known natural history of AVMs suggests that the rate of hemorrhage from an AVM is approximately 3% per year [1,2]. Each episode of bleeding is associated with a mean mortality rate of 10% and a mean rate of neurologic morbidity of 20%. Examining these numbers actuarially leads to the conclusion that the younger a patient is and the lower the surgical risk, the more likely the patient is to benefit from treatment. In children and younger patients, we are aggressive about surgical removal, especially because it avoids complications related to applying radiation to the young brain. Symptomatic patients are more likely to benefit, because surgery often eliminates the risks of rebleeding and vascular steal and can improve headache and, in some cases, seizures. As for the characteristics of the AVM itself, a higher risk of bleeding is associated with small AVMs; the presence of a feeding artery, nidus, or venous aneurysm; or impaired venous drainage [3]. For this reason, we favor treating most small lesions because they are easier to remove and more likely to bleed than larger aneurysms. Conversely, some evidence suggests that larger lesions are less likely to bleed than smaller ones. Because they are more formidable to remove, conservative management is a more reasonable option in such cases. Similarly, AVMs located in eloquent brain and with deep venous drainage are technically more difficult to remove without morbidity, relatively favoring their nonsurgical management. If a given AVM has already hemorrhaged and caused a fixed deficit or if recurrent hemorrhages, steal, or venous hypertension is producing a stepwise decline, we favor surgical removal.

Improvements in endovascular therapy and radiosurgery have resulted in welcome additions

* Corresponding author. c/o Neuroscience Publications, Barrow Neurological Institute, St. Joseph's Hospital and Medical Center, 350 West Thomas Road, Phoenix, AZ 85013, USA.

E-mail address: neuropub@chw.edu (R.F. Spetzler).

1042-3680/05/$ - see front matter
doi:10.1016/j.nec.2004.08.016

to the armamentarium of therapeutic modalities available for this disease. Endovascular embolization has rendered many previously difficult AVMs much easier to remove surgically. In general, endovascular embolization is most useful for grade III AVMs, although we also often use it for AVMs of lesser grades. Although there are anecdotal reports of permanent occlusion of AVMs through endovascular embolization alone, endovascular obliteration is not considered definitive treatment as a stand-alone therapy. The rate of complete occlusion associated with endovascular therapy alone is estimated at 10% [4]. The durability of the occlusion in this setting is unknown. In contrast, stereotactic radiosurgery produces an angiographic and clinical cure for many lesions. Optimally, the lesion should be small (<10 mL in total volume). The efficacy of radiosurgical treatment of lesions less than 2.5 cm in diameter ranges from 74% to 80% and is approximately 50% for lesions between 2.5 and 3 cm in diameter [5,6]. Two years or more may be required for the full protective effect of radiotherapy to be seen. We prefer surgery for accessible lesions and recommend radiosurgery for lesions when the associated approach-related morbidity is high (eg, AVMs in basal ganglia or thalamus). Endovascular embolization has been used to reduce the size of the nidus of a difficult AVM so that it can be treated with radiosurgery. The benefit of this strategy has not been substantiated, however. For large lesions (>4 cm in diameter), surgery typically offers the most realistic hope of cure.

There has been an increasing trend toward conservative management of high-grade AVMs (Spetzler-Martin grades IV and V), although some surgeons still advocate an aggressive approach [7,8]. The microsurgical removal of these lesions involves substantial risk. The possibility of achieving surgical cure is attractive, particularly when it can be achieved without morbidity in some cases. In our opinion, however, critical analysis of the risk-benefit ratio for a large number of patients does not support the routine treatment of grade IV and V lesions. Expectant care, even with the attendant rates of hemorrhage that the natural history of AVMs inevitably incurs, is still likely to produce an outcome as good as or better than that which can be achieved surgically. Incomplete treatment of an AVM seems to increase rather than decrease the risk of hemorrhage. This does not mean that surgery on high-grade AVMs is never justified. Each AVM needs to be evaluated individually. In equivocal cases, the patient's preference may drive the decision to pursue or forgo excision.

In summary, the best candidates for surgical treatment are patients in good medical condition, with a good life expectancy, who harbor small to medium-sized AVMs located in anatomically accessible parts of the brain. Indications further favoring surgery include significant symptoms, AVMs with a higher bleeding risk (eg, those associated with aneurysms or venous outflow obstruction), and AVMs that have failed treatment with radiotherapy or endovascular embolization. Any residual AVM should be considered to have at least the same risk of bleeding as a native lesion and should be treated. Once the decision to treat has been made, for many AVMs, the choice between radiosurgery and microsurgery depends on the patient's attitude about surgery and radiation and on the patient's willingness to wait for the protective effect of radiotherapy to be realized.

If surgery is chosen, multimodality therapy with combined endovascular embolization and surgery typically is preferred. Both therapies should be staged when appropriate.

References

[1] ApSimon HT, Reef H, Phadke RV, et al. A population-based study of brain arteriovenous malformation: long-term treatment outcomes. Stroke 2002;33:2794–800.

[2] Fults D, Kelly DL Jr. Natural history of arteriovenous malformations of the brain: a clinical study. Neurosurgery 1984;15:658–62.

[3] Spetzler RF, Hargraves RW, McCormick PW, et al. Relationship of perfusion pressure and size to risk of hemorrhage from arteriovenous malformations. J Neurosurg 1992;76:918–23.

[4] Gobin YP, Laurent A, Merienne L, et al. Treatment of brain arteriovenous malformations by embolization and radiosurgery. J Neurosurg 1996;85:19–28.

[5] Pollock BE, Gorman DA, Schomberg PJ, et al. The Mayo Clinic gamma knife experience: indications and initial results. Mayo Clin Proc 1999;74:5–13.

[6] Sasaki T, Kurita H, Saito I, et al. Arteriovenous malformations in the basal ganglia and thalamus: management and results in 101 cases. J Neurosurg 1998;88:285–92.

[7] Chang SD, Marcellus ML, Marks MP, et al. Multimodality treatment of giant intracranial arteriovenous malformations. Neurosurgery 2003;53:1–11.

[8] Heros RC. Spetzler-Martin grades IV and V arteriovenous malformations. J Neurosurg 2003;98:1–2.

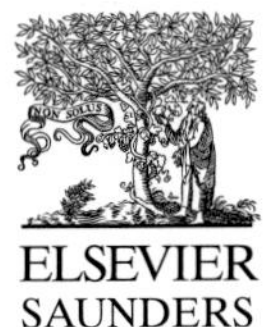
ELSEVIER
SAUNDERS

Neurosurg Clin N Am 16 (2005) 367–380

NEUROSURGERY
CLINICS
OF NORTH AMERICA

Endovascular Treatment of Cerebral Arteriovenous Malformations: Indications, Techniques, Outcome, and Complications

Kevin M. Cockroft, MD, MSc, FACS[a], Sung-Kyun Hwang, MD[b,c], Robert H. Rosenwasser, MD, FACS[c,*]

[a]*Department of Neurosurgery, MC H110, M.S. Hershey Medical Center, Pennsylvania State University, PO Box 850, Hershey, PA 17033, USA*

[b]*Department of Neurosurgery, Ewha Women's University School of Medicine, 70 Changro 6 KR, Changro-gu, Seoul 110-783, South Korea*

[c]*Division of Cerebrovascular Surgery and Interventional Neuroradiology, Department of Neurosurgery, Thomas Jefferson University Hospital, 909 Walnut Street, Third Floor, Philadelphia, PA 19107, USA*

In 1960, Luessenhop and Spence [1] reported the first case of the endovascular treatment of a cerebral arteriovenous malformation (AVM). In the early cases subsequently reported, plastic microspheres were often injected through direct access from the cervical carotid artery. Emboli were guided solely by flow and often ended up in the lungs. Over the years, endovascular therapy for cerebral AVMs has advanced greatly, although the basic principles and goals have remained similar. Microcatheters are now flow directed, and liquid embolic agents have replaced particles for the most part, but the eventual angiographic obliteration of the AVM remains the ultimate goal. In the following article, we review the basic indications, techniques, and complications associated with the current endovascular treatment of cerebral (pial) AVMs.

Cerebral arteriovenous malformations

Cerebral vascular malformations are commonly classified as belonging to one of four categories: (1) AVMs, (2) cavernous angiomas (ie, cavernomas, cavernous malformations), (3) capillary telangiectasias, and (4) venous angiomas (ie, developmental venous anomalies) [2]. Based on McCormick's autopsy series of 5743 consecutive patients [3], the incidence of venous angiomas seems to be the highest of the group at approximately 3%, followed by capillary telangiectasias at 0.9%, AVMs at 0.5%, and cavernous angiomas at 0.3%. Capillary telangiectasias and venous angiomas are almost always incidental or asymptomatic; as such, they rarely require treatment. In contrast, AVMs and cavernous angiomas commonly present with hemorrhage, seizures, or progressive neurologic deficit, and treatment is often required.

Like the other types of cerebral vascular malformations, high-flow pial AVMs are thought to be congenital lesions that arise during the first trimester of fetal development. Unlike cavernous angiomas, which are collections of low-flow venous sinusoids, AVMs are composed of multiple, primitive, high-flow arteries connected directly to the venous system without an intervening capillary network. Dysplastic brain tissue is present between the vessels of the AVM nidus. Because cavernous angiomas are, by definition, angiographically occult, no endovascular role is available for their management. AVMs, conversely, show a typical pattern of arteriovenous shunting on angiography, with venous outflow usually provided by one or two dilated and arterialized veins. This appearance makes cerebral AVMs quite amenable to all major forms of treatment,

* Corresponding author.
E-mail address: robert.rosenwasser@mail.tju.edu (R.H. Rosenwasser).

1042-3680/05/$ - see front matter
doi:10.1016/j.nec.2004.08.001

including endovascular embolization, microsurgical resection, and stereotactic radiosurgery.

Natural history

Approximately 50% to 60% of patients with AVMs come to medical attention after intracerebral hemorrhage (Fig. 1), making hemorrhage the most common—and, arguably, the most devastating—presenting symptom of cerebral AVMs [4–6]. Seizures, the next most common presenting symptom, have been reported to occur in approximately 30% of patients with supratentorial AVMs [6]. The hemorrhage rate for cerebral AVMs has been estimated at between 2% and 4% per year [7–13]. The most often quoted yearly hemorrhage rate for symptomatic lesions is probably that of 4% per year, based on the review by Ondra et al [12] of 166 symptomatic patients with AVMs who were followed prospectively for an average of 20 years without surgical treatment. Although the yearly rate of hemorrhage may be lower in asymptomatic patients, equal rates of hemorrhage have been reported [7]. In addition, although Ondra et al [58] did not find that the rehemorrhage risk was higher than that of the initial hemorrhage risk in patients harboring AVMs, other authors have noted higher rebleeding rates, especially in the first year [8–11,13]. The risks of morbidity and mortality associated with a particular hemorrhage are estimated at 10% and 30%, respectively [13,14].

Over the years, considerable effort has been spent in trying to stratify further the risk of hemorrhage according to various patient and AVM characteristics. The relation between AVM

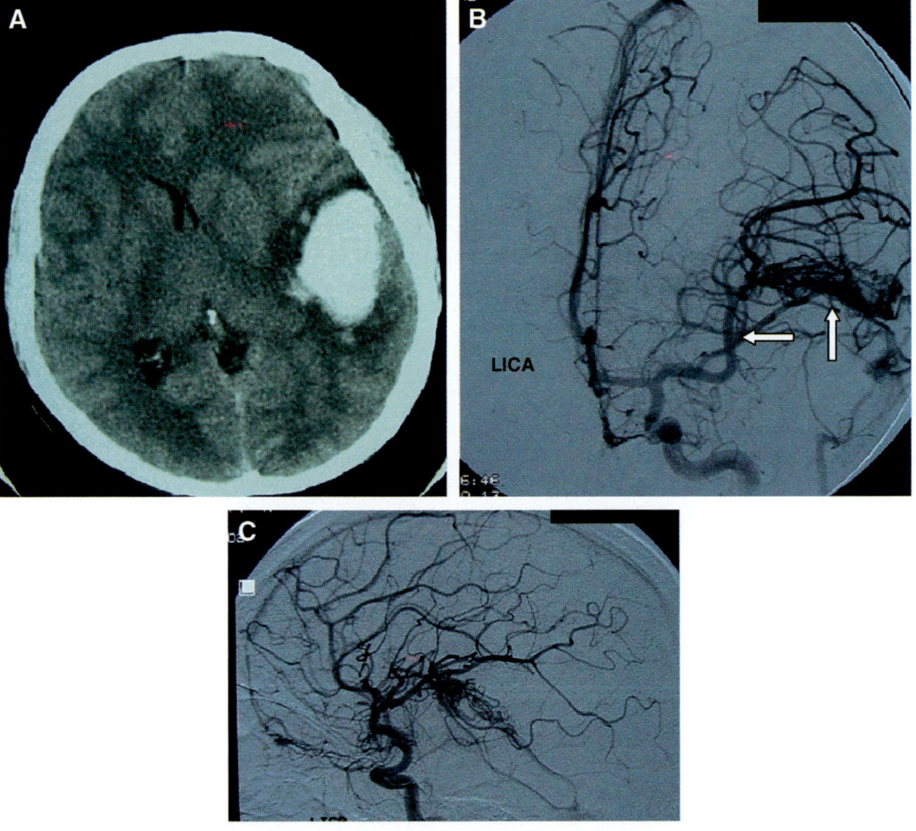

Fig. 1. (*A*) An axial noncontrast CT scan performed on a 27-year-old-man, who presented with the sudden onset of a severe headache and right hemiparesis, shows an acute left intracerebral hemorrhage with associated mass effect and shift. (*B, C*) A subsequent angiogram demonstrates an arteriovenous malformation located in the right posterior temporal lobe and fed by branches of the right middle cerebral artery (MCA). Note medial and upward displacement of the MCA (*arrows*) from the hematoma.

size and the risk of hemorrhage is controversial. A preponderance of evidence seems to suggest that small AVMs bleed more frequently than larger ones [11,15–21]. This may possibly result from increased feeding artery pressures in smaller AVMs [22,23]. Many studies have shown no association with size [18,24–27] or an increased risk of hemorrhage with increasing AVM size [28,29], however. On the venous side, deep venous drainage as well as venous outflow stenosis has been highlighted by several authors as a risk factor for hemorrhage [30–35]. The location of an AVM as it relates to the bleeding risk has also been controversial, but some reports suggest that infratentorial or deep (periventricular) lesions may be at increased risk for hemorrhage [6,32,36,37]. For infratentorial AVMs, this may be at least partially a result of the fact that posterior fossa lesions do not produce seizures, thereby leading to a selection bias in favor of hemorrhage for malformations in this location.

AVMs are known to be associated with aneurysms at a rate greater than that of chance alone, with various reports putting this association between 2.7% and 14% [18,38–42]. Furthermore, the presence of an associated aneurysm, particularly an intranidal aneurysm, seems to increase the risk of hemorrhage [32,34,37,38,42,43]. AVM-associated aneurysms may be located on feeding arteries, at remote sites, or within the AVM nidus itself; the wide-ranging estimate of prevalence is most likely a result of the inconsistent definitions of aneurysms used in the literature.

Management of AVM-associated aneurysms has been the subject of much discussion. Although the regression of some AVM-associated aneurysms after treatment of the AVM has been reported [41], other factors lend support to strategies of early intervention. In particular, it has been shown that in instances of intracranial hemorrhage in which an AVM and an aneurysm are present, the aneurysm is the lesion more likely to have bled [37]. Such evidence, combined with the higher morbidity and mortality associated with aneurysm hemorrhage, has led many to recommend that the aneurysm be treated first if at all possible.

Patient factors that influence hemorrhage are less well understood. Increasing age may contribute to an increased risk of hemorrhage [44]. Other characteristics, such as gender, hypertension, pregnancy, and tobacco use, may not be associated, however.

Various grading scales for cerebral AVMs have been proposed to aid in the prediction of patient morbidity or mortality with or without treatment. The most commonly applied grading scale is that proposed by Spetzler and Martin [45] in 1986 (Table 1). Based on a review of 100 consecutive surgically treated AVM patients, the grading system was designed to predict the risk of operative treatment. Three categories are described, and a "grade" is assigned based on point totals from each category. In the location category, a patient receives one point for an AVM located in eloquent brain and no points for a noneloquent location. Similarly, an AVM with deep venous drainage is assigned one point, whereas one with superficial venous drainage receives no points in this category. Size is broken down into three groups: less than 3 cm, 3 to 6 cm, and greater than 6 cm, with one to three points assigned as size increases. By categories, the maximum point total that can be assigned is five; however, an AVM may be given a grade of VI if it is deemed "unresectable." Because this grading scale is based on patients who were treated primarily with surgical resection, its applicability to endovascular therapy may be questionable. At present, however, there is no widely accepted grading scale for the endovascular treatment of cerebral AVMs.

Indications for treatment and treatment outcome

Given the natural history of these lesions, treatment is frequently recommended, particularly in those patients who are relatively young, demonstrate symptoms, or have angiographic or clinical risk factors that may predispose to hemorrhage. Treatment is undertaken to prevent future neurologic injury or to improve current

Table 1
Spetzler-Martin surgical grading scale for cerebral (pial) arteriovenous malformations

Category	Point value
Size (maximal dimension)	
<3 cm	1
3–6 cm	2
>6 cm	3
Location	
Noneloquent brain	0
Eloquent brain	1
Venous drainage	
Superficial only	0
Deep	1

From Spetzler RF, Martin NA. A proposed grading system for arteriovenous malformations. J Neurosurg 1986;65:476–83; with permission.

neurologic status. To this end, the goal of any single treatment modality or combination of modalities is the ultimate obliteration of the AVM. Each treatment modality may have its own specific role in the overall treatment plan, however. Endovascular embolization as a treatment modality usually assumes one of three roles: adjunctive, curative, or palliative.

Adjunct to microsurgery

The most commonly used role of endovascular embolization is that of an adjunct to microsurgical resection or stereotactic radiosurgery. For patients with surgically accessible lesions, microsurgical removal can provide an immediate cure. A large nidus, deep-feeding vessels, and high-flow shunts can make surgical resection more challenging, however. In such patients, the added risks of endovascular treatment may compare favorably with the risks of surgery alone (Fig. 2). In a comparison of patients undergoing embolization with N-butyl-cyanoacrylate (NBCA) before surgical resection versus patients undergoing surgery alone, Jafar et al [46] found that rates of complications and good or excellent outcomes were similar in both

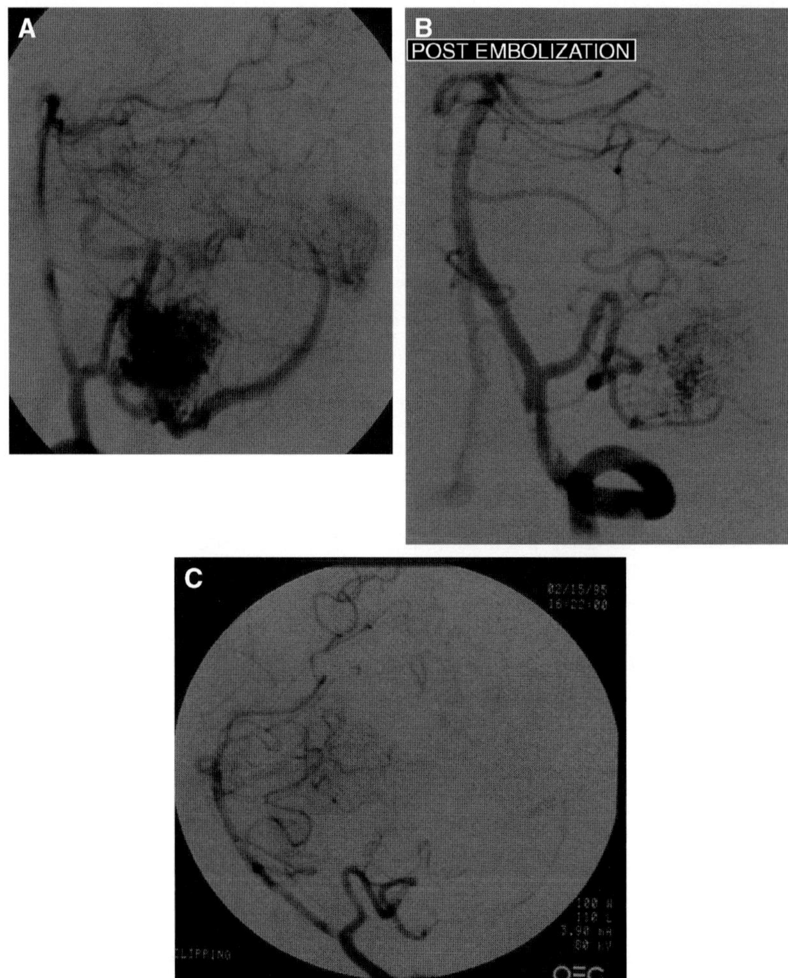

Fig. 2. (*A*) Initial cerebral angiogram from a 20-year-old woman, who presented with a small intraparenchymal hemorrhage, shows an arteriovenous malformation (AVM) located in the inferior portion of the left cerebellar hemisphere. (*B*) A control angiogram performed after a single session of N-butyl-cyanoacrylate embolization shows a considerable reduction in the nidus size. Given the patient's previous history of hemorrhage, the small size of the residual AVM, and the surgically accessible location, the patient underwent microsurgical excision of the lesion. (*C*) An intraoperative angiogram shows no residual nidus and no persistent early venous drainage.

groups despite the fact that the embolized patients had higher Spetzler-Martin grade lesions. Embolization shortened operative time and reduced blood loss. Similar findings have been reported by other practitioners [47–54].

The degree of volume reduction necessary before surgery to effect a difference in surgical resection is debatable. It has been suggested that although elimination of more than 75% of the AVM nidus facilitates surgical resection, occlusion of less than 50% does little to aid operative removal [55]. In cases in which less than 50% obliteration is likely with endovascular therapy and surgical resection is planned, benefit can still be achieved if deep-feeding arteries are occluded. It should be remembered that endovascular embolization is not without risk. Therefore, in general, the risks of embolization for surgically accessible small AVMs (<3 cm in diameter, Spetzler-Martin grade I or some grade II) probably outweigh the benefits.

Adjunct to radiosurgery

In patients with AVMs located in eloquent cortex or deep structures, stereotactic radiosurgery may be a preferable alternative to microsurgical resection when the risk of morbidity and mortality may be unacceptably high. In such patients, endovascular embolization may be used to reduce the size of the AVM before radiosurgery or to eliminate certain angiographic features, such as intranidal aneurysms, that may provide for elevated risk while the patient is awaiting AVM obliteration after radiosurgery (Fig. 3).

It is well known that the rate of AVM cure after stereotactic radiosurgery decreases as the volume of the AVM being treated increases [56–63]. Therefore, the role of endovascular embolization in this setting is to reduce the nidus size such that a cure after radiosurgery is more likely [58,60,64]. Case series have shown a greater percentage of radiosurgical cure for those patients with a reduction in AVM volume to below 10 cm^3 [65,66]. In preradiosurgery patients, it is helpful but not essential for the AVM nidus to be reduced to a smaller single focus. If this is not possible, a volume-staged approach may be used to treat two or more areas of residual AVM separately [67]. Alternatively, for those patients in whom the lesion does not proceed to obliteration after stereotactic radiosurgery, repeated embolization or surgical resection may still be used, often with greater success [68,69].

Curative treatment

The primary goal of AVM treatment is the eventual obliteration of the lesion. Only after the AVM has been obliterated can the treating physician have any confidence that the patient's future risk of hemorrhage has been eliminated. For endovascular embolization to be curative, there must be no residual filling of the nidus and the angiographic shunt or abnormal early venous drainage must be eliminated (Fig. 4). For most cerebral AVMs, however, endovascular embolization alone is unable to provide complete occlusion. The most common reason for this is probably the inability to catheterize and thereby embolize many of the small arterial feeders associated with most brain AVMs.

Published endovascular cure rates are difficult to interpret. Because embolization evolved primarily as a therapeutic adjunct, many published series suffer from considerable referral bias, whereby only "large" AVMs incapable of being treated with radiosurgery or open microsurgery alone are referred for embolization and smaller lesions with only one or two feeding pedicles are treated without endovascular intervention. In addition, the lack of a widely accepted endovascular grading scale makes comparison between various studies problematic. Nevertheless, in a series of 465 patients, Vinuela et al [70] reported a 9.7% rate of complete AVM occlusion with embolization alone. Gobin et al [65] reported a similar cure rate of 11.2% in a cohort of patients scheduled for radiosurgery who had undergone embolization initially as an "adjunctive" therapy. Both series found cure to be more likely in patients with small AVMs. Gobin et al [65] also found that the rate of cure was inversely related to the number of feeding pedicles. In contrast, other authors have reported much higher rates of cure with endovascular therapy when patients were selected specifically for embolization as a primary modality. After selecting a subgroup of patients on the basis of angiographic features they thought were likely to promote endovascular obliteration, Valavanis and Yasargil [71] noted a cure rate of 74% (or 35% of their overall series) with embolization alone. Factors that predisposed to complete occlusion included the presence of dominant feeders without perinidal angiogenesis, a single nidus, and a more fistulous than plexiform nidus.

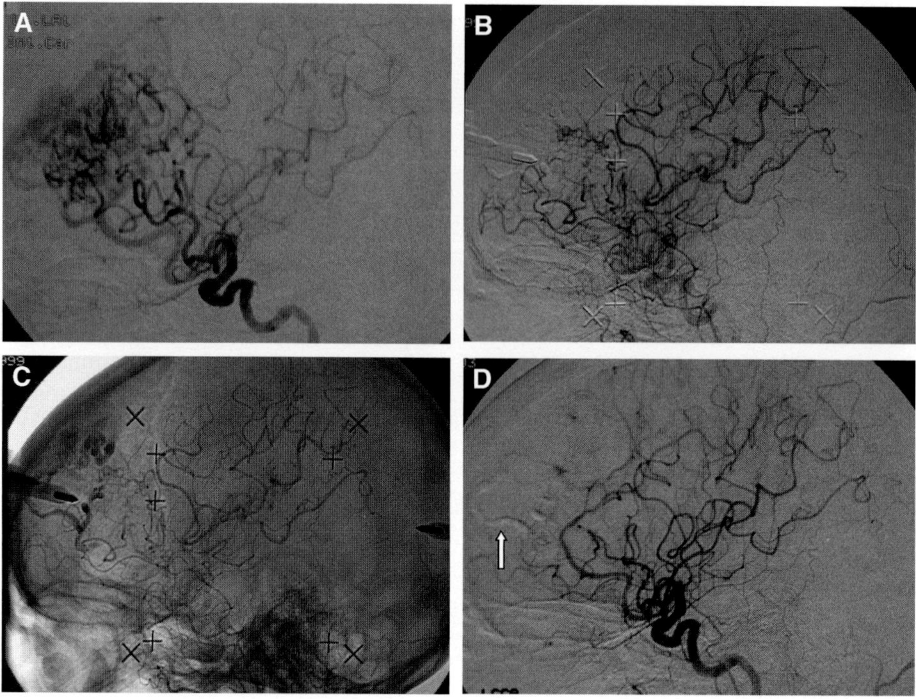

Fig. 3. (*A*) Pretreatment angiogram, performed on a 56-year-old woman with new-onset seizures, reveals a left frontal arteriovenous malformation (AVM) fed by branches of the left anterior cerebral artery and middle cerebral artery. After the nidus volume was reduced with multiple sessions of glue embolization, the patient was scheduled for gamma knife stereotactic radiosurgery. (*B*) An angiogram performed for gamma knife treatment planning shows a small area of residual AVM (*arrow*). (*C*) In an unsubtracted image from the same study, the glue cast is visible (*arrow*) as well as the skull pins and markers (+ marks) of the Leksell gamma knife head frame. (*D*) A follow-up angiogram performed approximately 3 years after radiosurgery shows no persistent filling of the AVM. A glue cast is still visible in the left frontal lobe (*arrow*).

Palliative treatment

Although only complete elimination of the AVM constitutes a true cure, palliative treatment may be used in selected cases. Specifically, patients who are symptomatic with large or deep-seated AVMs that are unlikely to be cured with any combination of modalities may benefit from subtotal endovascular embolization. Whether partial treatment of an AVM is at all beneficial, however, remains somewhat controversial, with some authors reporting a similar or worse natural history in incompletely treated patients [72,73].

In patients with repeated hemorrhages, embolization may be used to eliminate angiographic risk factors for hemorrhage, such as intranidal aneurysms. For those with intractable headaches or progressive neurologic deficits, the benefits of partial treatment are less certain. Nonetheless, embolization to reduce the arteriovenous shunt, and thereby decrease the amount of "steal" or venous hypertension associated with a lesion, has been reported to cause clinical improvement [74,75].

Surgical versus endovascular perspectives on treatment

Intellectual controversy exists between neurosurgeons and endovascular therapists in their approach to the indications for AVM treatment. As neurosurgeons who perform all three of the major modalities of AVM treatment, we prefer to view indications for treatment from a multidisciplinary perspective, with treatment tailored to the individual patient and AVM.

The first decision of the treating physician should be whether the AVM needs to be treated. Once that question has been answered in the affirmative, the process of tailoring a treatment plan may begin. For patients who have sustained a hemorrhage, every effort should be made to eliminate the risk of future bleeding as soon as

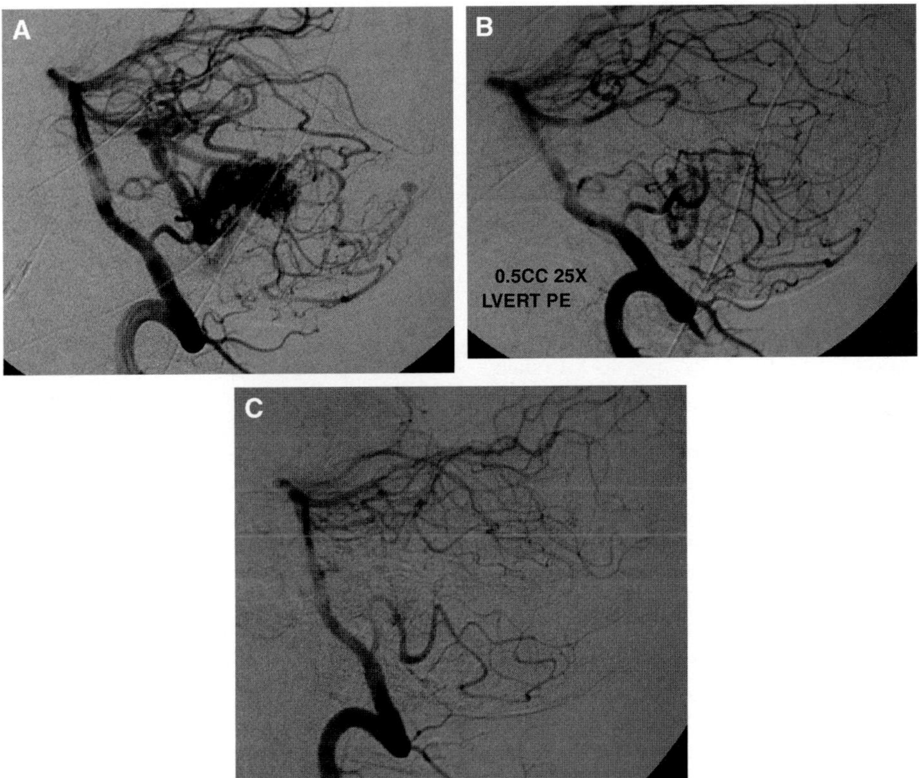

Fig. 4. Lateral projections of vertebral artery angiograms (*A,B,C*) from a 48-year-old woman with a cerebellar arteriovenous malformation (AVM) treated with N-butyl-cyanoacrylate embolization show progressive obliteration of the AVM after endovascular therapy alone.

possible. For such patients, this may mean a combination of surgical resection or endovascular embolization. If the morbidity or mortality associated with these treatments is likely to be greater than that of the natural history of the untreated AVM over the next few years, a combination of stereotactic radiosurgery or embolization may be desirable. Traditionally, surgical resection alone has been favored for patients with mass effect symptoms from a sizable acute intracerebral hemorrhage. Even in many of these patients, however, we have used emergent aggressive embolization before surgery to reduce intraoperative blood loss or simply evacuated the hematoma and left the AVM for later treatment with any combination of modalities. In general, however, most AVMs seen at our institution (a tertiary care referral center) are large and arise within or partially within eloquent brain. As a result, more than 50% of the patients with AVMs treated in the senior author's series were treated with stereotactic radiosurgery and embolization.

In the end, success is most likely to be achieved by a multidisciplinary approach tailored to the individual patient and the characteristics of the lesion itself. Such an approach may be best delivered at a tertiary care institution, where practitioners experienced in the latest microsurgical, radiosurgical, and endovascular techniques are readily available.

Endovascular techniques

The first reports of endovascular AVM treatment involved the nonselective use of particles; it was not until 1972 that Zanetti and Sherman [76] reported the first use of a liquid embolic acrylate polymer to treat cerebral AVMs. Today, liquid cyanoacrylate glue derivatives delivered through superselective microcatheterization are the most commonly used embolic agents for the treatment of cerebral AVMs.

At our institution, almost all AVM embolizations are performed under general endotracheal anesthesia with pharmacologic paralysis. This essentially eliminates patient movement and facilitates road-mapping for intravascular navigation. Tight blood pressure control is maintained. To minimize the risk of a neurologic deficit in patients treated under general anesthesia, we routinely use intraoperative neurophysiologic monitoring in the form of somatosensory evoked potentials and electroencephalography. Brainstem auditory evoked responses are used for lesions requiring access through the posterior circulation.

Arterial access is generally achieved through a transfemoral route. In adults, a 5- to 8-French guide catheter is usually used. The use of a 7-French sheath with a 6-French guide catheter allows for continuous blood pressure monitoring through the sheath, eliminating the need for a separate arterial line. In addition, the 6-French guide catheter provides for easy contrast injection such that a selective angiogram may be performed even with a microcatheter in place. Flow-directed microcatheters (rather than braided wire-driven catheters) are optimal for accessing AVM pedicles and delivering liquid embolic agents. Commonly used brands approved for use in the United States include the Spinnaker Elite (1.5- or 1.8-French; Boston Scientific-Neurovascular, Fremont, California) and the Regatta (1.8-French; Cordis Neurovascular, Miami, Florida). Although these catheters are flow directed, a hydrophilic guidewire (usually 0.10 in) is still required to facilitate the flow-independent movements often required for selecting a specific arterial pedicle. Aggressive manipulation with the wire, however, should be avoided so as to minimize the risk of vascular perforation.

After the appropriate first- or second-order vessel is selected and catheterized, a pretreatment biplane angiogram, including capillary and venous phases, should be obtained to serve as a reference. We attempt to place our guide catheter as distal as safely possible so as to provide added support for the microcatheter. A digital roadmap can then be created and used to navigate the flow-directed microcatheter into an appropriate pedicle (Fig. 5A). Larger pedicles are usually selected during initial sessions, because smaller pedicles may subsequently dilate as the flow characteristics of the AVM change with treatment. Once a specific pedicle has been selected, contrast injection through the microcatheter can then be used to judge flow through the nidus, assess the proximity of the draining vein(s), and determine whether any normal arterial branches are being supplied. In some instances, particularly in awake patients, selective barbiturate injections through the microcatheter may be used to assess the eloquence of brain served by the vascular territory in question ("Amytal testing") [44,77–79]. For patients under general anesthesia, superselective barbiturate injection may lead to changes in neurophysiologic parameters. The lack of certainty with regard to flow distribution of the barbiturate in the presence of an AVM may limit the usefulness of this method. As a result, a negative Amytal test result does not necessarily guarantee a good outcome.

Occlusion of the AVM is achieved with an embolic agent. Over the years, various types of embolic agents have been used to treat cerebral AVMs. Many earlier treatments were performed using particles, particularly polyvinyl alcohol (PVA). Today, liquid embolic derivatives of cyanoacrylate have largely supplanted PVA as the agent of choice for most practitioners. The results of a prospective randomized trial comparing NBCA with PVA for the preoperative embolization of cerebral AVMs were published in 2002 and demonstrated equivalence for both agents, at least in terms of the percentage of nidus reduction and number of pedicles embolized [80]. PVA particles are unlikely to provide permanent arterial occlusion, however; as such, they should only be used as an adjunct to timely surgical extirpation [81]. Occasionally, in lesions with fistulous components, the injection of glue may be facilitated by the use of pushable platinum coils to reduce flow [82].

Several liquid embolic agents have been used in the endovascular occlusion of cerebral AVMs, and these agents are discussed in an article elsewhere in this issue. The most popular liquid embolic agents are cyanoacrylate derivatives, including Trufill (Cordis Neurovascular) and Histocryl (Braun-Aesculap, Tuttlingen, Germany). Absolute ethyl alcohol has also been used as an embolic agent for vascular malformations, primarily those of the extracranial circulation. The treatment of cerebral AVMs with absolute alcohol has been reported [83], but its use remains controversial. Currently, the only "glue" approved by the US Food and Drug Administration for use in cerebral AVMs is Trufill (NBCA).

NBCA glue is a clear, colorless, and radiolucent liquid and comes packaged in single-concentration 1-mL vials. The glue begins to polymerize on contact with ionic material, such as blood, saline, and ionic contrast media. To alter the polymerization properties of the glue and make it visible during injection on angiography,

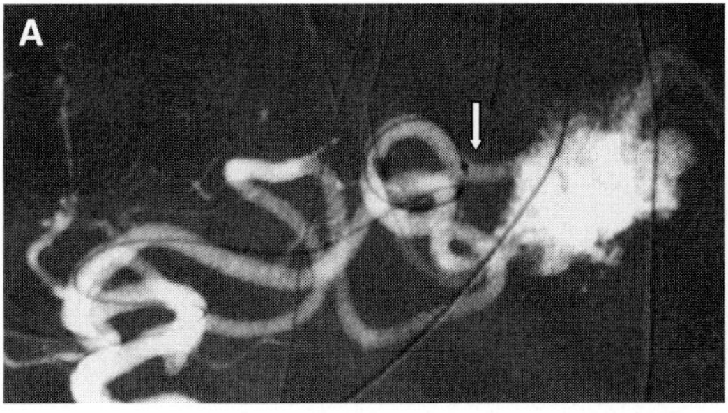

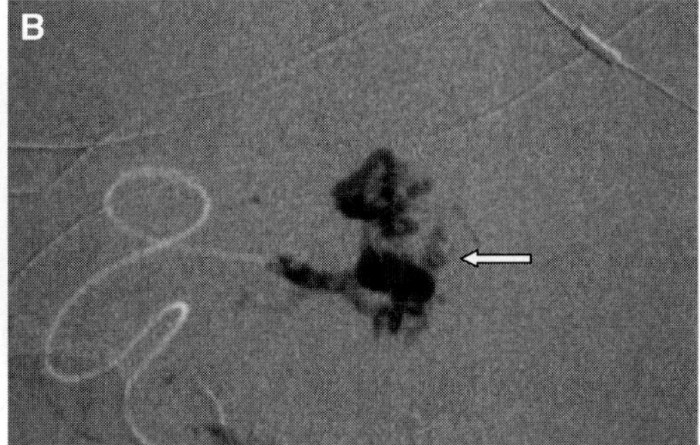

Fig. 5. (*A*) Lateral projection of a roadmap image obtained after internal carotid artery injection showing a microcatheter and microwire within a middle cerebral artery pedicle in close proximity to the arteriovenous malformation (AVM) nidus (*arrow*). (*B*) After N-butyl-cyanoacrylate embolization under roadmap ("mask") conditions, a glue cast can be seen within the AVM nidus (*arrow*). The path of the microcatheter as it was rapidly withdrawn appears as a bright line against the background of the mask.

NBCA may be combined with Ethiodol (Cordis-Neurovascular) (oil-based nonionic contrast), nonionic water-soluble contrast, or tantalum powder. Trufill is packaged with Ethiodol for dilution, although many have found the behavior of various Ethiodol-NBCA concentrations to be inconsistent in terms of viscosity and polymerization. Nevertheless, NBCA concentrations between 20% and 70% are commonly used depending on the proximity of the microcatheter to the nidus and the rapidity of the arteriovenous shunt. Some authors have advocated the use of glacial acetic acid as the diluting agent for NBCA, believing that its effects are more reproducible [53]. Because acetic acid is also radiolucent, the glue must be combined with tantalum powder (also packaged with Trufill) to make it radiopaque. Tantalum, however, also adds viscosity to the mixture.

With the microcatheter in optimal position, the embolic agent may then be prepared. The appropriate glue concentration should be mixed on a separate table to avoid contamination with blood or other ionic substances that may cause premature polymerization. Unfortunately, determining the appropriate glue concentration is not an exact science. Observation of the AVM flow characteristics and angioarchitecture after contrast injection through the microcatheter is critical. In the end, however, there is no substitute for experience with a specific embolic agent.

At our institution, moderate hypotension (mean arterial pressure of approximately 50 mm Hg) is induced before embolization. The microcatheter is flushed with dextrose (5%) to prevent premature polymerization in the catheter. The glue is then injected under road-mapping to enhance visualization (see Fig. 5B). After glue administration, the microcatheter must be rapidly pulled from the site of injection to prevent the catheter from being glued in place. If necessary, in a patient under general anesthesia, a Valsalva maneuver may be performed by the anesthesiologist to increase venous pressure to help prevent the embolic agent from reaching the draining vein(s).

After glue injection and removal of the microcatheter, the microcatheter should be checked to ensure that the entire catheter has been removed. Because of the possibility of residual glue in the catheter, we prefer to discard the microcatheter after every glue injection. The guide catheter should be thoroughly flushed and then may be reused. A postembolization angiogram should be performed to assess the degree and location of AVM obliteration obtained during the embolization.

After surgery, our patients are observed in a monitored intensive care or intermediate care unit. Mild hypotension (mean arterial pressure <80 mm Hg) is maintained for approximately 24 hours to minimize the risk of breakthrough hemorrhage. Dexamethasone is used during surgery to control the inflammatory response that may occur secondary to the NBCA. We do not routinely use any anticoagulation during the procedure. Femoral sheaths are usually removed the evening after embolization, and most patients are discharged home the following day.

There are no specific guidelines as to the percentage volume or number of pedicles that should be embolized at any given sitting. It has been suggested that major alterations in the hemodynamic characteristics of an AVM may occur after the rapid occlusion of a large percentage of its volume, thus increasing the risk of a hemorrhagic complication. This, however, continues to be controversial. In this regard, we prefer a conservative approach to endovascular AVM treatment, and we frequently embolize only one pedicle at any given session. Larger AVMs may thus require three or more sessions of embolization, usually spaced 4 to 5 weeks apart.

Complications and complication avoidance

The risks of endovascular AVM treatment are not insignificant. Because AVM embolization alone is not usually curative, it is important to weigh the risks of an adjunctive procedure against the potential benefits that such a procedure may have in improving cure with another modality.

Complications related to endovascular AVM treatment usually fall into one of two broad categories: ischemic or hemorrhagic. Ischemic complications may result from errant glue emboli in physiologic vessels or catheter/wire manipulation causing dissection and vascular occlusion. Careful review of the pre-embolization superselective angiogram is essential to prevent the inadvertent occlusion of normal distal branches or en passage vessels. Selecting the appropriate glue concentration to avoid early polymerization around the catheter tip and subsequent showering of emboli when the catheter is removed is likewise important. Some practitioners also administer anticoagulants to patients during embolization to reduce the risk of thromboembolic complications [84]. We have not found this to be necessary, however.

Hemorrhagic complications are perhaps more common and may be equally devastating. Too dilute a glue concentration can cause glue to travel through the nidus and occlude the draining vein(s); hemorrhage may then ensue as a result of venous outflow obstruction. Some believe that too rapid an alteration in the hemodynamics of an AVM, such as through the embolization of multiple pedicles at a single sitting, may also promote hemorrhage. Finally, catheter/wire manipulation may cause a vascular perforation, resulting in intracerebral or subarachnoid hemorrhage. Newer, softer, flexible-tipped microwires and more pliable flow-directed catheters have reduced the risk of this complication. Guidewire use should still be minimized, however. Whenever possible, the microwire should be used only for selecting the desired proximal pedicle while letting the natural flow characteristics of the AVM carry the microcatheter to the appropriate distal position for embolization.

Complication rates

The literature is replete with case series reporting rates of morbidity and mortality for endovascularly treated AVMs. Studies published in the 1980s, using mostly liquid embolic agents, documented rates of morbidity and mortality in the range of 10% to 22% and 2% to 6%, respectively [43,47,85,86]. In the late 1990s, Gobin et al [65] reported similar numbers, with a morbidity rate of 12.8% and a mortality rate of 1.6%. That there has been little change in the risk of embolization over the last several years was further confirmed by Frizzel and Fisher [87], who published a review of 32 case series that included 1246 patients treated over 35 years. The overall rates of permanent and temporary morbidity in their series were 8% and 10%, whereas the rate of mortality was 1%. When broken down into cohorts treated before and after 1990, the permanent morbidity rate went from 9% to 8%, respectively (not statistically significant), and the mortality rate changed from 2% to 1%, respectively (also not statistically significant).

Thomas Jefferson University Hospital experience

In the senior author's personal series covering a period from October 1995 to August 2003, a total of 448 AVMs were embolized, 225 underwent gamma knife radiosurgery, and 135 were surgically removed. An additional 164 patients have had no treatment and are being followed because of age or medical comorbidities. In a subset of 170 patients from this series, all treated with endovascular embolization and with complete follow-up at 36 months, permanent morbidity was noted in only 7 patients (4.1%). In this group, there were no cases of postembolization hemorrhage and no deaths after embolization. Most patients (125 [73%]) underwent one or two sessions of embolization. Twenty-six (15%) and 9 (5%) patients had three and four sessions, respectively, whereas 10 patients underwent five or more embolizations. The overall cure rate to date, including all modes of treatment, is 24.7%.

The cure rate for patients treated with endovascular embolization alone (49 of 170 patients or 28.8% of the total series) stands at 14.3% (7 patients). Those cured with embolization alone all harbored AVMs with a Spetzler-Martin grade of III or lower. None of these lesions had a maximal dimension over 6 cm.

Cure rates

As discussed previously, cure rates after endovascular embolization are difficult to interpret. This is at least partially a result of the lack of prospective, randomized, controlled studies comparing various treatment modalities. Given the current trend toward the multidisciplinary treatment of AVMs, it is doubtful that such studies will ever be performed. A multidisciplinary approach must thus be critically compared with the natural history of these lesions, and attention must be paid to clinical outcome in terms of functional status, quality of life, and patient satisfaction.

Summary

Untreated cerebral AVMs carry a significant risk of long-term morbidity and mortality. Endovascular embolization has evolved into an important treatment option for most AVMs, whether it is used as an adjunct or as the primary therapy. Although sometimes a challenge to use, liquid cyanoacrylate derivatives have become the material of choice for most practitioners performing endovascular AVM embolization. In addition, advances in flow-guided microcatheter technology have enabled safer access to ever more hard-to-reach areas of the cerebral vasculature. In the current era, the treatment of cerebral AVMs seems to be best approached from a multidisciplinary standpoint at facilities where the major treatment modalities of microsurgery, stereotactic radiosurgery, and endovascular embolization are all available.

References

[1] Luessenhop AJ, Spence WT. Artificial embolization of cerebral arteries: report of use in a case of arteriovenous malformation. JAMA 1960;172:1153–5.

[2] McCormick WF. The pathology of vascular ("arteriovenous") malformations. J Neurosurg 1966;24: 807–16.

[3] McCormick WF. Pathology of vascular malformations of the brain. In: Wilson C, Stein B, editors. Intracranial vascular malformations. Baltimore: Williams & Wilkins; 1984. p. 44–63.

[4] Drake CG. Cerebral arteriovenous malformations: considerations for and experience with surgical treatment in 166 cases. Clin Neurosurg 1979;26: 145–208.

[5] Mast H, Mohr JP, Osipov A, et al. "Steal" is an unestablished mechanism for the clinical presentation of cerebral arteriovenous malformation. Stroke 1995;26:1215–20.

[6] Perret G, Nishioka H. Report on the cooperative study of intracranial aneurysms and subarachnoid hemorrhage: arteriovenous malformations. J Neurosurg 1966;25:467–90.

[7] Brown RD, Wiebers DO, Forbes GS, et al. The natural history of unruptured intracranial arteriovenous malformations. J Neurosurg 1988;68:352–7.

[8] Crawford PM, West CR, Chadwick DW, et al. Arteriovenous malformations of the brain: natural history in unoperated patients. J Neurol Neurosurg Psychiatry 1986;49:1–10.

[9] Forster DMC, Steiner L, Hakanson S. Arteriovenous malformations of the brain. A long-term clinical study. J Neurosurg 1972;37:562–70.

[10] Fults D, Kelly DL Jr. Natural history of arteriovenous malformations of the brain: a clinical study. Neurosurgery 1984;15:658–62.

[11] Graf CJ, Perret GE, Torner JC. Bleeding from cerebral arteriovenous malformations as part of their natural history. J Neurosurg 1983;58:331–7.

[12] Ondra S, Troupp H, George E, et al. The natural history of symptomatic arteriovenous malformations of the brain: a 24-year follow-up assessment. J Neurosurg 1990;73:387–91.

[13] Wilkins RH. Natural history of intracranial vascular malformations of the brain: a review. Neurosurgery 1985;16:421–30.

[14] Hartmann A, Mast H, Mohr JP, et al. Morbidity of intracranial hemorrhage in patients with cerebral arteriovenous malformation. Stroke 1998;29:931–4.

[15] Henderson WR, Gomez RD. Natural history of cerebral angiomas. BMJ 1967;4:571–4.

[16] Moody RA, Poppen JL. Arteriovenous malformations. J Neurosurg 1970;32:502–11.

[17] Parkinson D, Bachers G. Arteriovenous malformations. Summary of 100 consecutive supratentorial cases. J Neurosurg 1980;53:285–99.

[18] Paterson JH, McKissock W. A clinical survey of intracranial angiomas with special reference to their mode of progression and surgical treatment: a report of 110 cases. Brain 1956;79:233–66.

[19] Pelletieri L. Surgical versus conservative treatment of intracranial arterio-venous malformations. Acta Neurol Scand 1980;29:1–86.

[20] Pia HW. The acute treatment of cerebral arteriovenous angiomas associated with hematomas. In: Pia H, Gleave J, Grate E, editors. Cerebral angiomas. Advances in diagnosis and therapy. New York: Springer-Verlag; 1975. p. 155–71.

[21] Stehbens WE. Pathology of the cerebral blood vessels. St. Louis: CV Mosby; 1972.

[22] Miyasaka Y, Kurata A, Irikura K, et al. The influence of vascular pressure and angiographic characteristics on haemorrhage from arteriovenous malformations. Acta Neurochir (Wien) 2000;142: 39–43.

[23] Spetzler RF, Hargraves RW, McCormick PW, et al. Relationship of perfusion pressure and size to risk of hemorrhage from arteriovenous malformations. J Neurosurg 1992;76:918–23.

[24] Albert P, Salgado H, Polaina M, et al. A study on the venous drainage of 150 cerebral arteriovenous malformations as related to haemorrhagic risks and size of the lesion. Acta Neurochir (Wien) 1990;103: 30–4.

[25] Duong DH, Young WL, Vang MC, et al. Feeding artery pressure and venous drainage pattern are primary determinants of hemorrhage from cerebral arteriovenous malformations. Stroke 1998;29: 1167–76.

[26] Karlsson B, Lindquist C, Johansson A, et al. Annual risk for the first hemorrhage from untreated cerebral arteriovenous malformations. Minim Invasive Neurosurg 1997;40:40–6.

[27] Mast H, Young WL, Koennecke HC, et al. Risk of spontaneous haemorrhage after diagnosis of cerebral arteriovenous malformation. Lancet 1997;350: 1065–8.

[28] Hirai S, Mine S, Yamakami I, et al. Angioarchitecture related to hemorrhage in cerebral arteriovenous malformations. Neurol Med Chir (Tokyo) 1998;38:165–70.

[29] Jomin M, Lesoin F, Lozes G. Prognosis for arteriovenous malformations of the brain in adults bases on 150 cases. Surg Neurol 1985;23:362–6.

[30] Albert P. Personal experience in the treatment of 178 cases of arteriovenous malformations of the brain. Acta Neurochir (Wien) 1982;61: 207–26.

[31] Fry DL. Acute vascular endothelial changes associated with increased blood velocity gradients. Circ Res 1968;22:165–97.

[32] Marks MP, Lane B, Steinberg GK, et al. Hemorrhage in intracerebral arteriovenous malformations: angiographic determinants. Radiology 1990;176: 807–13.

[33] Miyasaka Y, Yada K, Ohwada T, et al. An analysis of the venous drainage system as a factor in hemorrhage from arteriovenous malformations. J Neurosurg 1992;76:239–43.

[34] Muller-Forell W, Valavanis A. Neuroradiologic exploration of cerebral arteriovenous malformations. Radiologe 1991;31:269–73.

[35] Nataf F, Meder JF, Roux FX, et al. Angioarchitecture associated with haemorrhage in cerebral arteriovenous malformations: a prognostic statistical model. Neuroradiology 1997;39:52–8.

[36] Andoh T, Sakai N, Yamada H, et al. Cerebellar AVM–clinical analysis of 14 cases. No To Shinkei 1990;42:913–21.

[37] Brown RD, Wiebers DO, Forbes GS. Unruptured intracranial aneurysms and arteriovenous malformations: frequency of intracranial hemorrhage and relationship of lesions. Neurosurgery 1990;73: 859–63.

[38] Batjer H, Suss RA, Samson D. Intracranial arteriovenous malformations associated with aneurysms. Neurosurgery 1986;18:29–35.

[39] Cockroft KM, Thompson RC, Steinberg GK. Aneurysms and arteriovenous malformations. Neurosurg Clin N Am 1998;9:565–76.

[40] Higashi K, Hatano M, Yamashita T, et al. Coexistence of posterior inferior cerebellar artery aneurysm and arteriovenous malformation fed by the same artery. Surg Neurol 1979;12:405–8.

[41] Suzuki J, Onuma T. Intracranial aneurysms associated with arteriovenous malformations. J Neurosurg 1979;50:742–6.

[42] Thompson RC, Steinberg GK, Levy RP, et al. The management of patients with arteriovenous malformations and associated intracranial aneurysms. Neurosurgery 1998;43:202–11.

[43] Lasjaunias P, Manelfe C, Terbrugge K, et al. Endovascular treatment of cerebral arteriovenous malformations. Neurosurg Rev 1986;9:265–75.

[44] Kondziolka D, McLaughlin MR, Kestle JR. Simple risk predictions for arteriovenous malformation hemorrhage. Neurosurgery 1995;37:851–5.

[45] Spetzler RF, Martin NA. A proposed grading system for arteriovenous malformations. J Neurosurg 1986;65:476–83.

[46] Jafar JJ, David AJ, Berenstein A, et al. The effect of embolization with N-butyl-cyanoacrylate prior to surgical resection of cerebral arteriovenous malformations. J Neurosurg 1993;78:60–9.

[47] Debrun GM, Aletich V, Ausman JI, et al. Embolization of the nidus of brain arteriovenous malformations with N-butyl cyanoacrylate. Neurosurgery 1997;40:112–21.

[48] DeMerritt JS, Pile-Spellman J, Mast H. Outcome analysis of preoperative embolizations with N-butyl cyanoacrylate in cerebral arteriovenous malformations. AJNR Am J Neuroradiol 1995;16:1801–7.

[49] Deruty R, Pelissou-Guyotat I, Mottolese C, et al. The combined management of cerebral arteriovenous malformations. Experience with 100 cases and review of the literature. Acta Neurochir (Wien) 1993;123:101–12.

[50] Fournier D, TerBrugge KG, Willinsky R, et al. Endovascular treatment of intracerebral arteriovenous malformations: experience in 49 cases. J Neurosurg 1995;75:228–33.

[51] Grzyska U, Westphal M, Zanella F. A joint protocol for the neurosurgical and neuroradiologic treatment of cerebral arteriovenous malformations: indications, technique and results in 76 cases. Surg Neurol 1993;40:476–84.

[52] Pasqualin A, Scienza R, Cioffi F, et al. Treatment of cerebral arteriovenous malformations with a combi-

nation of preoperative embolization and surgery. Neurosurgery 1991;3:358–68.

[53] Pelz DM, Fox AJ, Vinuela F, et al. Preoperative embolization of brain AVMs with isobutyl-2 cyanoacrylate. AJNR Am J Neuroradiol 1988;9:757–64.

[54] Spetzler RF, Martin NA, Carter LP, et al. Surgical management of large AVM's by staged embolization and operative excision. J Neurosurg 1987;67: 17–28.

[55] Vinuela F, Dion JE, Duckwiler G, et al. Combined endovascular embolization and surgery in the management of cerebral arteriovenous malformations: experience with 101 cases. J Neurosurg 1991;75: 856–64.

[56] Colombo F, Pozza F, Chierego G, et al. Linear accelerator radiosurgery of cerebral arteriovenous malformations: an update. Neurosurgery 1994;34: 14–21.

[57] Friedman WA, Bova FJ, Bollampally S, et al. Analysis of factors predictive of success or complications in arteriovenous malformation radiosurgery. Neurosurgery 2003;52:296–307.

[58] Friedman WA, Bova FJ, Mendenhall WM. Linear accelerator radiosurgery for arteriovenous malformations: the relationship of size to outcome. J Neurosurg 1995;82:180–9.

[59] Karlsson B, Lindquest C, Steiner L. Prediction of obliteration after gamma knife surgery for cerebral arteriovenous malformations. Neurosurgery 1997; 40:425–31.

[60] Lunsford LD, Kondziolka D, Flickinger JC, et al. Stereotactic radiosurgery for arteriovenous malformations of the brain. J Neurosurg 1991;75:512–24.

[61] Pollock BE, Flickinger JC, Lunsford LD, et al. Factors associated with successful arteriovenous malformation radiosurgery. Neurosurgery 1998;42: 1239–44.

[62] Schlienger M, Atlan D, Lefkopoulos D, et al. LINAC radiosurgery for cerebral arteriovenous malformations: results in 169 patients. Int J Radiat Oncol Biol Phys 2000;46:1135–42.

[63] Steinberg GK, Fabrikant JI, Marks MP, et al. Stereotactic heavy-charged-particle Bragg-peak radiation for intracranial arteriovenous malformations. N Engl J Med 1990;323:96–101.

[64] Steiner L, Lindquist C, Adler JP, et al. Clinical outcome of radiosurgery for cerebral arteriovenous malformations. J Neurosurg 1992;77:1–8.

[65] Gobin YP, Laurent A, Merienne L, et al. Treatment of brain arteriovenous malformations by embolization and radiosurgery. J Neurosurg 1996;85: 19–28.

[66] Mathis JA, Barr JD, Horton JA, et al. The efficacy of particulate embolization combined with stereotactic radiosurgery for treatment of large arteriovenous malformations of the brain. AJNR Am J Neuroradiol 1995;16:299–306.

[67] Firlik AD, Levy EI, Kondziolka D, et al. Staged volume radiosurgery followed by microsurgical resection: a novel treatment for giant cerebral arteriovenous malformations: technical case report. Neurosurgery 1998;43:1223–8.

[68] Marks MP, Lane B, Steinberg GK, et al. Endovascular treatment of cerebral arteriovenous malformations following radiosurgery. AJNR Am J Neuroradiol 1993;14:297–303.

[69] Steinberg GK, Chang SD, Levy RP, et al. Surgical resection of large incompletely treated intracranial arteriovenous malformations following stereotactic radiosurgery. J Neurosurg 1996;84:920–8.

[70] Vinuela F, Duckwiler G, Gobin YP, et al. Contribution of Guglielmi detachable coil technique in the treatment of intracranial aneurysms. J Stroke Cerebrovasc Dis 1997;6:268–71.

[71] Valavanis A, Yasargil MG. The endovascular treatment of brain arteriovenous malformations. Adv Tech Stand Neurosurg 1998;24:131–214.

[72] Han PP, Ponce FA, Spetzler RF. Intention-to-treat analysis of Spetzler-Martin grades IV and V arteriovenous malformations: natural history and treatment paradigm. J Neurosurg 2003;98:3–7.

[73] Pollock BE, Flickinger JC, Lunsford LD, et al. Hemorrhage after stereotactic radiosurgery of cerebral arteriovenous malformations. Neurosurgery 1996;38:659–61.

[74] Fox AJ, Girvin JP, Vinuela F, et al. Rolandic arteriovenous malformations: improvement in limb function by IBC embolization. AJNR Am J Neuroradiol 1985;6:575–82.

[75] Kusske JA, Kelly WA. Embolization and reduction of the "steal" syndrome in cerebral arteriovenous malformations. J Neurosurg 1974;40:313–21.

[76] Zanetti PH, Sherman FE. Experimental evaluation of a tissue adhesive as an agent for the treatment of aneurysms and arteriovenous anomalies. J Neurosurg 1972;36:72–9.

[77] Moo LR, Murphy KJ, Gailloud P, et al. Tailored cognitive testing with provocative amobarbital injection preceding AVM embolization. AJNR Am J Neuroradiol 2002;23:416–21.

[78] Rauch RA, Vinuela F, Dion J, et al. Preembolization functional evaluation in brain arteriovenous malformations: the ability of superselective Amytal test to predict neurologic dysfunction before embolization. AJNR Am J Neuroradiol 1992;13: 309–14.

[79] Rauch R, Vinuela F, Dion J, et al. Preembolization functional evaluation in brain arteriovenous malformations: the superselective Amytal test. AJNR Am J Neuroradiol 1992;13:303–8.

[80] Tomsick TA, Purdy P, Horowitz M, et al. Investigators N-BCA trial: N-butyl cyanoacrylate embolization of cerebral arteriovenous malformations: results of a prospective, randomized, multi-center trial. AJNR Am J Neuroradiol 2002;23:748–55.

[81] Sorimachi T, Koike T, Takeuchi S, et al. Embolization of cerebral arteriovenous malformations achieved with polyvinyl alcohol particles:

angiographic reappearance and complications. AJNR Am J Neuroradiol 1999;20:1323–8.

[82] Richling B, Killer M. Endovascular management of patients with cerebral arteriovenous malformations. Neurosurg Clin N Am 2000;11:123–45.

[83] Yakes WF, Krauth L, Ecklund J, et al. Ethanol endovascular management of brain arteriovenous malformations: initial results. Neurosurgery 1997;40: 1145–52.

[84] Marks MP. Endovascular therapy for arteriovenous malformations. In: Marks M, Do H, editors. Endovascular and percutaneous therapy of the brain and spine. Philadelphia: Lippincott Williams & Wilkins; 2002. p. 243–75.

[85] Deruty R, Lapras C, Pierluca P, et al. Perioperative embolization of cerebral arteriovenous malformations with butylcyanoacrylate (18 cases). Neurochirurgie 1985;31:21–9.

[86] Merland JJ, Rufenacht D, Laurent A, et al. Endovascular treatment with isobutyl cyanoacrylate in patients with arteriovenous malformation of the brain. Indications, results and complications. Acta Radiol Suppl 1986;369:621–2.

[87] Frizzel RT, Fisher WS. Cure, morbidity, and mortality associated with embolization of brain arteriovenous malformations: a review of 1246 patients in 32 series over a 35-year period. J Neurosurg 1995; 37:1031–40.

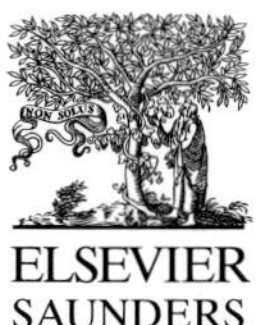

ELSEVIER
SAUNDERS

Neurosurg Clin N Am 16 (2005) 381–393

NEUROSURGERY
CLINICS
OF NORTH AMERICA

Treatment of Dural Arteriovenous Malformations and Fistulae

Henry H. Woo, MD*, Thomas J. Masaryk, MD, Peter A. Rasmussen, MD

Section of Cerebrovascular and Endovascular Neurosurgery, Departments of Neurosurgery and Radiology, The Cleveland Clinic Foundation, 9500 Euclid Avenue, S-80, Cleveland, OH 44195, USA

Dural arteriovenous malformations or dural arteriovenous fistulae (DAVFs) are acquired lesions consisting of one or more fistulous connections within the leaflets of the dura mater. They account for 10% to 15% of intracranial arteriovenous malformations [1,2]. We believe that the term *malformation* is a misnomer for two reasons: the term *malformation* implies a congenital etiology when, in fact, most if not all of these lesions are acquired; and the term *malformation* also implies that there is a true nidus, and although these lesions often have a complex angiographic appearance because of the recruitment of numerous arterial pedicles, they can frequently be isolated to a single or a few discrete fistulous sites of arteriovenous shunting.

Etiology and pathogenesis

Given the variable locations and complexity of dural fistulae, there are multiple etiologies responsible for fistula formation. Specific factors are known to predispose to fistula formation, however, including sinus thrombosis, trauma, and surgery. There are several cases of documented sinus thrombosis with subsequent fistula formation associated with the involved sinus [3–6]. In such cases, the primary cause of sinus thrombosis may be a generalized hypercoagulable state or an infection of the mastoid or sphenoid sinus. It is thought that the fistula occurs during the phase of attempted recanalization and neovascularization within the sinus.

Conversely, not all DAVFs are associated with thrombosis or stenosis of a major dural sinus. Subsequent sinus occlusion may then occur because of turbulence and venous hypertension within the sinus, ultimately leading to occlusion. Experimentally, rats in a carotid-jugular fistula venous hypertension model have been shown to develop DAVFs, suggesting that thrombosis in and of itself may not be the primary event [7–9]. A recent histopathologic study of DAVFs describes 30-μm "crack-like" vessels within the dural sinus wall and postulates that steno-occlusive disease of the venous sinuses triggers the development of these vessels. Subsequent sinus thrombosis is then an epiphenomenon that occurs because of turbulent flow and sinus wall thickening [10].

Finally, conditions associated with vascular fragility, such as fibromuscular dysplasia, neurofibromatosis type I, and Ehlers-Danlos syndrome, have been associated with DAVFs [11–15]. As a whole, despite the variety of potential factors that may be responsible for DAVF formation, it seems that pathologic findings on the venous side are probably the major contributor. Furthermore, most of the management and treatment decisions are primarily determined by the pathologic findings within the venous system.

Clinical presentation and angiographic considerations

The clinical presentation of DAVFS is highly varied and is primarily determined by the location of the fistula and the subsequent pattern of venous

* Corresponding author.

E-mail address: wooh@ccf.org (H.H. Woo).

doi:10.1016/j.nec.2004.08.012

drainage. Other factors include the degree of arteriovenous shunting, venous hypertension, and presence of venous stenoses or ectasias. The two most common locations are the transverse or sigmoid sinus and the cavernous sinus [16,17], followed by the following sites: deep venous, superior sagittal sinus, superior petrosal sinus, ethmoidal, marginal sinus, and inferior petrosal sinus. The reason for this discordant distribution has not been clearly established. A delay in the development of the external carotid territory and numerous emissary veins near the skull base have been proposed as two possible mechanisms [18]. Theoretically, any site along the dura is a potential source for fistula formation. The primary factor in determining the aggressive behavior of DAVFs, however, is the presence of leptomeningeal venous drainage, which can engender venous hypertension, progressive neurologic deficit, infarction, and hemorrhage [19].

Lesions involving the transverse sinus are the most common (38%) (Fig. 2) [17]. The clinical presentation can range from asymptomatic to overt hemorrhage. Common symptoms may include a simple pulsatile bruit or headache. If there has been long-standing venous hypertension and swelling, the presentation can mimic transient ischemic attacks or ischemic infarcts of the involved temporal lobe [20]. The arterial supply typically occurs through transmastoid branches of the occipital artery; branches of the middle meningeal artery; neuromeningeal branches of the ascending pharyngeal artery; branches of the vertebral artery, including the posterior meningeal and artery of the falx cerebelli; and tentorial branches of the meningohypophyseal trunk. A complete evaluation of the venous drainage should include identifying downstream stenosis or occlusion of the ipsilateral sinus, the presence of flow across the torcula, and the presence of cortical venous drainage. Particular attention should paid to the direction of flow in the vein of Labbé and its point of insertion, because this information has significant implications for the endovascular options for treatment. If the vein of Labbé flows in a retrograde fashion, its origin in the sinus can be occluded from a transvenous approach. If the flow is antegrade, occlusion of its origin can exacerbate the venous hypertension, leading to a worsening of symptoms and possible hemorrhage.

Lesions involving the cavernous sinus frequently manifest with ocular pathologic changes. The classic signs of orbital venous hypertension include pulsatile exophthalmos, chemosis, and conjunctival injection. A progressive cavernous sinus syndrome can also include increased ocular pressure, extraocular muscle paresis (especially of the third and sixth cranial nerves), decline in visual acuity, optic neuropathy, and proptosis. These are all indications for treatment. Tinnitus and ocular bruits are also relative indications. The arterial supply can include branches from the inferolateral or meningohypophyseal trunk, branches of the middle or accessory meningeal artery, the artery of foramen rotundum, and the ascending pharyngeal artery, among others. A large draining superior ophthalmic vein can easily be identified on MRI, and surgical access into this vein provides a route for potential therapy. Access into the cavernous sinus via the inferior petrosal sinus provides yet another route for endovascular therapy. Again, particular attention should be paid to possible intracranial cortical venous drainage from the cavernous sinus into the superficial and deep sylvian systems.

Ethmoidal dural fistulae typically derive supply from the anterior and posterior ethmoidal branches of the ophthalmic artery and may recruit supply from the distal branches of the internal maxillary artery. The drainage is almost always into a pial vein along the floor of the anterior cranial fossa, which ultimately drains into the superior sagittal sinus. As a result, the most common presentation is a frontal lobe hemorrhage. Occasionally, drainage can occur into the cavernous sinus, resulting in chemosis, proptosis, and elevated intraocular pressures. Such DAVFs have a male preponderance, and surgical coagulation of the vein is the preferred method of treatment because of its low morbidity and high cure rate [21].

Superior sagittal sinus DAVFs are rare and are varied in their presentation (Fig. 1). Because of the distant location between the superior sagittal sinus and the auditory apparatus, early detection secondary to pulsatile tinnitus is rare. The presentation is thus predominantly secondary to hemorrhage, either subarachnoid, subdural or intraparenchymal; headache; or symptoms from venous hypertension. The arterial supply is generally derived from branches of the middle meningeal artery, the anterior falcine artery from the ophthalmic artery, or the posterior meningeal artery. Frequently, the arterial supply is bilateral. Should endovascular therapy fail to achieve complete obliteration, surgical excision can be contemplated, with care noted to identify the presence of collateral venous drainage to prevent exacerbation of the venous hypertension.

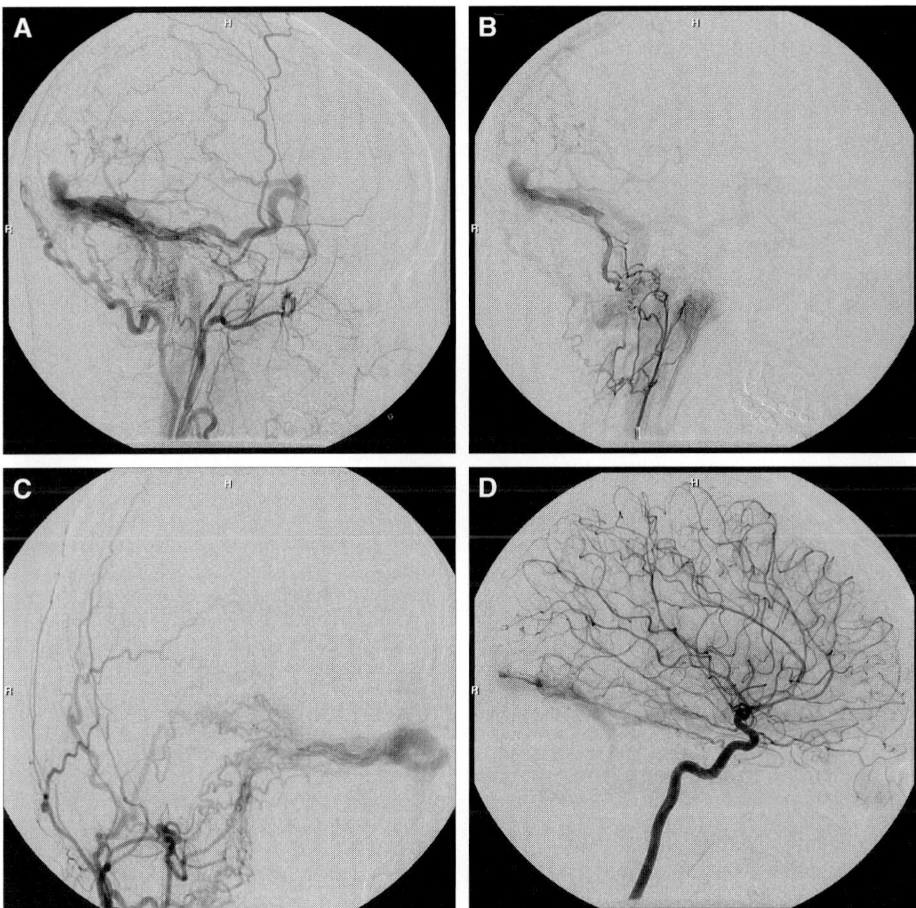

Fig. 1. A 29-year-old woman who presented with headaches and pulsatile tinnitus. On examination, she was noted to have a vigorous mastoid bruit. Radiographic evaluation documented this large transverse-sigmoid dural arteriovenous fistula. (*A*) Preprocedural lateral left external carotid angiogram demonstrates a vigorous left transverse sinus fistula with supply from the occipital, ascending pharyngeal, and middle meningeal arteries. Note the retrograde flow through the vein of Labbé and occlusion of the ipsilateral left jugular vein. (*B*) Preprocedural lateral ascending pharyngeal angiogram demonstrating the contribution from the neuromeningeal trunk. (*C*) Preprocedural anteroposterior (AP) right external carotid angiogram demonstrating the contribution from the right occipital and posterior auricular arteries. (*D*) Preprocedural lateral left internal carotid angiogram demonstrating the contribution from the meningohypophyseal trunk artery of Bernasconi and Cassinari. (*E*) Preprocedural AP left vertebral angiogram demonstrating extensive supply from the artery of the falx cerebelli and recruitment of pial supply from the posterior cerebral artery. (*F*) AP roadmap image demonstrating the position of the microcatheter traversing the contralateral jugular vein across the torcula and into the left transverse-sigmoid junction. (*G*, *H*) AP and lateral projections of a middle meningeal injection after coil occlusion of the transverse sinus. This is the position from which N-butyl-cyanoacrylate was injected. (*I*) AP roadmap image of the glue cast demonstrating liquid embolic not only in the sinus but in the proximal portion of the vein of Labbé and other arterial collaterals. (*J-M*) Postprocedural lateral angiograms of the left external carotid, occipital, ascending pharyngeal, and internal carotid arteries demonstrating complete angiographic obliteration of the fistula. (*N*, *O*) Postprocedural AP angiograms of the left vertebral and right external carotid arteries confirming an angiographic cure. The patient was discharged home on the following day neurologically intact. (*P*, *Q*) Three month follow-up lateral angiograms of the left common carotid artery and left pharyngo-occipital trunk demonstrating regression in the caliber of all the previously enlarged vessels. The complete angiogram demonstrated no evidence of recurrence.

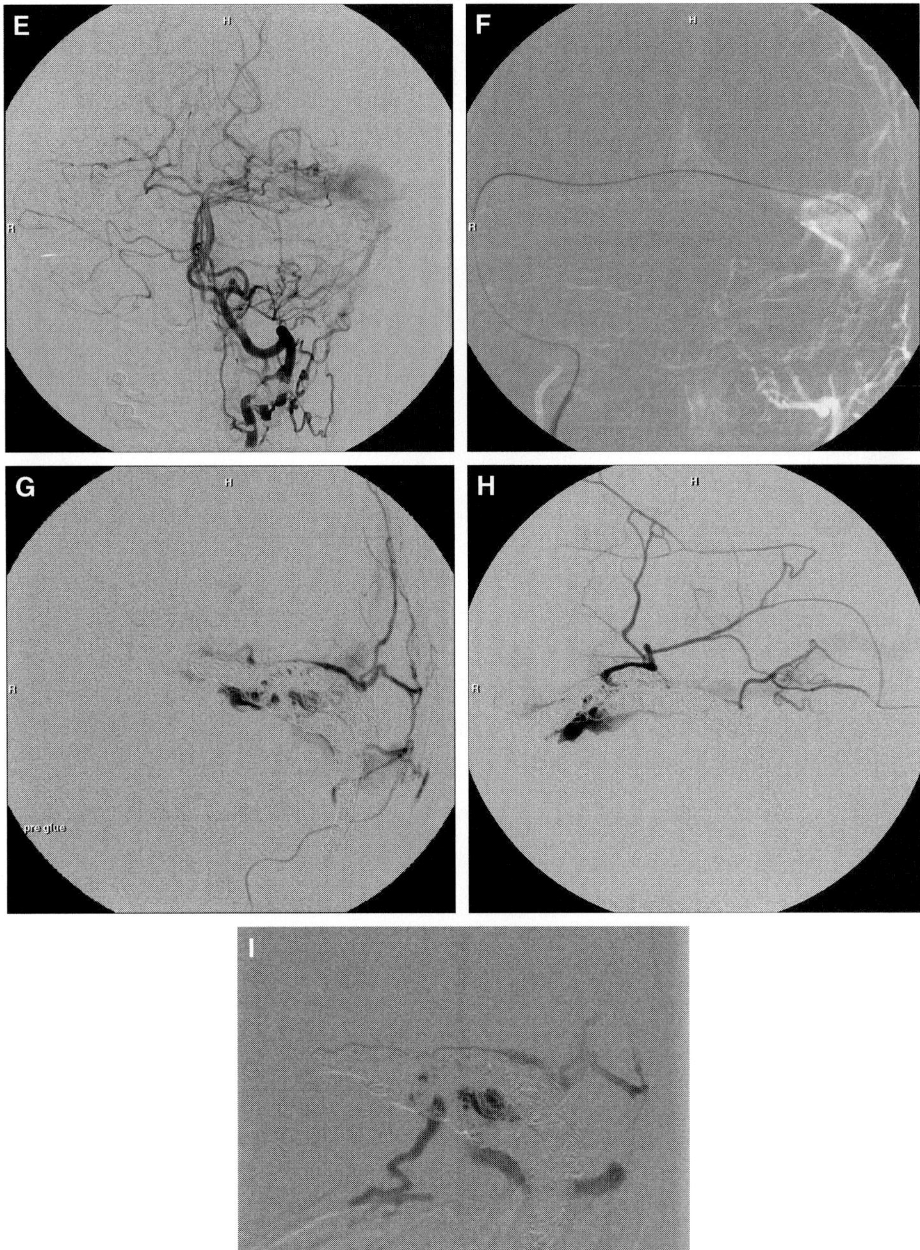

Fig. 1 (*continued*)

Lesions involving the superior petrosal sinus, also referred to as tentorial DAVFs, generally present with hemorrhage or mass effect from dilated veins (Fig. 3). The arterial supply typically arises from the artery of Bernasconi and Cassinari off of the meningohypophyseal trunk as well as from the petrosal and petrosquamosal branches of the middle meningeal artery. The venous drainage usually involves the superior petrosal sinus and the pontine and perimesencephalic veins. Even if endovascular treatment fails to obliterate the fistula, it can aid in localization of the fistula on postprocedure axial imaging and can minimize the blood loss during surgical resection [22].

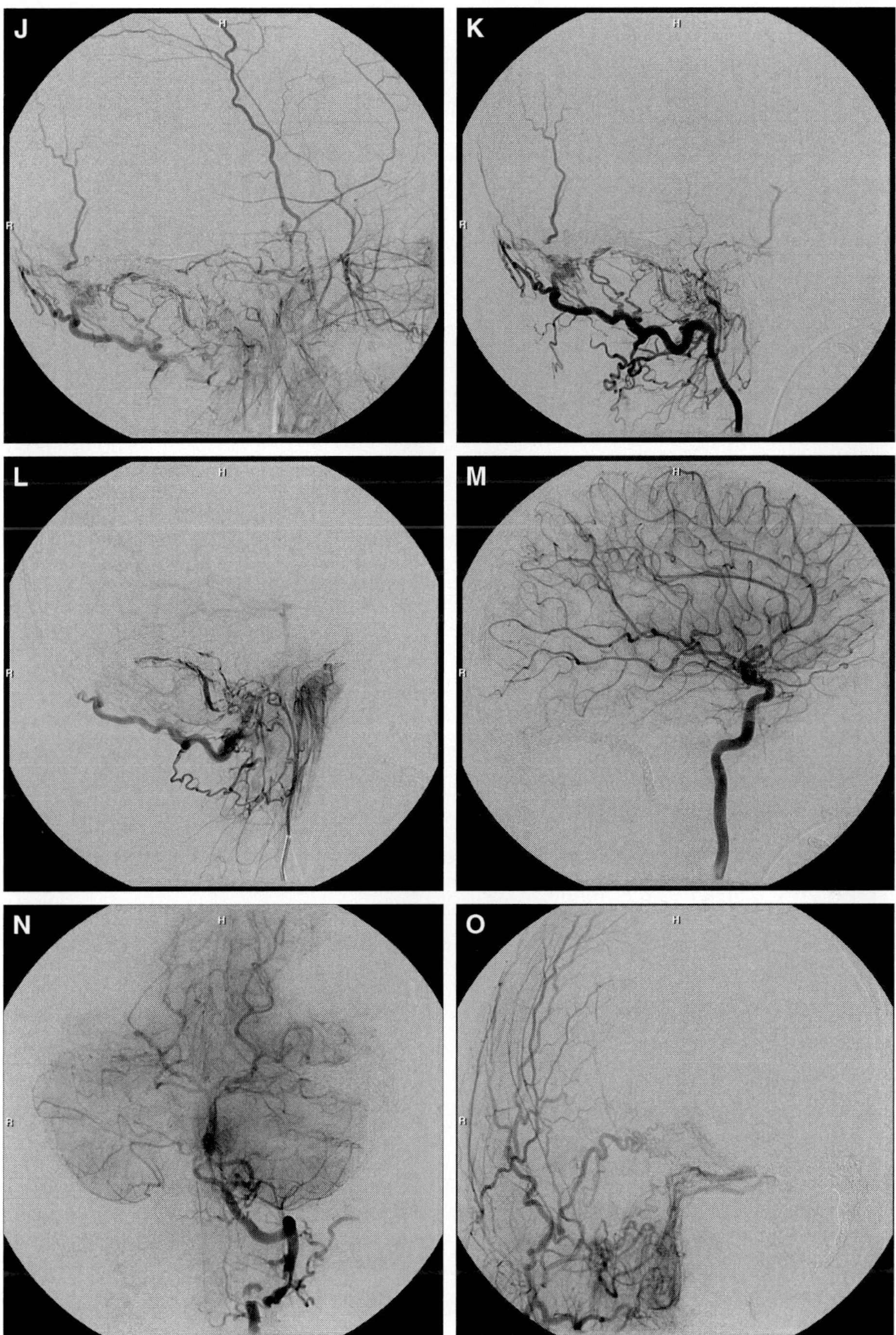

Fig. 1 (*continued*)

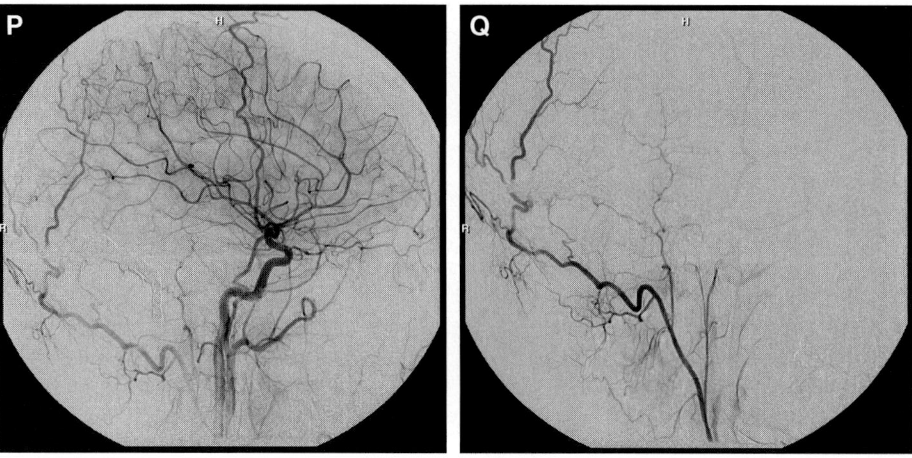

Fig. 1 (*continued*)

In summary, the location and pattern of venous drainage are the key components in determining the clinical presentation. The arterial supply is largely determined by the location of the fistula, and the venous drainage and degree of venous hypertension indicate the potential for a malignant clinical course. The overall angiographic anatomy aids in determining whether endovascular therapy by transarterial, transvenous, or a combined treatment can obliterate the fistula, and an endovascular approach is generally the first line of therapy for most of these lesions. Should endovascular therapy fail to cure the lesion, it can aid in localization of the fistula on axial CT imaging and minimize the blood loss during surgical resection.

Radiographic diagnosis

The preliminary diagnosis of a DAVF is based on clinical presentation. CT, CT angiography, MRI, and magnetic resonance angiography often support the clinical diagnosis by revealing engorged cortical veins, sinus stenosis or occlusion, hemorrhage, osseous changes from hypertrophied and ectatic vessels, or parenchymal abnormalities from venous hypertension [23]. All patients with clinical and radiographic evidence suggesting a DAVF should undergo cerebral angiography. If a DAVF is revealed, a thorough angiographic evaluation should delineate the fistula's location, arterial feeders, sinus drainage, cortical venous drainage, occlusions, stenoses, ectasias, and blood flow dynamics. A complete angiogram may require evaluation of internal and external carotid arteries, vertebral arteries, and possibly the ascending and deep cervical systems.

Classification

There are numerous classification schemes for DAVFs dating back to the initial scheme proposed by Djindjian and Merland in 1978 [24]. The most useful and modern are the revised Djindjian classification proposed by Cognard et al [25] and the classification proposed by Borden et al [26], both of which are based on that initial scheme. No matter the classification system, they all focus on the patterns of venous drainage and the clinical implications of presentation, treatment, and prognosis associated with them (Tables 1 and 2).

Treatment decision making

The decision to treat DAVFs depends primarily on the clinical presentation of the patient and the angiographic characteristics of the fistula, especially on the venous side. A simple fistula draining into a sinus in a patient with a mild bruit or who is asymptomatic is best served with conservative or compression therapy. It is important to continue to follow these patients, because DAVFs can progress to a more malignant state. If a pulsatile bruit resolves, it is an indication for repeat angiography, because the sinus may have thrombosed and the venous drainage may be redirected into the leptomeningeal or deep venous system, portending a more aggressive course.

There is a subset of patients who are symptomatic (most commonly a bruit) and whose activities of daily living are affected but do not harbor aggressive angiographic features. In these cases, subtotal obliteration can palliate the

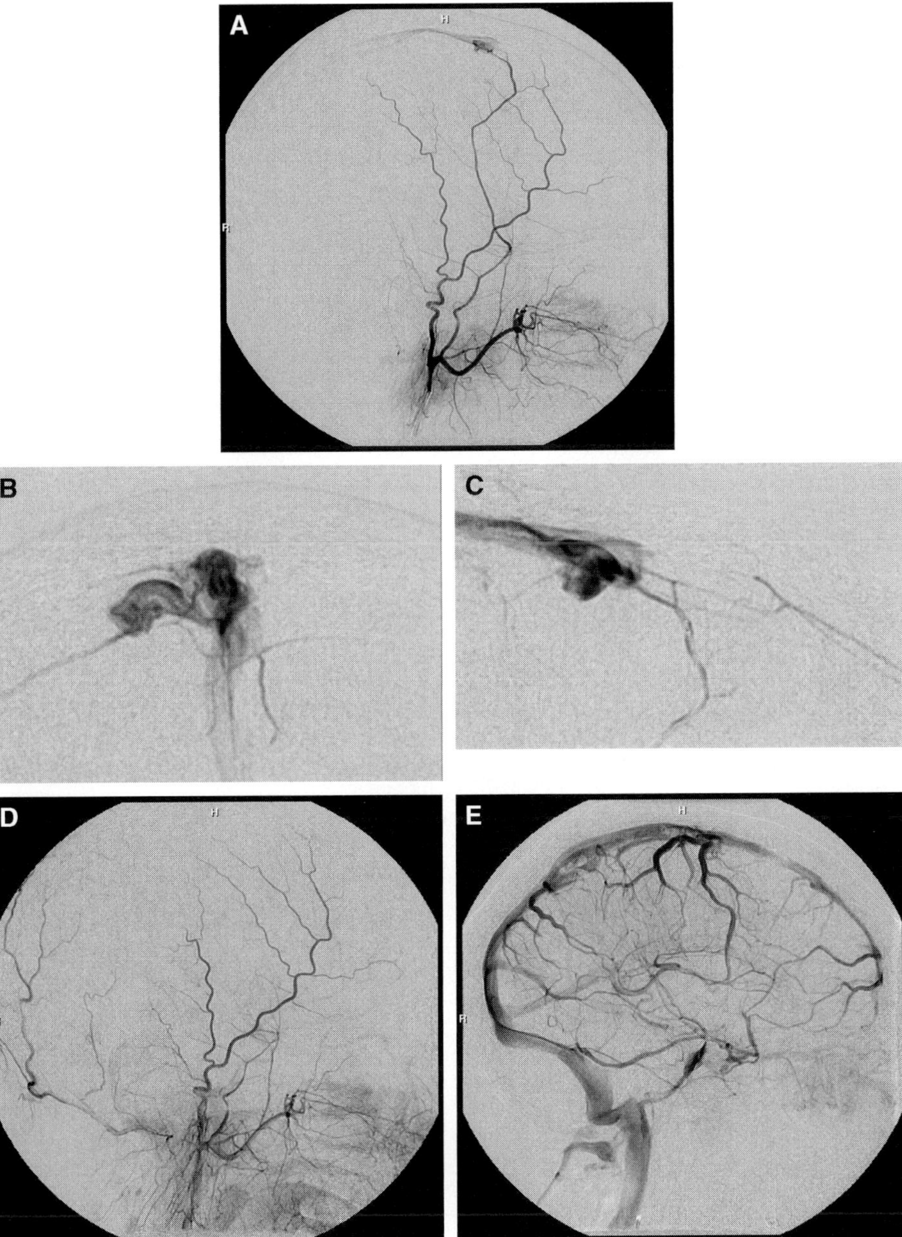

Fig. 2. A 49-year-old woman who, during evaluation of a left facial droop, was noted to harbor this sagittal sinus dural arteriovenous fistula. (*A*) Preprocedural right external carotid angiogram demonstrates supply from the middle meningeal artery. (*B*, *C*) Anteroposterior and lateral projections of a superselective middle meningeal injection demonstrate drainage into a cortical vein and, ultimately, the superior sagittal sinus. N-butyl-cyanoacrylate was injected from this position. (*D*) Postprocedural right external carotid angiogram demonstrates angiographic obliteration of the fistula. (*E*) Postprocedural venous phase of a right internal carotid injection demonstrates patency of the superior sagittal sinus. The patient was discharged home the following day neurologically intact.

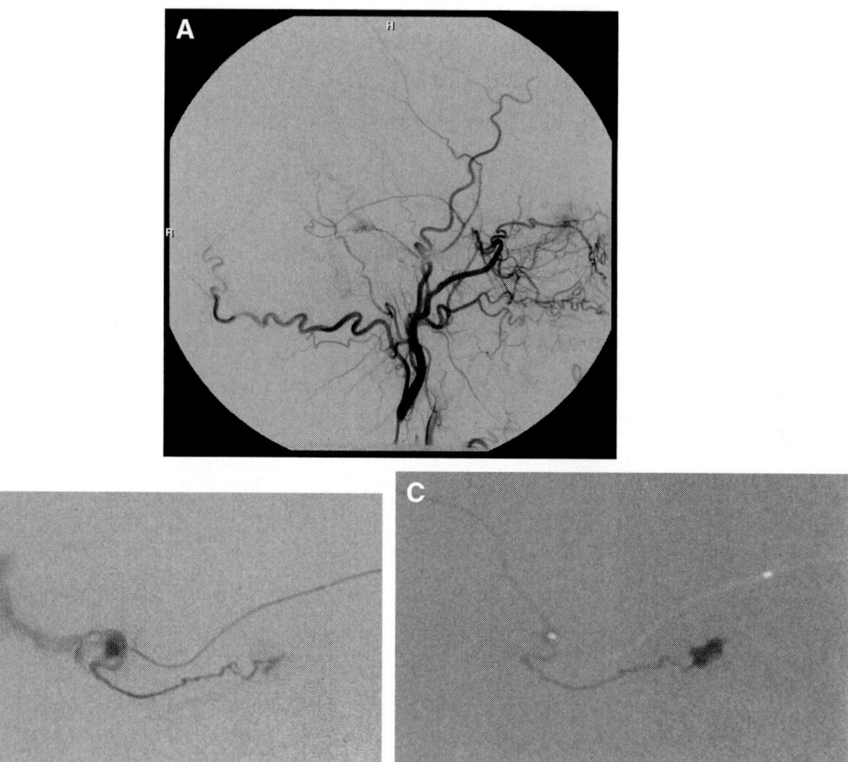

Fig. 3. A 60-year-old man with an incidentally discovered superior petrosal dural arteriovenous fistula (DAVF) during an evaluation for seizures. (*A*) Preprocedural lateral left external carotid angiogram demonstrating a small fistula supplied by the petrosquamosal and petrosal branches of the middle meningeal artery. (*B*) Superselective lateral angiogram of the petrosquamosal branch of the middle meningeal artery. Note the small amount of extravasation caused by attempts to navigate the severe tortuosity. Fortunately, a flow arrest position was obtained, and N-butyl-cyanoacrylate (NBCA) was injected from this position, sealing the defect and preventing an epidural hematoma. (*C*) Glue cast from the middle meningeal embolization. (*D*) Lateral left internal carotid angiogram demonstrating the remainder of the fistula supply from the meningohypophyseal trunk draining into the superior petrosal sinus and the petrosal vein, and, ultimately, into the vein of Galen via the lateral mesencephalic vein. (*E*) To catheterize the meningohypophyseal trunk, a balloon was inflated in the cavernous segment of the internal carotid so that the microcatheter would deflect off of the balloon and into the meningohypophyseal trunk. (*F*) Microcatheter injection of the meningohypophyseal trunk. Note the presence of reflux into the carotid artery. The balloon was then positioned over the origin of the meningohypophyseal trunk and inflated during the injection of NBCA. (*G*) Glue cast from meningohypophyseal trunk embolization. (*H*, *I*) Postprocedural lateral angiograms of the left internal and external carotid arteries demonstrating complete occlusion of the DAVF and angiographic cure without evidence of glue emboli in the intracranial circulation.

symptoms effectively. An aggressive angiographic cure may not be required and may even impose unnecessary risks [27,28].

The treatment goal for any patient presenting with hemorrhage, symptoms of cortical venous hypertension, or significant ocular pathologic findings should be complete obliteration. Even the asymptomatic patient whose fistula demonstrates significant cortical venous pathologic findings should be considered for aggressive treatment. In this high-risk population, there is little evidence to support the possibility that incomplete obliteration reduces the risk of hemorrhage, venous infarction, or visual loss.

Treatment methods

Compression therapy

A small percentage of DAVFs involving the transverse or sigmoid sinus or cavernous sinus can

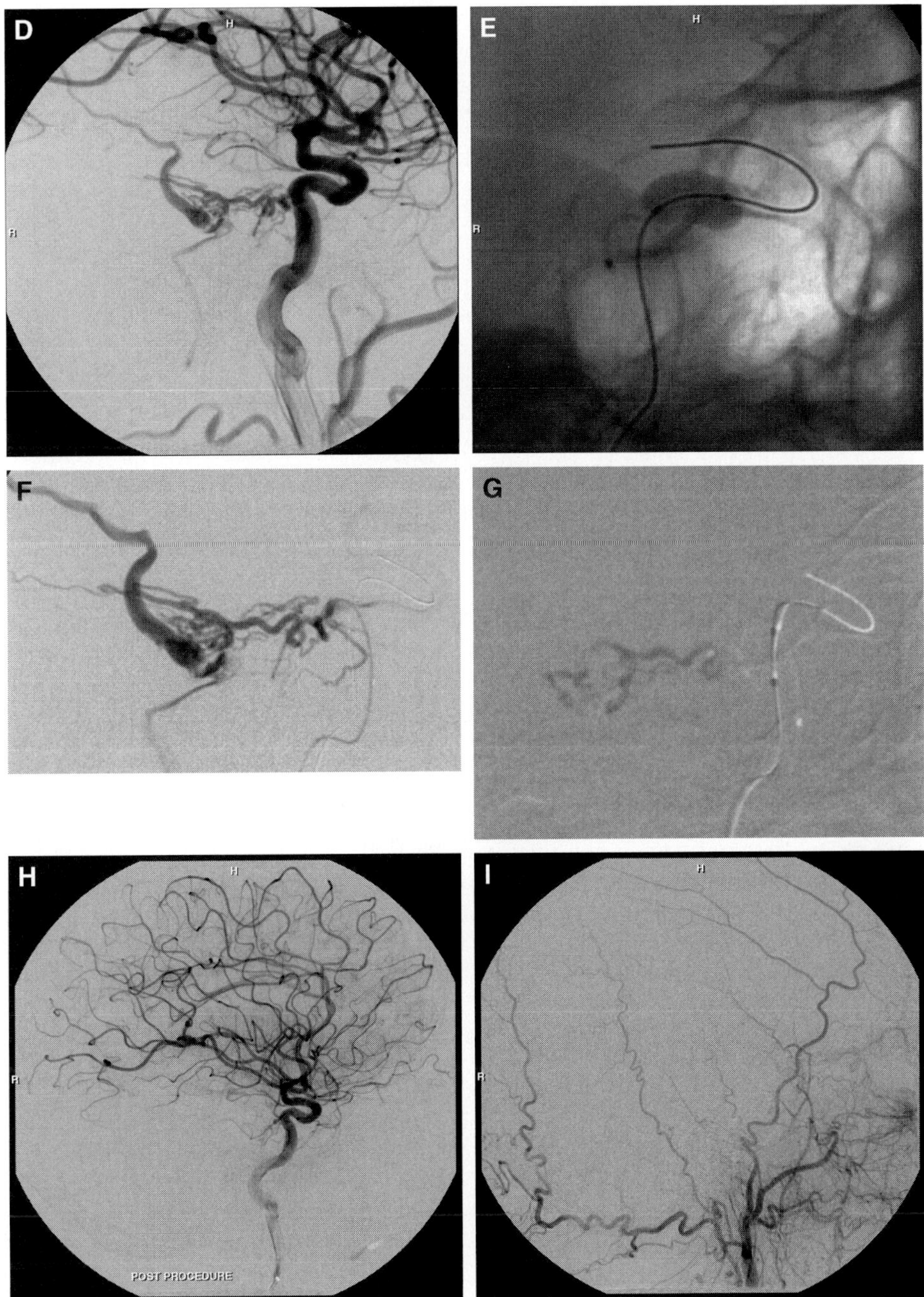

Fig. 3 (*continued*)

be treated with compression therapy. This involves compression of the involved occipital artery or the carotid artery (carotid atherosclerosis must be excluded) with the contralateral hand for 30 minutes several times a day. For small fistulae, this may promote thrombosis in up to 30% of the cases [20,29,30].

Endovascular treatment

Transvenous embolization of fistulae has historically been used with good success and is especially effective in the treatment of transverse sinus DAVFs. Venous access into the transverse sinus is generally not an issue, and even if the

Table 1
Classification schemes of venous drainage and the clinical application: revised Djindjian classification

Type I	Antegrade drainage into a sinus
Type IIa	Reflux into the sinus (retrograde flow)
Type IIb	Reflux into cortical veins
Type IIa+b	Reflux into both sinus and cortical veins
Type III	Direct cortical venous drainage without venous ectasia
Type IV	Direct cortical venous drainage with venous ectasias
Type V	Spinal venous drainage

Data from Djindjian R, Merland J. Meningeal arteriovenous fistula. Superselective arteriography of the external carotid artery. New York: Springer-Verlag; 1978. p. 405–6.

Cognard C, Gobin YP, Pierot L, Bailly AL, Houdart E, Casasco A, et al. Cerebral dural arteriovenous fistulas: clinical and angiographic correlation with a revised classification of venous drainage. Radiology 1995;194(3):671–80.

sinus is occluded at the level of the sigmoid sinus or jugular bulb, access into the involved sinus can be obtained by crossing the torcula. Consideration of the venous drainage of the fistula itself as well as the drainage of normal cerebral tissue is paramount in minimizing risk. Care must be taken not to reroute the pattern of venous drainage into the cortical veins, which can exacerbate venous hypertension. For transverse sinus fistulae, particular attention must be paid to the vein of Labbé. If the flow in the vein of Labbé is antegrade, embolization cannot proceed across the origin of the vein of Labbé without compromising normal venous drainage. If it is retrograde, however, occlusion across the vein of Labbé is well tolerated and may be required to provide a definitive cure.

There are many methods of occluding the sinus with balloons or coils. Advocates of balloon occlusion [31] espouse the advantage of possible balloon test occlusion of the sinus. Unlike arterial infarction, however, venous infarction generally does not occur for hours, and occasionally for days, after the permanent occlusion. A short temporary period of balloon occlusion therefore does not suggest that the patient will tolerate long-term occlusion. Furthermore, placement of a detachable balloon against the blood flow into a sinus may not be technically feasible in every case and certainly is not possible for Borden type III DAVFs, where the drainage occurs directly into subarachnoid veins. The other option to balloons is coil occlusion. Unfortunately, even dense packing with coils may not permanently occlude the fistula and may require further thrombosis within the coil mass itself. Currently, we favor coil embolization of the sinus, which decreases the degree of shunting, followed by transarterial N-butyl-cyanoacrylate (NBCA) embolization through a preselected arterial pedicle.

Table 2
Classification schemes of venous drainage and the clinical application: Borden classification

Type I	Drainage into the dural venous sinus
Type II	Drainage into the dural venous sinus with retrograde drainage into subarachnoid veins
Type III	Drainage into subarachnoid veins
Subtype a	Simple fistula
Subtype b	Multiple fistulas

Data from Borden JA, Wu JK, Shucart WA. A proposed classification for spinal and cranial dural arteriovenous fistulous malformations and implications for treatment. J Neurosurg 1995;82(2):166–79.

The initial results of transarterial treatment of DAVFs were suboptimal because of the low rates of cure and the subsequent recruitment of collaterals [20,29,32]. The difficulty in curing DAVFs transarterially probably resulted from the use of polyvinyl alcohol (PVA) particles and proximal occlusion of feeding pedicles during NBCA injections [33,34]. It is well known that embolization with PVA ultimately results in recanalization. In addition, NBCA embolization that does not traverse the fistulous connection into the venous side will, over time, recruit collaterals that are certain to be more difficult to catheterize selectively. With the advances in microcatheter and microguidewire technology, greater distal access can be established; however, the potential for dangerous overt or occult external carotid–to–internal carotid or vertebral anastomoses or ischemic cranial nerve palsies could preclude safe and effective embolization. A recent series of 21 patients treated transarterially under flow arrest conditions demonstrated cures in all fistulae without complications [35]. Although the definite curative embolization occurred under flow arrest conditions, a significant portion of these patients underwent adjunctive embolization with PVA or NBCA or prior transvenous coiling of the recipient venous structure. This served to devascularize the collateral inflow to minimize NBCA fragmentation, prevent systemic venous embolization, and increase the probability of polymerization within the pathologic shunt itself. This illustrates the complex angioarchitectural spectrum of DAVFs and the expertise in multimodality treatments required to engender safe and effective outcomes.

Surgical treatment

Unlike pial arteriovenous malformations of the brain or spinal cord, the venous drainage of a DAVF can frequently be safely ligated, excised, or occluded before occlusion of all the arterial pedicles [36]. Profuse bleeding can occur during the exposure and bone flap elevation, however, because of the arterialized dura, pedicles, and drainage into the intradiploic vascular channels [37]. Sinus skeletonization or excision of DAVFs should be reserved for those cases in which endovascular therapy has failed to effect a cure but has at least decreased the flow to reduce blood loss. Surgical access of a recipient venous structure, such as the superior ophthalmic vein for cavernous DAVFs, to deliver endovascular materials continues to play a significant role. As previously mentioned, for ethmoidal fistulae [21] and some petrosal sinus fistulae, surgical excision of the draining vein is the primary treatment modality.

In a recent series, 34 patients with primarily transverse or sigmoid, superior sagittal, or superior petrosal sinus DAVFs were cured by surgical treatment [36]. The authors separated their patient population into two groups depending on whether the fistulous drainage occurred purely through leptomeningeal veins (nonsinus fistulae) or whether the fistula drained into a sinus with retrograde flow into the leptomeningeal circulation (sinus fistulae). In the former scenario, the surgical treatment required disconnection of the draining veins at the point where they exited the dural wall of the sinus. In the latter, surgical excision of the involved sinus segment after preoperative embolization represented a safe and definitive treatment, because this segment did not serve to drain the normal cerebrovasculature. Their cure rate was 100%, and there were no instances of mortality or permanent morbidity. Again, the treatment goals were determined by a careful evaluation of the venous anatomy, and the importance of preoperative embolization was emphasized.

Radiosurgery

The role of stereotactic radiosurgery in the treatment of DAVFs is continuing to develop, and the experience with this modality is growing [38–44]. Because of the complex nature of DAVFs and the relatively small number of patients in each series, the rate of angiographic obliteration is still uncertain. It does appear, however, that the complication rates of the initial treatment are relatively low. There is the possibility of hemorrhage or symptomatic clinical events that could occur from the time of treatment until obliteration is obtained, however. This may be untenable for patients who present with hemorrhage, significant venous hypertension, or high-risk angiographic profiles.

Because of the relative efficacy of endovascular and surgical treatment of these lesions, we view stereotactic radiosurgery as the third-line treatment modality. There is, however, a relatively small patient population in which endovascular or surgical treatment may be extremely difficult or risky, as is the case for the elderly population with significant comorbidities, where stereotactic radiosurgery may play a role.

Summary

DAVFs comprise a highly complex series of lesions clinically and angiographically. The clinical presentation can range from asymptomatic to devastating intracranial hemorrhage. The location of the fistula is a primary factor in determining the method of presentation. Angiographically, the pattern of venous drainage is the main factor in determining the ultimate prognosis. The goal of treatment of any DAVF that exhibits cortical venous drainage should be angiographic obliteration and cure. The method of treatment should be highly individualized to the angiographic architecture of each DAVF and can comprise endovascular, surgical, or a combination of methods to achieve the appropriate treatment goal and to minimize risk. In general, we think that the endovascular approach is the primary mode of therapy for transverse sinus, cavernous, superior sagittal, or petrosal sinus fistulae and that surgery is the primary mode of therapy for ethmoidal fistulae. Stereotactic radiosurgery should be reserved for lesions in which endovascular or surgical options have failed or would subject the patient to inordinate risk. The importance of a multidisciplinary approach to these highly complex lesions cannot be overemphasized and engenders the safest and most effective outcomes.

References

[1] Newton TH, Cronqvist S. Involvement of dural arteries in intracranial arteriovenous malformations. Radiology 1969;93(5):1071–8.

[2] Nishijima M, Takaku A, Endo S, Kuwayama N, Koizumi F, Sato H, et al. Etiological evaluation of dural arteriovenous malformations of the lateral and sigmoid sinuses based on histopathological examinations. J Neurosurg 1992;76(4):600–6.

[3] Chaudhary M, Sachdev V, Cho S. Dural arteriovenous malformations of the major venous sinuses, and acquired lesion. AJNR Am J Neuroradiol 1982;3:13–9.

[4] Houser OW, Campbell JK, Campbell RJ, Sundt TM Jr. Arteriovenous malformation affecting the transverse dural venous sinus—an acquired lesion. Mayo Clin Proc 1979;54(10):651–61.

[5] Kuhner A, Krastel A, Stoll W. Arteriovenous malformations of the transverse dural sinus. J Neurosurg 1976;45(1):12–9.

[6] Obrador S, Soto M, Silvela J. Clinical syndromes of arteriovenous malformations of the transverse-sigmoid sinus. J Neurol Neurosurg Psychiatry 1975;38(5):436–51.

[7] Herman JM, Spetzler RF, Bederson JB, Kurbat JM, Zabramski JM. Genesis of a dural arteriovenous malformation in a rat model. J Neurosurg 1995; 83(3):539–45.

[8] Lawton MT, Jacobowitz R, Spetzler RF. Redefined role of angiogenesis in the pathogenesis of dural arteriovenous malformations. J Neurosurg 1997;87(2): 267–74.

[9] Terada T, Higashida RT, Halbach VV, Dowd CF, Tsuura M, Komai N, et al. Development of acquired arteriovenous fistulas in rats due to venous hypertension. J Neurosurg 1994;80(5):884–9.

[10] Hamada Y, Goto K, Inoue T, Iwaki T, Matsuno H, Suzuki S, et al. Histopathological aspects of dural arteriovenous fistulas in the transverse-sigmoid sinus region in nine patients. Neurosurgery 1997;40(3): 452–6.

[11] Bahar S, Chiras J, Carpena JP, Meder JF, Bories J. Spontaneous vertebro-vertebral arterio-venous fistula associated with fibro-muscular dysplasia. Report of two cases. Neuroradiology 1984;26(1):45–9.

[12] Deans WR, Bloch S, Leibrock L, Berman BM, Skultety FM. Arteriovenous fistula in patients with neurofibromatosis. Radiology 1982;144(1):103–7.

[13] Graf CJ. Spontaneous carotid-cavernous fistula. Ehlers-Danlos syndrome and related conditions. Arch Neurol 1965;13(6):662–72.

[14] Halbach VV, Higashida RT, Dowd CF, Barnwell SL, Hieshima GB. Treatment of carotid-cavernous fistulas associated with Ehlers-Danlos syndrome. Neurosurgery 1990;26(6):1021–7.

[15] Schievink WI, Piepgras DG. Cervical vertebral artery aneurysms and arteriovenous fistulae in neurofibromatosis type 1: case reports. Neurosurgery 1991;29(5):760–5.

[16] Malek A, Halbach V, Higashida R, Phatouros C, Meyers P, Dowd C. Treatment of dural arteriovenous malformations and fistulas. Neurosurg Clin N Am 2000;11(1):147–66.

[17] McDougall C, Halbach V, Higashida R. Treatment of dural arteriovenous fistulas. Neurosurgery Quarterly 1997;7:110–34.

[18] Houser O, Baker H, Rhoton A, Okazaki H. Intracranial dural arteriovenous malformations. Radiology 1972;105:55–64.

[19] Awad IA, Little JR, Akarawi WP, Ahl J. Intracranial dural arteriovenous malformations: factors predisposing to an aggressive neurological course. J Neurosurg 1990;72(6):839–50.

[20] Halbach VV, Higashida RT, Hieshima GB, Goto K, Norman D, Newton TH. Dural fistulas involving the transverse and sigmoid sinuses: results of treatment in 28 patients. Radiology 1987;163(2): 443–7.

[21] Halbach VV, Higashida RT, Hieshima GB, Wilson CB, Barnwell SL, Dowd CF. Dural arteriovenous fistulas supplied by ethmoidal arteries. Neurosurgery 1990;26(5):816–23.

[22] Tomak PR, Cloft HJ, Kaga A, Cawley CM, Dion J, Barrow DL. Evolution of the management of tentorial dural arteriovenous malformations. Neurosurgery 2003;52(4):750–60.

[23] Halbach V, Higashida R, Hieshima G. Diagnosis and treatment of dural arteriovenous fistulae. In: Margulis A, Gooding C, editors. Diagnostic radiology. San Francisco: University of California Press; 1987. p. 303–14.

[24] Djindjian R, Merland J. Meningeal arteriovenous fistula. Superselective arteriography of the external carotid artery. New York: Springer-Verlag; 1978. p. 405–6.

[25] Cognard C, Gobin YP, Pierot L, Bailly AL, Houdart E, Casasco A, et al. Cerebral dural arteriovenous fistulas: clinical and angiographic correlation with a revised classification of venous drainage. Radiology 1995;194(3):671–80.

[26] Borden JA, Wu JK, Shucart WA. A proposed classification for spinal and cranial dural arteriovenous fistulous malformations and implications for treatment. J Neurosurg 1995;82(2):166–79.

[27] Cognard C, Houdart E, Casasco A, Jhaveri H, Chapot R, Merland J. Endovascular therapy and long-term results for intracranial dural arteriovenous fistulae.. In: Connors J, Wojak J, editors. Interventional neuroradiology. Philadelphia: WB Saunders; 1999. p. 198–214.

[28] Barnwell SL, Halbach VV, Higashida RT, Hieshima G, Wilson CB. Complex dural arteriovenous fistulas. Results of combined endovascular and neurosurgical treatment in 16 patients. J Neurosurg 1989;71(3):352–8.

[29] Halbach VV, Higashida RT, Hieshima GB, Reicher M, Norman D, Newton TH. Dural fistulas involving the cavernous sinus: results of treatment in 30 patients. Radiology 1987;163(2):437–42.

[30] Higashida RT, Hieshima GB, Halbach VV, Bentson JR, Goto K. Closure of carotid cavernous sinus fistulae by external compression of the carotid artery

and jugular vein. Acta Radiol Suppl 1986;369: 580–3.

[31] Roy D, Raymond J. The role of transvenous embolization in the treatment of intracranial dural arteriovenous fistulas. Neurosurgery 1997;40(6): 1133–41.

[32] Grossman RI, Sergott RC, Goldberg HI, Savino PJ, Zimmerman RA, Bilaniuk LT, et al. Dural malformations with ophthalmic manifestations: results of particulate embolization in seven patients. AJNR Am J Neuroradiol 1985;6(5):809–13.

[33] Marks MP, Do HM. Endovascular therapy for dural arteriovenous fistulas. In: Chaloupka J, editor. Endovascular and percutaneous therapy of the brain and spine. Philadelphia: Lippincott Williams & Wilkins; 2002. p. 277–315.

[34] Quisling RG, Mickle JP, Ballinger W. Small particle polyvinyl alcohol embolization of cranial lesions with minimal arteriolar-capillary barriers. Surg Neurol 1986;25(3):243–52.

[35] Nelson PK, Russell SM, Woo HH, Alastra AJ, Vidovich DV. Use of a wedged microcatheter for curative transarterial embolization of complex intracranial dural arteriovenous fistulas: indications, endovascular technique, and outcome in 21 patients. J Neurosurg 2003;98(3):498–506.

[36] Collice M, D'Aliberti G, Arena O, Solaini C, Fontana R, Talamonti G. Surgical treatment of intracranial dural arteriovenous fistulae: role of venous drainage. Neurosurgery 2000;47:56–67.

[37] Sundt TM Jr, Piepgras DG. The surgical approach to arteriovenous malformations of the lateral and sigmoid dural sinuses. J Neurosurg 1983;59(1):32–9.

[38] Friedman JA, Pollock BE, Nichols DA, Gorman DA, Foote RL, Stafford SL. Results of combined stereotactic radiosurgery and transarterial embolization for dural arteriovenous fistulas of the transverse and sigmoid sinuses. J Neurosurg 2001;94(6):886–91.

[39] Guo WY, Pan DH, Wu HM, Chung WY, Shiau CY, Wang LW, et al. Radiosurgery as a treatment alternative for dural arteriovenous fistulas of the cavernous sinus. AJNR Am J Neuroradiol 1998;19(6): 1081–7.

[40] Lewis AI, Tomsick TA, Tew JM Jr. Management of tentorial dural arteriovenous malformations: transarterial embolization combined with stereotactic radiation or surgery. J Neurosurg 1994;81(6):851–9.

[41] Maruyama K, Shin M, Kurita H, Tago M, Kirino T. Stereotactic radiosurgery for dural arteriovenous fistula involving the superior sagittal sinus. Case report. J Neurosurg 2002;97(5 Suppl):481–3.

[42] O'Leary S, Hodgson TJ, Coley SC, Kemeny AA, Radatz MW. Intracranial dural arteriovenous malformations: results of stereotactic radiosurgery in 17 patients. Clin Oncol (R Coll Radiol) 2002;14(2): 97–102.

[43] Onizuka M, Mori K, Takahashi N, Kawahara I, Hiu T, Toda K, et al. Gamma knife surgery for the treatment of spontaneous dural carotid-cavernous fistulas. Neurol Med Chir (Tokyo) 2003;43(10): 477–82.

[44] Pan DH, Chung WY, Guo WY, Wu HM, Liu KD, Shiau CY, et al. Stereotactic radiosurgery for the treatment of dural arteriovenous fistulas involving the transverse-sigmoid sinus. J Neurosurg 2002; 96(5):823–9.

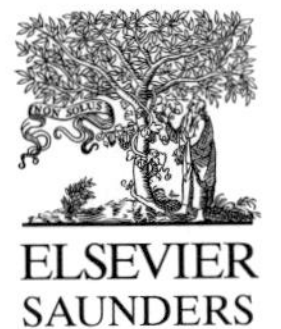
ELSEVIER
SAUNDERS

Neurosurg Clin N Am 16 (2005) 395–410

NEUROSURGERY
CLINICS
OF NORTH AMERICA

Endovascular Techniques for Vascular Malformations of the Spinal Axis

Cameron G. McDougall, MD*, Vivek R. Deshmukh, MD, David J. Fiorella, MD, Felipe C. Albuquerque, MD, Robert F. Spetzler, MD

Division of Neurological Surgery, Barrow Neurological Institute, St. Joseph's Hospital and Medical Center, 350 West Thomas Road, Phoenix, AZ 85013, USA

The purpose of this article is to discuss the use of endovascular techniques in the management of vascular lesions of the spinal axis. As with any other therapeutic modality, in deciding whether endovascular treatment is indicated, it is essential that the treating physician have a clear understanding of the pathologic entity in question, a clear understanding of the overall treatment plan, and a realistic understanding of the capabilities and limits of endovascular therapy. Without such an understanding, appropriate patients may be denied valuable treatment options and inappropriate patients may undergo procedures that are not in their best interest.

The use of percutaneous catheter-based embolization for treating conditions of the craniospinal axis began to be reported in the early 1960s, but applications were limited until improved devices began to become available in the 1970s and 1980s. Most important in driving this development was the introduction of variable stiffness "microcatheters" and, subsequently, suitable embolic materials. A variable stiffness catheter is a catheter that is stiffer at the proximal end than it is at the distal end. This design resulted in a catheter with a small soft tip that could be safely navigated within the vascular system much more distally than was previously possible. With these microcatheters, it became possible to access vascular territories percutaneously that otherwise could be reached only through direct surgical exploration. Indeed, it became possible to access vascular territories that may not normally be safely approached surgically. In turn, this improved access created the opportunity to deliver embolic agents in a "superselective" manner. It has been less than 20 years since high-quality variable stiffness microcatheters became readily available, but in this brief time, there has been rapid evolution of technology and techniques. These advances have allowed embolization to play a more prominent role in the treatment of many neurovascular conditions.

Endovascular anatomy

Spinal cord

The spinal cord receives its nourishment from one anterior spinal artery (ASA) and two posterior spinal arteries. The ASA lies in the anterior median sulcus, and the paired posterior spinal arteries lie on either side of the dorsolateral surface of the spinal cord. The numerous branches of the ASA travel within the anterior median sulcus and are responsible for providing supply to greater than two thirds of the spinal cord, including the anterior and lateral corticospinal tracts. The posterior spinal arteries primarily supply the posterior columns.

Anterior spinal artery

Paired ASAs originate at the craniovertebral junction as branches of the fourth segment of the

* Corresponding author. c/o Neuroscience Publications, Barrow Neurological Institute, 350 West Thomas Road, Phoenix, AZ 85013, USA.

E-mail address: neuropub@chw.edu (C.G. McDougall).

1042-3680/05/$ - see front matter
doi:10.1016/j.nec.2004.08.011

vertebral artery. The takeoff of the ASAs is distal to the origin of the posterior inferior cerebellar arteries. The two ASAs then converge to form a single ASA ventral to the caudal brain stem or rostral spinal cord. The ASA then continues within the anterior median sulcus for the entire extent of the cord and conus medullaris. In the cervical region, the ASA receives further contribution via branches of the vertebral artery as well as the ascending cervical branch of the thyrocervical trunk. One anatomically constant radicular artery at the C5 or C6 level is known as the artery of cervical enlargement. Radiculomedullary branches of the supreme intercostal artery and the thoracic/lumbar radicular arteries supply the ASA in the thoracic and lumbar region. The most prominent of these radicular vessels is known as the arteria radicularis magna, more commonly referred to eponymously as the artery of Adamkiewicz. This artery commonly arises from the lower intercostal or lumbar arteries, most frequently on the left side between the levels of T10 to L2. It is a slender midline vessel measuring 0.5 to 1 mm in diameter. On an anterior-posterior projection, the artery has an ascending segment that makes a characteristic hairpin turn into a descending ASA located in the midline. Whenever possible, the artery of Adamkiewicz should be identified angiographically before embolization of middle/lower thoracic and rostral lumbar lesions.

Posterior spinal artery

A pair of posterior spinal arteries supplies the posterolateral aspect of the spinal cord. They originate in the upper cervical region, typically branching from the vertebral arteries. They receive supply from the segmental radiculomedullary arteries, which form a hairpin configuration similar to the supply of the ASA. The ASA anastomoses with the posterior spinal arteries at the conus medullaris to form a luxuriant arterial network.

Spinal column

Supply to the anterior and lateral aspect of the vertebral body is primarily via branches of the vertebral artery and the ascending cervical branch of the thyrocervical trunk in the cervical spine. In the thoracic and lumbar spine, branches of the intercostal arteries and lumbar radicular arteries, respectively, are the predominant arteries. The epidural spaces ventral and dorsal to the spinal cord and thecal sac contain a rich plexus of vessels. In the ventral epidural space, these vessels lie beneath the posterior longitudinal ligament and contribute to the vascularity of the vertebral body. In the dorsal epidural space, these vessels richly supply the lamina and a portion of the posterior spinous process. A plexus from the main trunk of the dorsospinal artery lines the outer surface of the lamina and the posterior spinous process.

Endovascular techniques

The ability to carry out high-quality spinal angiography is an essential prerequisite to the embolization of spinal lesions. High-resolution, preferably biplane, angiography is required. As with cerebral angiography, "subtraction" techniques are used to provide detailed images of vascular structures. Subtraction techniques require that a "mask" image is first acquired; then, after contrast injection, the original mask image is "subtracted" from the postcontrast images, resulting in greatly enhanced visibility of the contrast agent. When there is patient movement between the time of the initial or mask image and the time when the contrast-injected images are acquired, the mask no longer matches the new position and image quality is markedly degraded. Similarly, motion artifact can be problematic when catheters and devices are being maneuvered. When manipulating catheters and endovascular devices, progress is visually monitored using real-time subtracted fluoroscopic images known as "roadmaps." As long as there is no motion, these images remain clear, but even subtle movements render the roadmaps useless. Motion from breathing or intestinal peristaltic movements can also make the images uninterpretable. The importance of minimizing this motion artifact is further exaggerated when interventions are undertaken. It is crucial, for example, that there be no patient motion during the injection of an embolic agent, because any significant motion results in poor visualization of the embolic material being delivered. Spinal embolizations can be lengthy procedures, and it is difficult for the awake or sedated patient to remain adequately still. Because of these issues with patient motion, the authors prefer having their patients under general anesthesia for all but the most straightforward of spinal embolizations. Under general anesthesia, patient motion is largely eliminated. Likewise, ventilation can easily and reliably be suspended during key periods of image acquisition or during delivery of embolic agents. Glucagon can be administered to reduce intestinal motility, again helping to minimize motion artifact and enhance image quality.

In the process of optimizing image quality, it remains equally important that patients and staff are protected from excessive exposure to radiation. Appropriate attention must be paid to radiation shielding, fluoroscopy time, and other issues relating to radiation exposure.

When endovascular neurosurgical procedures are performed with the patient under general anesthesia, many advocate using electrophysiologic monitoring to compensate for the inability to carry out clinical monitoring. Motor evoked potentials have been anecdotally reported to be particularly useful [1].

Microcatheters are categorized as one of two broad types. Catheters may be "over the wire" or "flow directed." Over-the-wire systems are advanced toward their target using a fine curved guidewire that is steered toward the target area using torque to direct the wire and then advancing the catheter over the wire. Flow-directed catheters are generally softer and more flexible. As the operator advances the proximal end of the catheter, the distal tip is carried forward passively with the arterial blood flow. Because of their dependence on flow, these catheters are best suited for use in the treatment of high-flow lesions, such as arteriovenous malformations (AVMs). These catheters are generally of smaller diameter and thus more restricted in their capacity to deliver embolic agents. The development of extremely fine guidewires (ie, 0.008-in diameter) has meant that to some extent, a flow-directed catheter can be delivered by flow but with some guidewire assistance. Within each class of catheter, there are a multitude of commercially available variations.

Embolic agents may be classified as liquid or particulate. Liquid agents may be "glue" type agents, such as N-butyl-cyanoacrylate (NBCA), or sclerosing agents, such as ethanol. Recently, ethylene vinyl alcohol copolymer dissolved in dimethyl sulfoxide (Onyx liquid embolic system; Micro Therapeutics, Irvine, California) has been reported in the treatment of spinal AVMs with good results [2]. This material is not yet approved for use in the United States. Particulate agents may be larger particulates, such as metallic coils (generally platinum), or smaller injected particles, such as polyvinyl alcohol. In general, the larger the particle is, the larger is the size of vessel that will be occluded. This may be desirable, or it may result in an occlusion more proximal to the target lesion than is desired.

Classification of spinal vascular malformations

Spinal vascular malformations are relatively uncommon, and the role of embolization varies depending on the type of malformation and the practice patterns of a given institution. Many different classification systems exist for spinal vascular malformations, but there remains widespread disagreement and confusion regarding nomenclature for these entities [3–11]. Recently, Spetzler et al [12] proposed an updated classification system clarifying the nomenclature and discussing a recently described and clinically distinct entity, the conus AVM. The conus malformation has also been discussed as a separate entity by Hurst et al [13]. The classification system proposed by Spetzler et al [12] is particularly helpful in that the nomenclature is clearly descriptive and replaces a bewildering array of overlapping and confusing names. Additionally, the classification system incorporates recent advances in imaging and new clinical insights enhancing understanding of these lesions, thereby permitting a more logical and easily understood framework. Box 1 from their publication lists the proposed replacement classification, whereas Tables 1 and 2 give the clinical summaries, respectively, for arteriovenous fistulas (AVFs) and AVMs as they occur in the spinal axis.

To summarize their classification, most vascular lesions relevant to this article are divided into AVFs or AVMs. Spinal aneurysms are separate

Box 1. Proposed classification of spinal cord vascular malformations by Spetzler and colleagues

- Neoplastic vascular lesions
  - Hemangioblastomas
  - Cavernous malformation
- Spinal aneurysms
- Arteriovenous fistulas
  - Extradural
  - Intradural
    - Ventral
    - Dorsal
- Arteriovenous malformations
  - Extradural-intradural
  - Intradural
    - Intramedullary
      - Compact
      - Diffuse
    - Conus

Table 1
Summary of clinical characteristics in arteriovenous fistulas

Characteristic	Extradural	Dorsal intradural	Ventral intradural
Pathophysiology	Spinal cord compression, venous congestion, vascular steal	Venous congestion, rare hemorrhage	Compression (venous aneurysm), hemorrhage, vascular steal
Presentation	Progressive myelopathy	Progressive myelopathy	Progressive myelopathy
Diagnostic modality	MRI, angiography	MRI, angiography	MRI, angiography
Previous nomenclature	Epidural	Dural AVF, long dorsal, type 1A, others	Types IVA (small), B (medium), and C (large), perimedullary

Abbreviation: AVF, arteriovenous fistula.

From Spetzler RF, Detwiler PW, Riina HA, Porter RW. Modified classification of spinal cord lesions. J Neurosurg (Spine 2) 2002;96:145–56; with permission.

but, of course, may exist in conjunction with high-flow spinal vascular lesions [14]. Fistulas may be extradural or intradural, and the intradural fistulas may be dorsal or ventral. AVMs may be intramedullary or combined extradural-intradural. The intramedullary lesions may be compact or diffuse. The conus AVM, as noted previously, is seen as a distinct entity. Again from this publication are included artist's illustrations of the AVFs and AVMs that afflict the spinal axis (Figs. 1–7) [12]. Information regarding the role of endovascular techniques in treating these lesions is considered below, grouped by lesion type. Discussion focuses on the AVFs and AVMs, because endovascular techniques are likely to play a key role in the treatment of these lesions. The rare spinal artery aneurysm that is not associated with a fistula or malformation may require surgical wrapping to ensure preservation of the artery [15].

Extradural spinal arteriovenous fistulas

Extradural spinal arteriovenous fistulas (ESAVFs) are rare. They are also known as epidural AVFs. Patients with these lesions most typically present with progressive neurologic deficits or pain. Symptoms may be secondary to direct compression of neural structures by the enlarged vascular channels or may occur as a result of venous hypertension or arterial steal [16]. Diagnosis is usually made by MRI or magnetic resonance angiography, but digital subtraction angiography is necessary for accurate characterization of the lesion.

ESAVFs may often be treated and cured by endovascular techniques alone. These lesions may have high flow rates. Endovascular closure of the fistula usually requires elimination of a small length of the distal feeding artery proximal to the fistula as well as the fistula itself and the proximal portion of the draining vein. To reduce the risk of the embolic material traveling beyond the target zone, it is preferable to use fibered detachable coils rather than liquid embolics. The disadvantage of using fibered coils is that larger catheters are required, and it may be more difficult to reach the target lesion with these larger catheters. Occasionally, a transvenous approach rather than a transarterial approach may facilitate endovascular access to the fistula [17].

Table 2
Summary of clinical characteristics in arteriovenous malformations

Characteristic	Extradural-intradural	Intramedullary	Conus medullaris
Pathophysiology	Compression, vascular steal, hemorrhage	Hemorrhage, compression, vascular steal	Venous hypertension, compression, hemorrhage
Presentation	Pain, progressive myelopathy	Acute myelopathy, pain, progressive myelopathy	Progressive myelopathy radiculopathy
Diagnostic modality	MRI, angiography, high-flow, multiple feeders	MRI, angiography	MRI, angiography
Previous nomenclature	Juvenile AVM, metameric AVM	Classic AVM, glomus type	None

From Spetzler RF, Detwiler PW, Riina HA, Porter RW. Modified classification of spinal cord lesions. J Neurosurg (Spine 2) 2002;96:145–56; with permission.

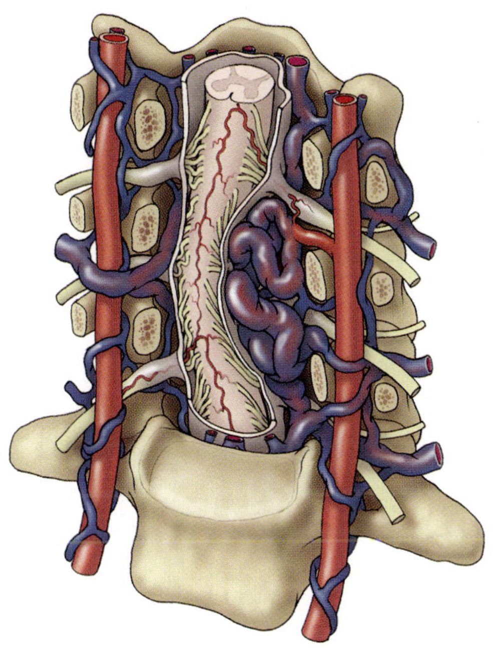

Fig. 1. Illustration of extradural arteriovenous fistula with thecal sac compression from venous engorgement. (*From* Spetzler RF, Zabramski JM, Flom RA. Management of juvenile spinal AVMs by embolization and operative excision: case report. J Neurosurg 1989;70(4): 628–32; with permission.)

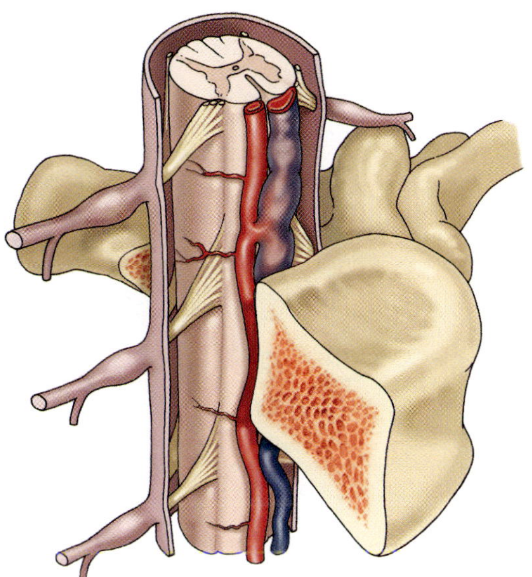

Fig. 2. Illustration of ventral arteriovenous fistula with significant venous engorgement. (Courtesy of Barrow Neurological Institute; with permission.)

Fig. 1 shows an artist's rendition of an ESAVF at the level of the cervical spine. Fig. 8 shows a clinical example of a large ESAVF identified in an 18-month-old girl after a vascular bruit was heard. This lesion was nicely demonstrated by magnetic resonance angiography. Coil embolization of the fistula resulted in angiographic cure of the lesion, elimination of the bruit, and continued normal neurologic function at the most recent follow-up 4 years after treatment.

Intradural dorsal spinal arteriovenous fistulas

These lesions have also been referred to as "spinal dural arteriovenous fistulas" or "type 1 spinal arteriovenous malformations." The treatment of intradural dorsal spinal arteriovenous fistulas (DSAVFs) is controversial. The urgency of this controversy is heightened because DSAVFs are well known as a preventable cause of paralysis, but it is also well known that the diagnosis is frequently delayed and that many patients present late to the neurosurgeon. Increased awareness and better imaging techniques have resulted in more frequent diagnosis of this problem. MRI and magnetic resonance angiography are proving highly useful in identifying the fistulas and documenting improvement of abnormal findings after successful treatment. For example, Lee et al [18] have shown that T2 imaging reliably shows signal hyperintensity in the spinal cord and that this hyperintensity diminishes after successful DSAVF treatment. They have also shown magnetic resonance angiography to be reliably diagnostic for DSAVFs.

As with intracranial dural AVFs, the key to the effective treatment of DSAVFs is the accurate identification of the AVF, followed by its complete and durable elimination. Whether this should be achieved by direct surgical obliteration or by endovascular embolization is at the core of the treatment controversy. If treatment is incomplete, DSAVFs are likely to cause a stepwise neurologic deterioration resulting in paralysis. The elimination of the fistula is likely to halt this progression; for this reason, cure rather than palliation must be the treatment goal. Indeed, with cure of DSAVFs, substantial neurologic recovery can occur, particularly if the duration of symptoms before cure is short [19]. At issue are the success rate, effectiveness, and durability of embolization as compared with open surgical treatment.

Careful analysis is required to understand the precise site of the arteriovenous connection,

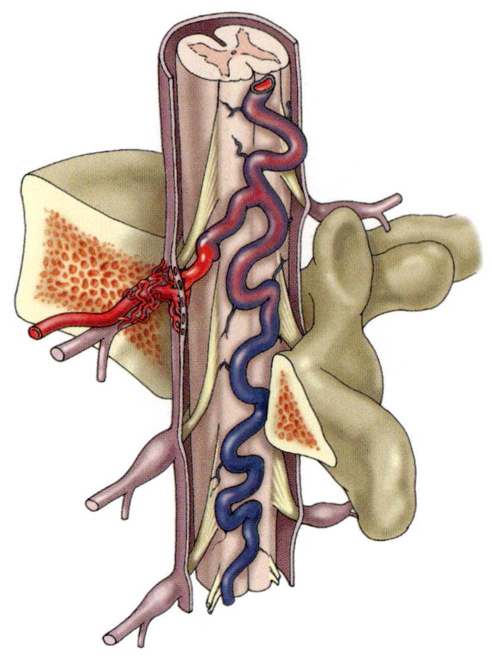

Fig. 3. Illustration of dorsal spinal arteriovenous fistula. The site of the fistula is intradural. (Courtesy of Barrow Neurological Institute; with permission.)

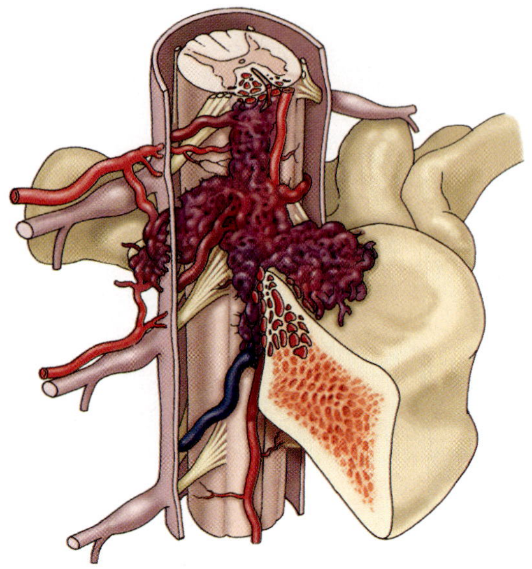

Fig. 4. Illustration of extradural-intradural arteriovenous malformation involving neural and bony elements. (*From* Spetzler RF, Detwiler PW, Riina HA, Porter RW. Modified classification of spinal cord vascular lesions. J Neurosurg (Spine 2) 2002;96:145–56; with permission.)

because recruitment of multiple feeding arteries and draining veins can present a confusing picture. Our understanding of the typical location of these fistulas was greatly enhanced by McCutcheon et al [20], who used microangiographic techniques on surgical specimens to demonstrate the characteristic anatomy of the lesions, specifically by demonstrating the intradural site of the AVF connection. Armed with this understanding and combining it with high-quality superselective angiographic techniques, these fistulas can be confidently identified, and percutaneous access to the fistula itself with a microcatheter is often straightforward. In this situation, embolization can be performed rapidly and safely. Similarly, superselective angiography through the microcatheter can also be valuable in identifying the spinal artery if it is associated with the arterial pedicle feeding the fistula. In this setting, embolization should not be used because of the risk of unintended embolization of the radiculomedullary arterial supply to the spinal cord. At other times, localization of DSAVFs can be challenging, particularly in elderly patients or patients with advanced atherosclerotic changes. In some instances, microcatheter access to the fistula is not possible. Large fistulas with multiple feeding arteries may also be difficult to treat endovascularly.

Higher rates of recurrence have been reported after treatment of DSAVFs by embolization compared with after treatment by open surgical obliteration. For this reason, some advocate embolization if it is technically feasible and reserve surgery for failure of or recurrence after embolization, whereas others advocate surgical obliteration as the primary modality of therapy. When a strategy of using embolization as the first line of treatment is used, published case series report DSAVF embolization cure rates of between 30% and 75%, depending on the series [15,21–25]. Song et al [26] reported that of 27 DSAVFs for which NBCA embolization was planned, treatment was technically feasible initially in 20 (75%) of 27 lesions. Of the 20 lesions actually embolized with NBCA, cure was achieved in 18, but recurrence of the fistula occurred in 3.

Despite the reported low morbidity of endovascular treatment for DSAVFs, some concerned about the risk of endovascular failure continue to advocate open surgical treatment as the primary mode of therapy [27–30].

Some of the recurrences of DSAVFs after embolization have been reported to occur because

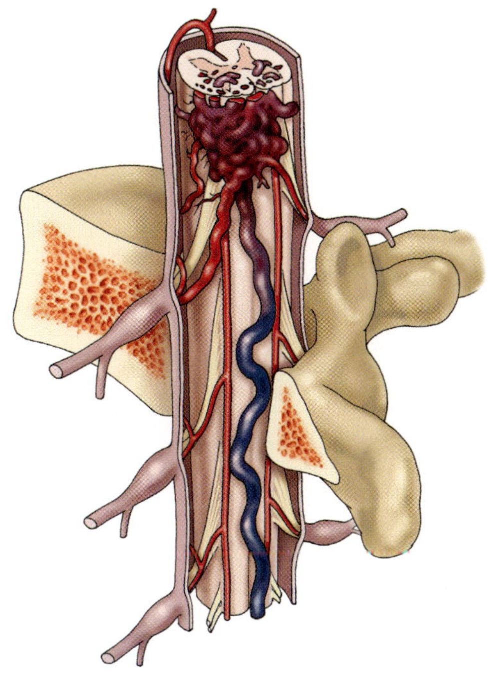

Fig. 5. Illustration of intramedullary compact arteriovenous malformation. Angiography is crucial in defining arterial supply. (Courtesy of Barrow Neurological Institute; with permission.)

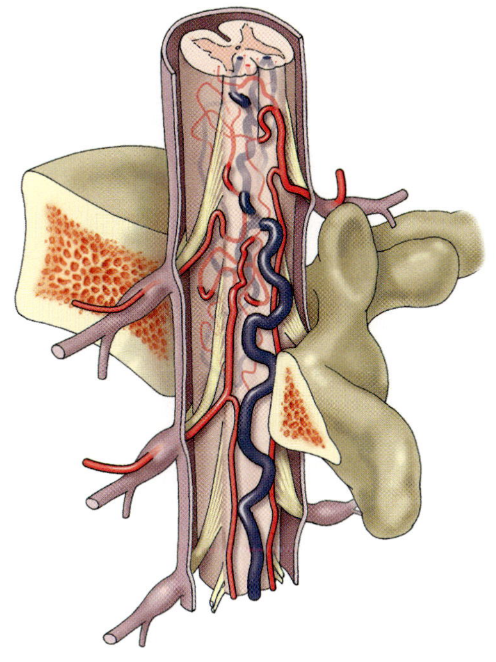

Fig. 6. Illustration of intramedullary diffuse arteriovenous malformation. (Courtesy of Barrow Neurological Institute; with permission.)

of partial embolization or embolization with particulate embolic materials. Partial embolization for treatment of DSAVFs is not helpful; in this regard, proximal embolization with particulate agents (eg, polyvinyl alcohol) is to be especially avoided [29,31]. Particulate embolizations carry the risk of proximal occlusion of the feeding arteries, obscuring the angiographic visualization of the fistula without improving the clinical condition. The fistula remains patent and the venous pressures pathologically elevated because the proximal feeding artery occlusion does not eliminate continued supply of the fistula through the rich collateral supply that typically exists more distally (ie, in the region of the fistula). Similarly, embolic agents that do not result in permanent occlusion of the fistula may permit recurrence of the condition. If endovascular treatment is to be considered, it is imperative that the fistula be thoroughly and permanently occluded. If any question in this regard persists, surgical exploration should be considered.

With liquid embolization materials, such as NBCA, DSAVFs can be treated effectively at the same session as the diagnostic angiography with little additional morbidity. Series reviewing endovascular treatment have found that NBCA embolization can be effective; however, as noted previously, there are treatment limitations. Adequate embolization must be achieved. "Adequate" embolization has been defined by Niimi et al [22] as (1) use of a liquid embolic material, (2) penetration of the embolic material to the fistulas or the draining vein, (3) angiographic disappearance of the fistulas or their drainage after embolization (determined by bilateral angiogram of two pedicles above and two pedicles below the level of the shunt as well as by angiography of the bilateral pedicles at the level of the shunt), and (4) no compromise of the venous drainage of the spinal cord after embolization. They reported adequate embolization in 87% of their patients after the introduction of variable stiffness microcatheters.

Fig. 9 illustrates a typical DSAVF treated endovascularly with NBCA, resulting in cure of the lesion.

Intradural ventral spinal arteriovenous fistulas

Intradural ventral spinal arteriovenous fistulas (IVSAVFs) are rare. This lesion was initially

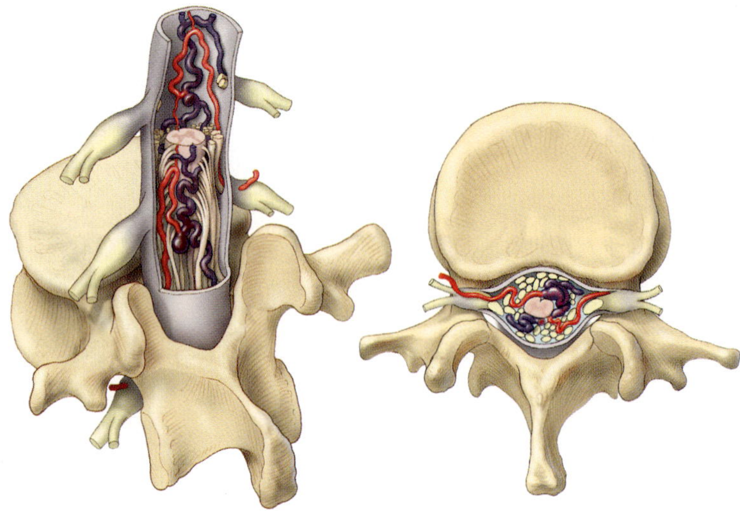

Fig. 7. Illustration of conus arteriovenous malformation. (*From* Spetzler RF, Detwiler PW, Riina HA, Porter RW. Modified classification of spinal cord vascular lesions. J Neurosurg (Spine 2) 2002;96:145–56; with permission.)

described by Djindjian et al [32] as an intradural extramedullary fistula. As the name implies, they are located ventral to the spinal cord, and their primary vascular supply is most often the ASA. They have previously been referred to as type IV lesions or perimedullary fistulas. These fistulas have been subdivided into three categories variously referred to as I, II, and III or a, b, and c in the literature, with the divisions being based on the volume of arteriovenous shunting [9,32–34]. They have been described in association with congenital syndromes, such as Rendu-Osler-Weber and Cobb's syndromes [9,32,35]. Clinical presentation is most often with hemorrhage, but patients may also present with progressive myelopathy, often secondary to compression from enlarged venous varices or venous hypertension [36].

Although IVSAVFs are rare, a clear understanding is important. Because there is no intramedullary component, there is a greater chance for cure and a lower treatment-related morbidity than is the case for intramedullary spinal arteriovenous malformations (ISAVMs). By contrast, the natural history poses significant risk for hemorrhage and neurologic disability. The involvement of the spinal medullary arteries can present major therapeutic challenges. While recognizing the critical vascular supply, these lesions can be accessed for endovascular treatment similar to an ESAVF. Again, because the ASA is frequently involved, the angioarchitecture must be well understood to be certain that closing the fistula will not compromise blood supply to the spinal cord distal to the fistula site. Excellent outcomes have been reported using embolization or surgical resection [36–38]. For larger lesions with relatively simple direct arteriovenous architecture, transvenous rather than transarterial catheterization is sometimes useful [35].

Extradural-intradural spinal arteriovenous malformations

Extradural-intradural spinal arteriovenous malformations (EISAVMs) are formidable lesions. They can rarely be cured without unacceptable morbidity [39]. They have been previously known by various names, such as type III, metameric, or juvenile AVMs. These lesions are characterized by the fact that they may involve multiple tissues (ie, they do not respect tissue boundaries). As a result, the AVM may extensively involve the neural elements, vertebral body, and adjacent cutaneous and soft tissues at the affected level. The moniker "metameric" stems from the fact that they are, in some instances, confined to a single segmental level. Fig. 3 is an illustration of this malformation.

As with other high-flow spinal lesions, symptoms may result from bleeding, direct compression, arterial steal, or venous hypertension [17]. Because these lesions are rarely curable, treatments are palliative and should be performed with

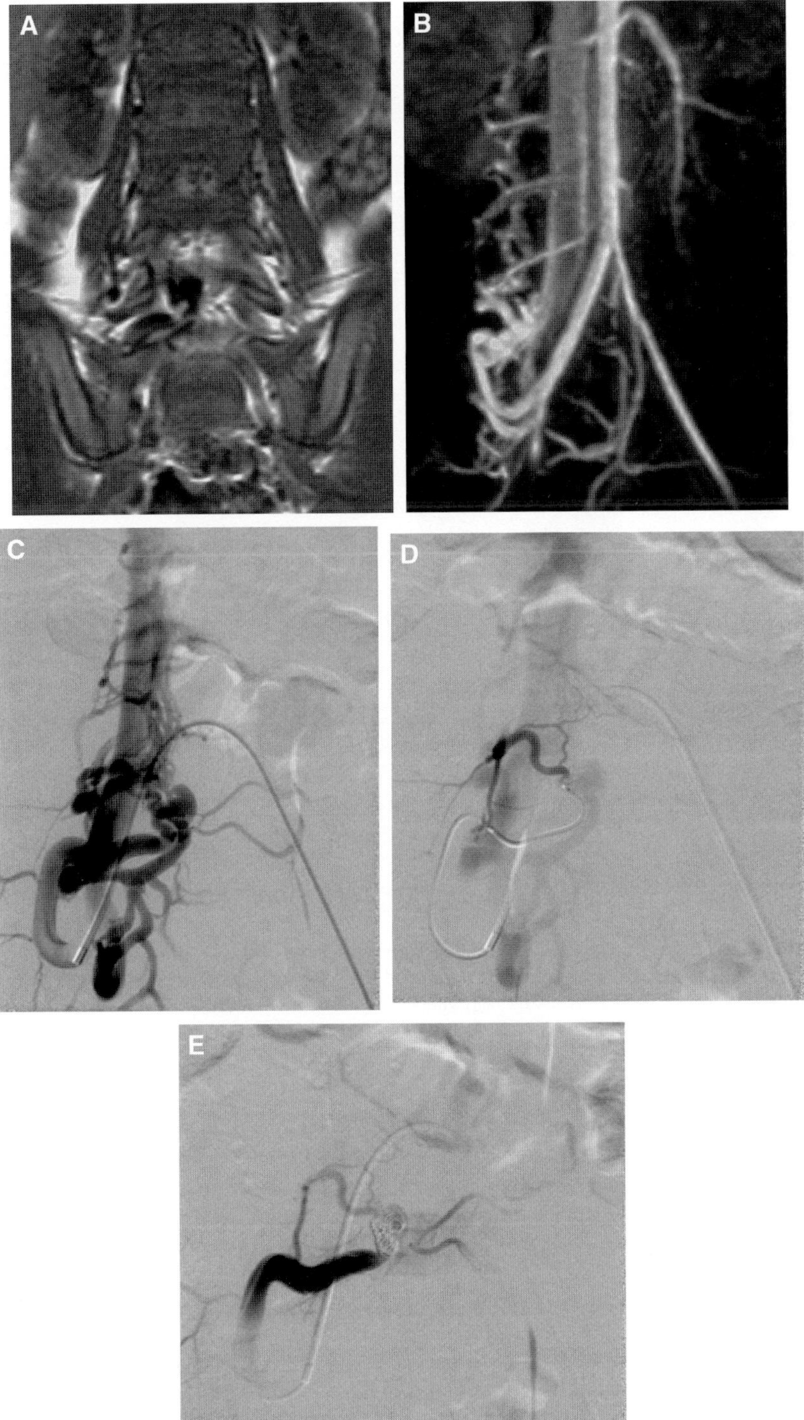

Fig. 8. (*A*) MRI and (*B*) magnetic resonance angiography demonstrate abnormally dilated extradural vessels in an 18-month-old girl. (*C*) Right internal iliac artery injection shows an extradural arteriovenous fistula. (*D*) The microcatheter is positioned on the venous side of the fistula. (*E*) Selective internal iliac artery injection after coil embolization of the fistula confirms its complete obliteration without venous shunting. The patient remains neurologically intact.

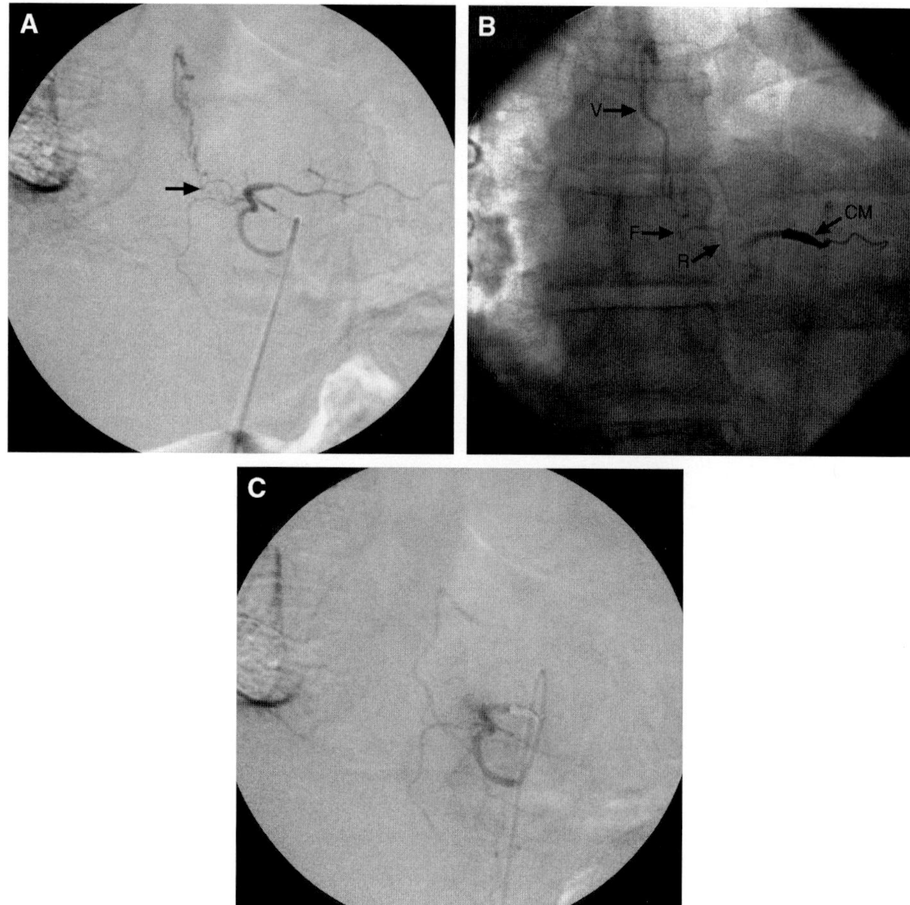

Fig. 9. (*A*) Intercostal artery injection in a 56-year-old man with progressive myelopathy shows an intradural dorsal arteriovenous fistula. (*B*) Unsubtracted image shows the coil mass (CM) within the intercostal branch. Glue is visible within the radiculomedullary feeder (R), fistula (F), and proximal vein (V). (*C*) Postembolization angiogram confirms complete obliteration of the fistula. The patient experienced immediate improvement in lower extremity paresthesias and weakness.

clearly identified goals in mind. The most straightforward situation is seen when symptoms and signs correlate well with a site of direct spinal cord compression by enlarged vascular structures. In this situation, the compressive lesion can be targeted with embolization to reduce or eliminate flow through this component of the malformation. This in itself may be adequate for the treatment goal or may be combined with subsequent surgical decompression. Fig. 10 illustrates a clinical example of an EISAVM. This 29-year-old man presented with progressive myelopathy. Angiography revealed an extensive AVM with large fistulas and high flow, resulting in marked engorgement of the draining veins. The arterial supply to the malformation was extensively embolized. This allowed surgical decompression of the compressing veins without concern for development of iatrogenic venous hypertension. After this staged combined therapy, the patient has enjoyed near-complete recovery from his myelopathy.

Intramedullary spinal arteriovenous malformations

ISAVMs have previously been known (among other names) as type II malformations and "classical" or "glomus" AVMs. The nidus may be discrete and compact, or it may be more diffuse. Angiography is essential to characterize the lesion and to identify potential associated aneurysms. These aneurysms are often identified as the source of subarachnoid hemorrhage in

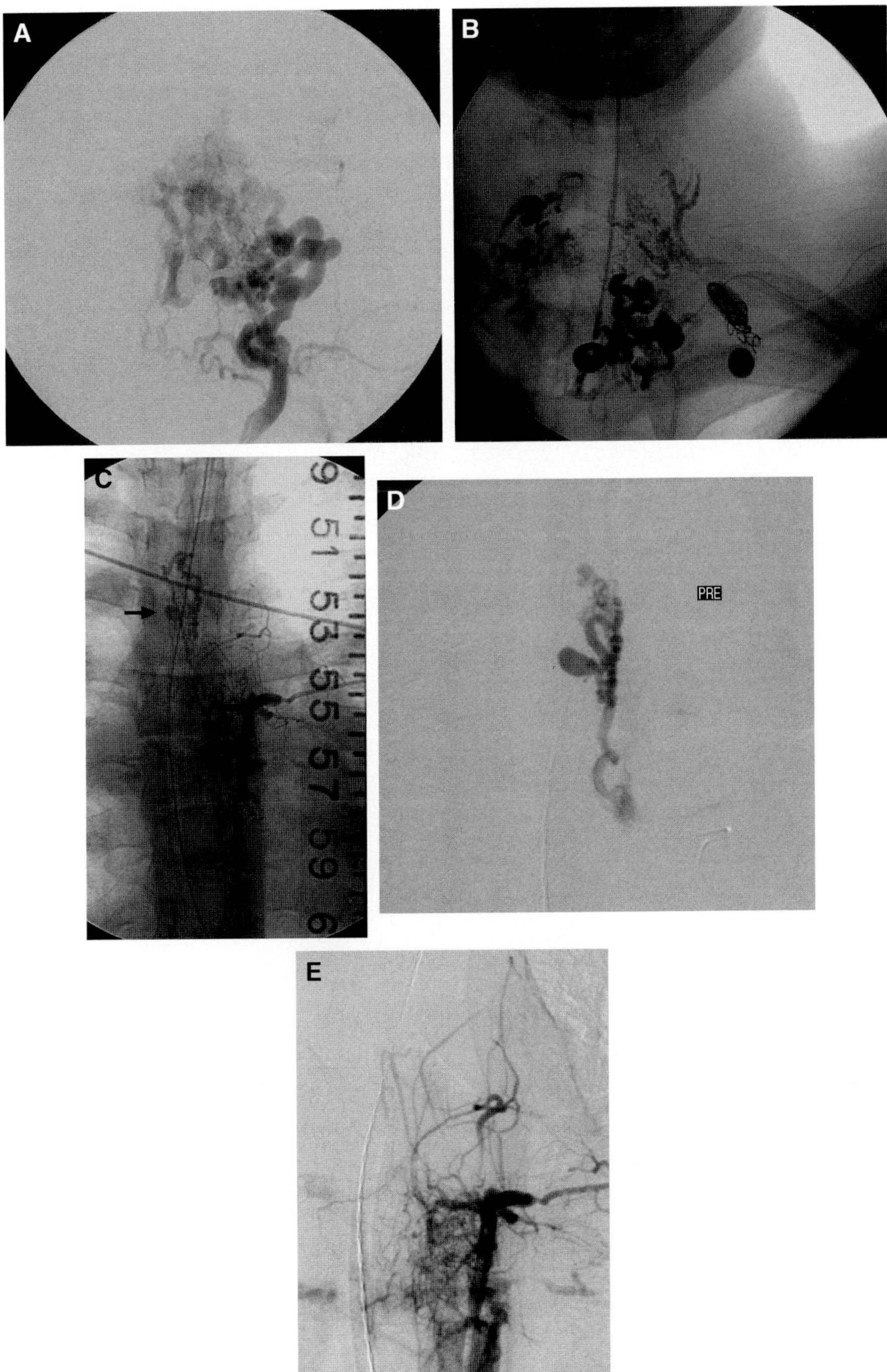

Fig. 10. (*A*) Angiogram shows a large cervicothoracic intradural-extradural (metameric) arteriovenous malformation (AVM) in a 29-year-old man. (*B*) Unsubtracted posterior-anterior view shows extensive coil and glue embolization of the anterior feeders and nidus. (*C*) Thoracic radicular injection shows residual AVM. (*D*) Microcatheter injection further defines the residual AVM and venous varix. (*E*) Posterior-anterior view confirms complete obliteration of the AVM and venous varix. The patient underwent complete resection of the AVM with improvement in myelopathy.

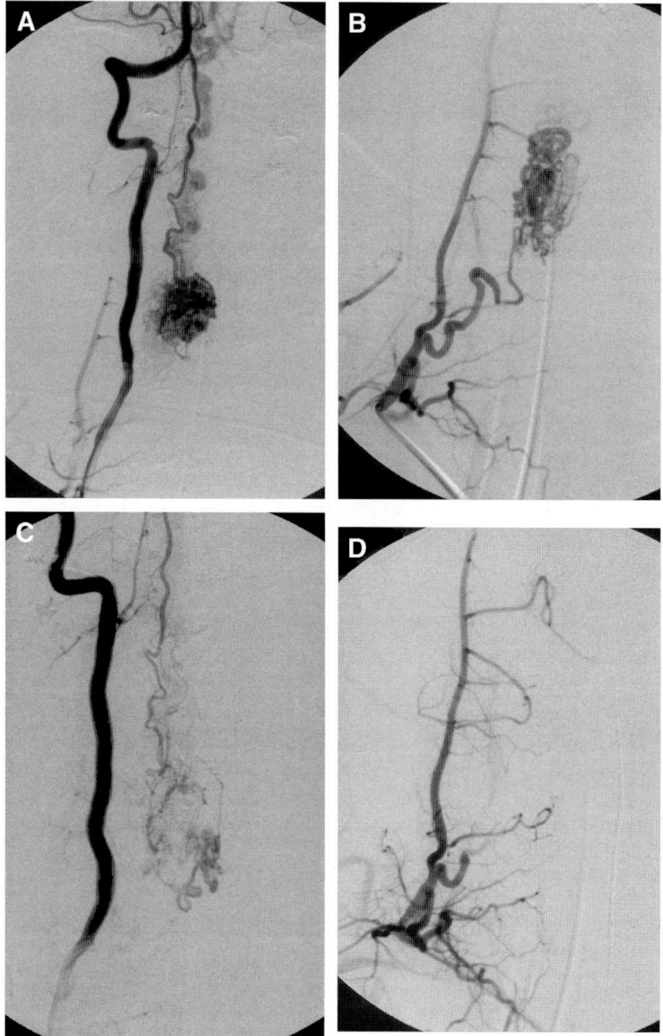

Fig. 11. (*A*) Right vertebral artery injection shows the blood supply to a diffuse intradural arteriovenous malformation (AVM) from the anterior spinal artery in an 18-year-old man with progressive weakness and myelopathy. (*B*) Thyrocervical trunk injection shows further blood supply via the ascending cervical and deep cervical branches. Postembolization vertebral (*C*) and thyrocervical trunk (*D*) injections show significant reduction in the arterial supply and size of the nidus. The patient underwent resection of the AVM, although a small anterior spinal artery feeder to the nidus remains.

patients with ISAVMs. When feeding artery aneurysms are identified, they should be seriously considered for treatment even if they have not produced hemorrhage. It has been reported that aneurysms on feeding arteries of spinal AVMs regress with treatment of the AVM itself in some cases [14,40].

Superselective catheterization is essential if embolization is to be undertaken. The ASA may be used to gain access to the malformation. The superselective angiogram must be carefully analyzed to ensure that no normal branches are put at risk. Embolization may be targeted to symptomatic components, such as ruptured feeding artery aneurysms, or may be used before surgery to facilitate surgical resection. Figs. 11 and 12 show examples of diffuse and compact ISAVMs involving the cervical spinal cord. Superselective

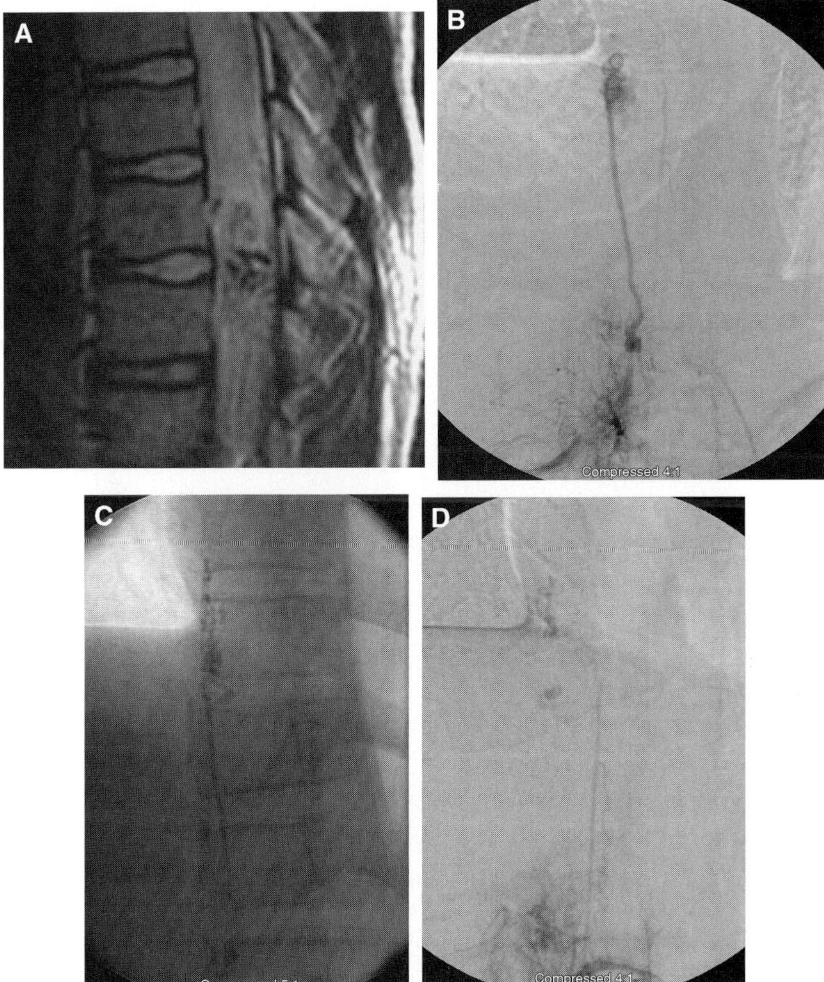

Fig. 12. (*A*) MRI shows a compact intradural arteriovenous malformation (AVM) at T9 to T10 in a 13-year-old boy with a gait disturbance. (*B*) Selective injection of the right T12 radicular branch shows the compact nidus. (*C*) Unsubtracted posterior-anterior view shows the glue cast within the arterial feeder and nidus. (*D*) Postembolization angiogram confirms minimal residual opacification of the AVM. The AVM was completely excised without complication.

angiography demonstrates typical positioning of the catheter before embolization. Recently, Molyneux and Coley [2] have reported excellent angiographic results in two cases treated with the new liquid embolic agent ethylene vinyl alcohol copolymer, which is delivered dissolved in dimethyl sulfoxide (Onyx).

Conus medullaris arteriovenous malformations

Conus medullaris arteriovenous malformations have been described as a distinct lesion by Hurst et al [13] and Spetzler et al [12]. This lesion may present like other conus lesions with combinations of myelopathy and cauda equina symptoms. A combination of a conus-based intramedullary AVM is seen together with multiple large direct AVFs [12]. This lesion is illustrated in Fig. 7. The extensive nature of these malformations makes them difficult to cure by embolization alone, but most flow may be eliminated by embolization, thereby greatly enhancing the chance for cure by surgical resection. Fig. 13 demonstrates a conus malformation embolized to an angiographic cure. This 47-year-old man presented with subarachnoid

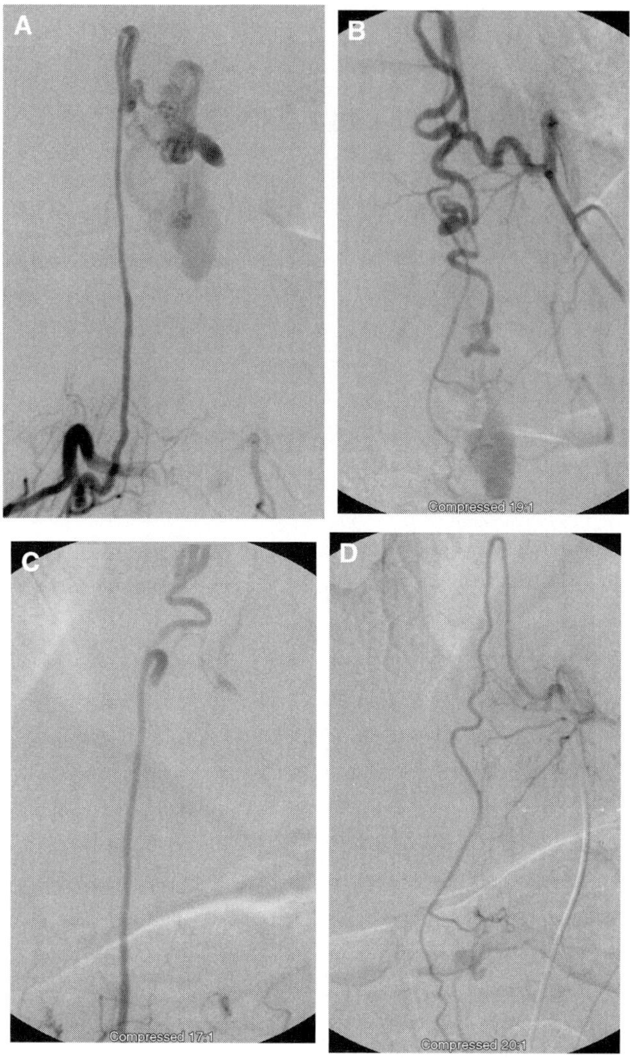

Fig. 13. (*A*) Right L2 injection shows the presence of a complex conus medullaris arteriovenous malformation (AVM) in a 47-year-old man with a history of subarachnoid hemorrhage and myelopathy. (*B*) Left T10 selective injection also shows the blood supply to the conus AVM. Postembolization right L2 (*C*) and left T10 (*D*) injections show almost complete obliteration of AVM supply. The patient underwent complete resection of the AVM. He is ambulatory and has retained bowel and bladder function.

hemorrhage. After embolization, surgical exploration and resection were performed. Interestingly, despite the postembolization impression of angiographic cure, components of patent malformation were identified at the time of surgical resection. For this reason, it may reasonable to consider surgical exploration even after the achievement of excellent embolization. Practically speaking, in most cases, embolization for this lesion is incomplete, and surgical excision should be performed after embolization. In most instances, cure of the lesion is possible and should be considered the treatment goal.

Summary

Endovascular techniques have evolved remarkably in the past 20 years since the advent of the variable stiffness microcatheter. Advances in imaging, embolic materials, and the ability to deliver embolic agents safely have facilitated dramatic improvements in our ability to care for patients with spinal axis vascular lesions. Even more important in this work has been the accompanying growth in our understanding of these lesions. It is hoped that continued progress will lead to even greater improvements in our ability to care for patients with these conditions.

References

[1] Sala F, Niimi Y, Krzan MJ, Berenstein A, Deletis V. Embolization of a spinal arteriovenous malformation: correlation between motor evoked potentials and angiographic findings: technical case report. Neurosurgery 1999;45(4):932–8.

[2] Molyneux AJ, Coley SC. Embolization of spinal cord arteriovenous malformations with an ethylene vinyl alcohol copolymer dissolved in dimethyl sulfoxide (Onyx liquid embolic system). Report of two cases. J Neurosurg 2000;93(2 Suppl):304–8.

[3] Aminoff MJ, Logue V. The prognosis of patients with spinal vascular malformations. Brain 1974;97: 211–8.

[4] Bao Y-H, Ling F. Classification and therapeutic modalities of spinal vascular malformations in 80 patients. Neurosurgery 1987;40:75–81.

[5] Borden JA, Wu JK, Shucart WA. A proposed classification for spinal and cranial dural arteriovenous malformations and implications for treatment. J Neurosurg 1995;82:166–79.

[6] Cahan LD, Higashida RT, Halbach VV, et al. Variants of radiculomeningeal vascular malformations of the spine. J Neurosurg 1987;66:333–7.

[7] Grote EH, Voigy K. Clinical syndromes, natural history and pathophysiology of vascular lesions of the spinal cord. Neurosurg Clin N Am 1999;10:17–45.

[8] Marsh WR. Vascular lesions of the spinal cord: history and classification. Neurosurg Clin N Am 1999; 10:1–8.

[9] Riche MC, Reizine D, Melki JP, Merland JJ. Classification of spinal cord vascular malformations. Radiat Med 1985;3:17–24.

[10] Rodesch G, Hurth M, Alvarez H, Tadie M, Lasjaunias P. Classification of spinal cord arteriovenous shunts: proposal for a reappraisal—the Bicetre experience with 155 consecutive patients treated between 1981 and 1999. Neurosurgery 2002;51:374–80.

[11] Rosenblum B, Oldfield EH, Doppman JL, et al. Spinal arteriovenous malformations: a comparison of dural arteriovenous fistulas and intradural AVMs in 81 patients. J Neurosurg 1987;67:795–802.

[12] Spetzler RF, Detwiler PW, Riina HA, Porter RW. Modified classification of spinal cord vascular lesions. J Neurosurg (Spine 2) 2002;96:145–56.

[13] Hurst RW, Bagley LJ, Marcotte P, Schut L, Flamm ES. Spinal cord arteriovenous fistulas involving the conus medullaris: presentation, management, and embryologic considerations. Surg Neurol 1999;52: 95–9.

[14] Konan AV, Raymond J, Roy D. Transarterial embolization of aneurysms associated with spinal cord arteriovenous malformations. Report of four cases. J Neurosurg 1999;90(1 Suppl):148–54.

[15] Westphal M, Koch C. Management of spinal dural arteriovenous fistulae using an interdisciplinary neuroradiological/neurosurgical approach: experience with 47 cases. Neurosurgery 1999;45:451–8.

[16] Asai J, Hayashi T, Fujimoto T, Suzuki R. Exclusively epidural arteriovenous fistula in the cervical spine with spinal cord symptoms: case report. Neurosurgery 2001;48:1372–5.

[17] Goyal M, Willinsky R, Montanera W, terBrugge K. Paravertebral arteriovenous malformations with epidural drainage: clinical spectrum, imaging features and results of treatment. AJNR Am J Neuroradiol 1999;20:749–55.

[18] Lee TT, Gromelski EB, Bowen BC, Green BA. Diagnostic and surgical management of spinal dural arteriovenous fistulas. Neurosurgery 1998;43(2):242–6.

[19] Song JK, Vinuela F, Gobin YP, Duckwiler GR, Murayama Y, Kureshi I, et al. Surgical and endovascular treatment of spinal dural arteriovenous fistulas: long-term disability assessment and prognostic factors. J Neurosurg 2001;94(2 Suppl): 199–204.

[20] McCutcheon IE, Doppman JL, Oldfield EH. Microvascular anatomy of dural arteriovenous abnormalities of the spine: a microangiographic study. J Neurosurg 1996;84:215–20.

[21] Eskandar EN, Borges LF, Budzik RF, Putman CM, Ogilvy CS. Spinal dural arteriovenous fistulas: experience with endovascular and surgical therapy. J Neurosurg 2002;96(2 Suppl):162–7.

[22] Niimi Y, Berenstein A, Setton A, Neophytides A. Embolization of spinal dural arteriovenous fistulae: results and follow-up clinical study. Neurosurgery 1997;40:675–83.

[23] Niimi Y, Berenstein A. Endovascular treatment of spinal vascular malformations. Neurosurg Clin N Am 1999;10(1):47–71.

[24] Symon L, Kuyama H, Kendall B. Dural arteriovenous malformations of the spine. Clinical and surgical results in 55 cases. J Neurosurg 1984;60(2): 238–47.

[25] Tacconi L, Lopez-Izquierdo BC, Symon L. Outcome and prognostic factors in the surgical treatment of spinal dural arteriovenous fistulas. A long-term study. Br J Neurosurg 1997;11(4):298–305.

[26] Song JK, Gobin YP, Duckwiler GR, Murayama Y, Frazee JG, Martin NA, et al. N-butyl 2-cyanoacrylate embolization of spinal dural arteriovenous fistulae. AJNR Am J Neuroradiol 2001; 22(1):40–7.

[27] Anson JA, Spetzler RF. Spinal dural arteriovenous malformations. In: Awad IA, Barrow DL, editors. Dural arteriovenous malformations. Park Ridge,

IL: American Association of Neurological Surgeons; 1995. p. 175–91.
[28] Hall WA, Oldfield EH, Doppman JL. Recanalization of spinal arteriovenous malformations following embolization. J Neurosurg 1989;70:714–20.
[29] Morgan MK, Marsh WR. Management of spinal dural arteriovenous malformations. J Neurosurg 1989;70(6):832–6.
[30] Watson JC, Oldfield EH. The surgical management of spinal dural vascular malformations. Neurosurg Clin N Am 1999;10(1):73–87.
[31] Nichols DA, Rufenacht DA, Jack CR Jr, Forbes GS. Embolization of spinal dural arteriovenous fistula with polyvinyl alcohol particles: experience in 14 patients. AJNR Am J Neuroradiol 1992;13(3): 933–40.
[32] Djindjian M, Djindjian R, Rey A, et al. Intradural extramedullary spinal arteriovenous malformations fed by the anterior spinal artery. Surg Neurol 1977; 8:85–93.
[33] Gueguen B, Merland JJ, Riche MC, Rey A. Vascular malformations of the spinal cord: intrathecal perimedullary arteriovenous fistulas fed by medullary arteries. Neurology 1987;37:969–79.
[34] Riche MC, Merland JJ. Embolization of spinal cord vascular malformations via the anterior spinal artery. AJNR Am J Neuroradiol 1983;4:378–81.
[35] Halbach VV, Higashida RT, Dowd CF, Fraser KW, Edwards MS, Barnwell SL. Treatment of giant intradural (perimedullary) arteriovenous fistulas. Neurosurgery 1993;33:972–80.
[36] Hida K, Iwasaki Y, Goto G, Miyasaka K, Abe H. Results of the surgical treatment of perimedullary arteriovenous fistulas with special reference to embolization. J Neurosurg (Spine 2) 1999;90:198–205.
[37] Barrow DL, Colohan ART, Dawson R. Intradural perimedullary arteriovenous fistulas (Type IV spinal cord arteriovenous malformations). J Neurosurg 1994;81:221–9.
[38] Mourier KL, Gobin YP, George B, Lot G, Merland JJ. Intradural perimedullary arteriovenous fistulae: results of surgical and endovascular treatment in a series of 35 cases. Neurosurgery 1993;32:885–91.
[39] Spetzler RF, Zabramski JM, Flom RA. Management of juvenile spinal AVMs by embolization and operative excision: case report. J Neurosurg 1989; 70(4):628–32.
[40] Biondi A, Merland JJ, Hodes JE, Aymard A, Reizine D. Aneurysms of spinal arteries associated with intramedullary arteriovenous malformations. II. Results of AVM endovascular treatment and hemodynamic considerations. AJNR Am J Neuroradiol 1992;13:923–31.

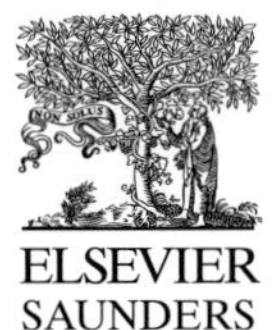
ELSEVIER
SAUNDERS

Neurosurg Clin N Am 16 (2005) 411–432

NEUROSURGERY
CLINICS
OF NORTH AMERICA

Preoperative Embolization of Central Nervous System Tumors

Vivek R. Deshmukh, MD, David J. Fiorella, MD, Cameron G. McDougall, MD, Robert F. Spetzler, MD, Felipe C. Albuquerque, MD*

Division of Neurological Surgery, Barrow Neurological Institute, St. Joseph's Hospital and Medical Center, 350 West Thomas Road, Phoenix, AZ 85013, USA

Surgical excision of hypervascular central nervous system (CNS) tumors can be daunting and is associated with the potential for staggering blood loss. The need to mitigate intraoperative tumoral hemorrhage has fostered the refinement of neuroendovascular techniques for preoperative embolization of tumors. Since these techniques were first described in the early 1970s, the field has matured rapidly, with advances in microcatheter technology and ongoing improvements in the design of embolisates. Nonetheless, the tenets fundamental to embolization of tumors are not novel. They include an understanding of neurovascular anatomy and of the natural history and behavior of tumors.

Principles of embolization

Tumor embolization is defined as the interruption of blood supply to a tumor. The goal of preoperative embolization is to decrease intraoperative blood loss. Embolization-induced tumor ischemia often softens a tumor, thereby facilitating its resection and reducing the compression exerted on nearby neural structures. Theoretically, tumor resection then becomes safer and more complete. Other purported goals of embolization are to reduce operating time, to relieve intractable pain, and to decrease the likelihood of a recurrence.

Pre-embolization procedure

If a patient is identified as having a hypervascular tumor on preoperative MRI, the surgical team should discuss the utility of preoperative embolization. In many cases, surgical resection may not be undertaken safely without embolization and vice versa. The tumor surgeon and the neuroendovascular surgeon must agree on the goals of embolization and on the degree of aggressiveness required. These goals are tailored to each patient.

Embolization procedure

Embolization may be transarterial via a transfemoral route or via direct puncture of the tumor. Embolization may be performed in a single session, or it may be staged. Typically, patients undergo angiography and particulate embolization under conscious sedation. Conscious sedation permits provocative testing of the cranial nerves and balloon test occlusion of the carotid artery as needed. The location of the tumor dictates the vessels to be examined. A thorough examination of the external carotid artery (ECA) is mandatory. If N-butyl cyanoacrylate (NBCA) glue is used, the patient may be placed under general anesthesia or conscious sedation. We prefer general anesthesia, because the hazards associated with patient movement are magnified during glue embolization. Somatosensory evoked potentials and

* Corresponding author. c/o Neuroscience Publications, Barrow Neurological Institute, 350 West Thomas Road, Phoenix, AZ 85013, USA.

E-mail address: neuropub@chw.edu (F.C. Albuquerque).

1042-3680/05/$ - see front matter
doi:10.1016/j.nec.2004.08.010

electroencephalography are monitored routinely by our group.

The size of the femoral sheath should be tailored to the surgical goals, and attention should be given to the necessity of a balloon delivery system. A coaxial Envoy (Cordis, Miami, Florida) guiding catheter and a UCSF-3 (Cordis) catheter are advanced to the ECA or internal carotid artery (ICA). The UCSF-3 catheter is removed or steered selectively into an ECA branch to provide further support of the microcatheter system.

Once an embolizable arterial supply is identified, a microcatheter is advanced coaxially through the guiding catheter to the feeding artery with the use of fluoroscopic roadmap guidance. The microcatheter is navigated to the most distal point. We prefer using the new-generation hydrophilic microcatheters and microwires (wire diameter is typically 0.014 or 0.010 mm). Embolization is performed with polyvinyl alcohol (PVA) particles or NBCA glue embolisate.

Before embolization begins, several anatomic factors should be assessed: the presence of extracranial-intracranial (EC-IC) anastomoses, shared arterial supply between tumor and normal structures, the caliber of tumor vessels, and the potential for embolisate to reflux into the parent vessel. These factors are best evaluated by careful superselective microcatheter angiography. Embolization is most beneficial for tumors primarily supplied by the ECA [1,2]. For particulates, the number of emboli that reach a vascular tumor depends on the blood flow to the lesion relative to the rest of the brain. Therefore, selective catheterization allows a maximal amount of embolisate to be delivered to the lesion.

Occlusion of the proximal feeding arteries only reduces blood flow to the tumor temporarily. Collateral supply quickly develops, and the beneficial effect of the embolization is short-lived. Occlusion of proximal arteries may, however, be considered if access to distal supply is poor. The logical end point for embolization is an angiographically demonstrated decrease in the vascularity of the tumor with preservation of normal arterial territories. The ideal barometers for efficacy of embolization include MRI-verified tumor infarction, histologic evidence of tumor necrosis, ease of surgical resection, and mitigation of intraoperative blood loss.

The introduction of variable stiffness and hydrophilic microcatheters has permitted microvascular selectivity. For tumors with significant blood supply from the cavernous ICA, embolization can be performed via direct microcatheterization of these small branches. If technically infeasible, another option [3,4] (used by C.G.M) is occlusion of the distal ICA with a nondetachable balloon and subsequent infusion of embolic material (typically PVA or ethanol) into the segment of the ICA supplying the tumor. Before the balloon is deflated, this region of the ICA must be flushed with heparinized saline (at least 20 mL). A similar volume is withdrawn from the guiding catheter to irrigate the ICA. Theron et al [4] believe that this balloon-assisted technique may be used for hypervascular lesions supplied by branches of the vertebral artery (ie, posterior inferior cerebellar artery [PICA]). Garcia-Cervinon et al [5], however, described four patients who developed balloon-related complications (balloon displacement/migration and failed balloon deflation). None of these patients suffered a permanent neurologic complication. Balloon-assisted embolization must be used judiciously because of the distal migration of embolic material on balloon deflation and because of potential vessel endothelial injury from ethanol.

Pial vessels are fragile and are thus associated with a high risk of arterial perforation and intracranial hemorrhage. The potential for stroke from thromboembolism within pial vessels is also higher than the risk of thromboembolic complications within the circulation of the ECA.

When a hypervascular tumor is supplied by the ophthalmic artery, embolization may be performed safely if a few principles are followed. First, embolization must be performed only if it is essential and only if the embolized vessel cannot readily be accessed surgically. The central retinal artery and choroidal blush must be visualized. Embolisates must not be allowed to enter the central retinal artery. A lidocaine or Amytal (sodium amobarbital) test may be performed to verify that occlusion of ophthalmic artery branches will not cause blindness. If the central retinal artery is thought to be at high risk, coils or larger diameter embolisates (>400 μm) may be used. Their use does not guarantee the integrity of the central retinal artery, however. Lefkowitz et al [6] embolized three anterior skull base meningiomas and one nasal angiofibroma via the ophthalmic artery. One patient experienced transient visual deterioration after embolization with PVA (700–1000-μm particles).

Intraoperative percutaneous tumor puncture has been advocated for tumors predominantly supplied by the ICA or pial vessels. Patients whose ECA has already been sacrificed are perhaps better served with direct tumor puncture. Casasco et al [7] recommended the use of intraoperative fluoroscopy to assist with the embolization. If reflux into the feeding arteries is visualized, embolization should cease. They also advocated using this technique for palliation in patients with inoperable tumors or for the treatment of elderly or debilitated patients. For lesions not readily amenable to endovascular therapy, George et al [8] delivered NBCA embolisate before or during surgery directly into superficial tumors with a standard 18- or 19-gauge needle and directly into deeply seated tumors with a 16-gauge Teflon sheath needle. Of 21 patients with tumors, such as juvenile nasopharyngeal angiofibromas, hemangiopericytomas, or metastases, who were treated with this technique, no patient suffered a permanent neurologic complication.

Postembolization procedure

After embolization, patients should be monitored in an intensive care unit for 24 hours. Particular attention must be paid to periprocedural stroke, cranial nerve deficits, or intracranial hemorrhage. Corticosteroids are recommended for large tumors associated with significant surrounding edema. Postembolization MRI is often obtained for the purpose of frameless stereotaxy. These images should be reviewed for intracranial hemorrhage or exacerbation of peritumoral edema. Such findings may warrant more urgent surgical excision.

Radiographic effects of embolization

Radiographic demonstration of tumor necrosis after particulate embolization seems to be indiscriminate. Terada et al [9] noted disappearance of tumor flow voids after embolization with Gelfoam or PVA. Most tumors showed a decrease in the level of contrast enhancement. Bendszus et al [10] found that more completely embolized tumors showed less contrast enhancement on postembolization MRI. Wakhloo et al [11], however, reported diminished enhancement on contrast MRI in only 2 of 14 patients after embolization with 150- to 300-μm particulates. They theorized that this disappointing radiographic result reflected proximal occlusion of the feeding arteries by larger particulates. Grand et al [12] described only a minimal decrease in tumor enhancement after embolization and attributed this discrepancy to vasospasm of the embolized vessels. Therefore, smaller particulates may allow embolization of more distal capillaries, increasing the likelihood of tumor necrosis after embolization.

Timing of embolization

The optimal timing for preoperative embolization is controversial [13–15]. Some authors recommend surgical resection 1 to 5 days after embolization [15–17], whereas others advocate waiting 1 to 2 weeks [13]. With time, embolization-induced necrosis shrinks and softens the tumor, thereby facilitating surgical resection. Compared with more proximal occlusion, delivering microemboli directly into the tumor maximizes this necrotic effect. The potential for recanalization of embolized vessels and collateral development increases if surgical resection is significantly delayed (>1 week). In contrast, Kai et al [18] retrospectively reviewed 45 patients with meningiomas embolized with cellulose porous beads. Resectability was greatest in tumors excised 7 to 9 days after embolization. The consensus remains, however, that the greatest benefit is derived from embolization if surgical resection is performed within a few days of embolization [2,17,19].

Embolisates

The ideal embolic agent should be permanent, easily deployed, and should not encumber tumor resection. Historically, various embolic agents have been used for the preoperative embolization of tumors. These permanent or temporary embolic agents include liquid tissue adhesives, such as NBCA and silicone rubber, and particulates, such as silastic beads, lyophilized dura mater, phenytoin, microspheres [20], microfibrillar collagen [21], oxidized cellulose, gelatin sponge, PVA [22], and fibrin glue [14]. Ethanol and detachable coils should also be included in this armamentarium.

Polyvinyl alcohol

PVA is the most common particulate agent used. It can be used for all tumors, including those with associated with high blood flow and arteriovenous shunting. PVA is shaved into precisely sized particles from an original block form [23–25]. The size of particles can range from 50 to 150 μm to 500 to 1200 μm.

Large embolisates do not penetrate deeply into tumor tissue, but they pose less risk of embolizing adjacent normal tissue. Smaller particulates and liquid agents penetrate deeply into the tumor but also have the potential to migrate into normal territory. PVA is delivered until stasis of contrast is noted in the embolized vessel. Should any reflux be visible, embolization should be discontinued.

PVA has several advantages. The particles are inert and water insoluble. They are absorbed slowly and are known to expand to occlude arteries with a diameter larger than the inner diameter of the microcatheter. They produce a vigorous inflammatory reaction. Polymorphonuclear proteins predominate at 2 weeks; a giant cell reaction occurs at 3 months; and an adherent, organized, partially calcified thrombus appears at 9 months [24,26]. PVA embolisate is long lasting but not permanent. Degradation occurs within several weeks to months. Technically, PVA is easy to deliver. The risk of stroke or cranial nerve palsy with the use of PVA particles diminishes as larger particles are used. PVA, however, has limitations. Early recanalization can occur when thrombus between the particles is dissolved by endogenous lytics. Furthermore, the high friction coefficient of PVA can lead to frequent catheter obstruction.

Tissue adhesive embolisate

NBCA glue embolisate is a stable, nonabsorbable, liquid polymerizing agent that is commonly used to treat arteriovenous malformations (AVMs) or fistulas and, less frequently, tumors. NBCA is mixed with an oil-based contrast agent (Ethiodol [ethiodized oil]), usually at a ratio of 1 mL to 2.5 mL. This formulation polymerizes immediately on contact with ionic solution or blood and occludes distal and proximal feeders almost simultaneously.

NBCA is a more permanent agent than PVA, and it immediately obliterates the feeding branch. NBCA is used with tumors less often than PVA because of its tendency to occlude distal and proximal vessels, which may be associated with a greater likelihood of cranial nerve injury or stroke. The delivery of NBCA has technical constraints that require experience to use it successfully. When used for ophthalmic lesions, NBCA can cause ocular myositis, resulting in ocular pain [6]. If acrylic glue is used for embolization, microcatheters can get caught or break, particularly if the microcatheter is bathed in the glue for an inordinate length of time [27].

Cellulose beads and microspheres

Cellulose porous beads also have been used for the preoperative embolization of tumors. Their favorable properties include a uniform size, a specific gravity similar to that of blood, and a positive charge that prevents clumping. Hamada et al [28] performed a prospective clinical trial in which 16 patients (13 with tumors) underwent embolization with cellulose porous beads measuring 150 or 200 μm. None of the patients suffered complications. Postembolization angiography showed satisfactory stasis in all cases. Histologic analysis of embolized vessels demonstrated no stretching of the embolized vessel and only mild inflammatory reactions. Trisacryl gelatin microspheres are a hydrophilic, nonabsorbable, collagen-coated agent, which is calibrated, deformable, and tends not to aggregate. Progressively larger embospheres may be used in the course of embolization. Bendszus et al [29] compared trisacryl gelatin microspheres with PVA particles in achieving distal microembolization and in mitigating intraoperative blood loss. Their most important finding was that the microspheres penetrated more distally than PVA particles. Further investigations are needed to establish the role of cellulose beads and microspheres in this arena.

Alcohol

Alcohol is a powerful sclerotic and cytotoxic agent that allows small-caliber arterial feeders to be obliterated. Its capacity to devascularize is potent. It causes anoxic cell damage, protein precipitation, and fibrinoid necrosis of the intimal lining [30]. Because its viscosity is low, alcohol can permeate more distally than other agents and cause sclerosis from within the tumor. The use of ethyl alcohol, however, is associated with a high risk of cranial nerve deficits or normal tissue infarction [3,22]. It also induces a robust inflammatory response that obliterates tissue planes and is directly toxic to the parent vessel and target tissue. Horowitz et al [31] embolized a carotid body tumor with ethanol in conjunction with distal balloon occlusion. They circumvented the limitations mentioned previously by reducing the dosing rate (4×10^{-5} mL/kg/s) and resecting the lesions within 24 hours of embolization. During surgery, alcohol injected intratumorally has yielded devascularization. Before alcohol is injected, aspiration is necessary to verify that a large vessel is not receiving this sclerotic agent. Lonser et al [32] treated three spinal epidural masses and one posterior fossa hemangioblastoma with direct intratumoral injection of ethanol. They avoided exposing normal tissues and used a small needle (28-gauge) to introduce the embolisate into the tumor. The end point was visible blanching of the tumor. They recommended intratumoral injection of ethanol as an inexpensive universally available method of augmenting preoperative embolization. Ethanol has proven to be a powerful embolisate with a well-defined, albeit limited, role.

Coils

The primary utility of coils in tumor embolization is their ability to augment or facilitate the effects of other embolisates. Liquid or fibered coils are most commonly used for tumor embolization. Liquid coils are soft and injectable. Fibered coils are pushed mechanically through the microcatheter with a coil pusher. Coils may be used to obliterate potentially dangerous EC-IC connections before embolization with particulates. After particulate embolization, they also can be used to obliterate the proximal aspect of a feeding artery to reduce the rate of recanalization.

Gelatin foam

Gelatin foam particles are typically 40 to 60 μm; therefore, their use achieves deep tissue penetration with subsequent necrosis. Gelfoam has the advantage of being easy to use; it is easily delivered through a microcatheter without friction or blockage. It is quickly degraded by native proteolytic mechanisms, however. Embolized vessels thus recanalize fairly rapidly. Furthermore, their small caliber increases the risks of embolization of the vaso vasorum of the cranial nerves and of unpredictable embolization via EC-IC collaterals. As with other embolisates, there is a learning curve in avoiding these complications.

Fibrin glue

Fibrin glue has been used successfully to embolize tumors. The radiopacity of the fibrin glue enables continuous monitoring during embolization. Probst et al [14] argue that fibrin allows the most distal loading of the vascular bed and decreases the potential for reflux. In their series of 80 patients in whom fibrin glue was used for embolization, 2 patients suffered permanent neurologic deficits (hypesthesia in the trigeminal nerve distribution and incomplete facial paresis).

Microfibrillar collagen

Microfibrillar collagen is prepared from purified bovine collagen. It is frequently used as a topical agent during surgery and effectively controls capillary hemorrhage. It promotes platelet aggregation and is effective even in the presence of underlying coagulopathies or heparinization. Kumar et al [21] contend that the semiliquid suspension readily passes through microcatheters and that the collagen can penetrate end arteries more effectively than PVA.

Phenytoin

Phenytoin is rarely used as an embolisate. Kasuya et al [33] demonstrated that phenytoin administered via a microcatheter at a dose of 250 to 500 mg resulted in ischemic and hemorrhagic necrosis with devascularization of meningiomas. They suggested that phenytoin has the added advantages of producing precapillary microthrombosis and more complete devascularization than other agents. They recommended the perioperative administration of steroids as prophylaxis against malignant edema.

Miscellaneous

Kubo et al [34] used hydroxyapatite ceramic microparticles to embolize meningiomas in 13 patients. They noted excellent biocompatibility, good injection control, and excellent occlusion of the distal capillary bed. No microcatheters became clogged. Histologic analysis revealed mild inflammation with lymphocytic infiltration. No patient suffered a hemorrhage after embolization.

Complications of embolization

Minor and major complications can be associated with preoperative embolization. Table 1 illustrates the complications that we have noted in patients treated since 1995 at our institution. The most common complications of embolization are fever and localized pain [35]. Potentially more devastating complications include inadvertent delivery of embolisate into the intracranial circulation, intracranial or intratumoral hemorrhage, and cranial nerve injury.

Embolization of ECA branches can be complicated by unrecognized collateral connections with the posterior circulation or ICA, resulting in delivery of embolisate into the intracranial circulation. EC-IC collaterals that warrant particular note include the anastomosis between the

Table 1
Complications of tumor embolization (Barrow Neurological Institute series: n = 52)

Complication	Number (%)
Death	0 (0)
Stroke	0 (0)
Postoperative fever	1 (2)
Arterial perforation (extracranial)	1 (2)
Cranial nerve deficits	(4)
Transient	2
Permanent	0
IC embolization through EC-IC collaterals (asymptomatic)	1 (2)

Abbreviations: EC, indicates extracranial; IC, intracranial.

ophthalmic artery and the meningolacrimal branch of the middle meningeal artery. Branches of the middle meningeal and accessory meningeal arteries can have reciprocal communications with branches of the cavernous segment of the ICA. The vertebral artery shares collaterals with the ascending pharyngeal artery and the occipital artery at the odontoid arterial arch and the interspaces of C1 to C2, respectively. The internal maxillary artery may have reciprocal connections with branches of the cavernous ICA, namely, between the artery of the foramen rotundum and the anterolateral branch of the inferolateral trunk, between the accessory meningeal artery and the posteromedial branch of the inferolateral trunk, and between the middle meningeal artery and the posterolateral branch of the inferolateral trunk.

In the presence of an unrecognized patent foramen ovale, Horowitz et al [36] showed that particulate embolization may result in paradoxic embolization and subsequent stroke. They recommended the liberal use of neurophysiologic monitoring in patients undergoing general anesthesia and frequent neurologic examinations in sedated patients. Intraoperative monitoring of somatosensory evoked potentials has increased the safety of embolization by enabling the early identification of ischemia [37].

Embolization can injure cranial nerves by interrupting the vascular supply of the cranial nerves (vaso vasorum), which is often derived from the ECA. A petrous branch of the middle meningeal artery may supply the facial nerve, and the neuromeningeal branch of the ascending pharyngeal artery frequently supplies the spinal accessory and hypoglossal nerves. The potential blood supply of a cranial nerve cannot readily be identified from the dynamic anatomic information provided by angiography; therefore, provocative testing with lidocaine has been used to determine if a potentially embolizable branch supplies a cranial nerve. Horton and Kerber [38] described 26 patients who underwent the injection of 2% lidocaine mixed in equal volumes with Conray 60 (Mallinckrodt, St. Louis, Missouri). The injection (30–70 mL) was monitored with continuous fluoroscopy to ensure that no reflux occurred into the ICA. Continuous cardiac monitoring was also performed. Patients with heart block did not undergo this lidocaine challenge. Patients underwent embolization with PVA and Gelfoam particles if cranial nerve function remained stable. If the lidocaine test result was positive, the catheter was removed from the vessel and the palsy was allowed to resolve. The use of provocative testing with lidocaine for potentially embolizable intracranial branches is not widespread, because the rates of false-positive and false-negative results are high and because reflux of lidocaine intracranially can cause seizures.

Applications of preoperative embolization

The principles of embolization, choice of embolic agents, and potential complications associated with commonly embolized tumors, namely, meningiomas, hemangiopericytomas, hemangioblastomas, paragangliomas, and juvenile nasopharyngeal angiofibromas, are discussed next. An abbreviated list of hypervascular CNS tumors is given in Box 1. The variety of hypervascular tumors embolized at our institution is demonstrated in Table 2, the Barrow Neurological Institute experience since 1995.

Meningiomas

Meningiomas are typically benign and potentially curable tumors. The cell of origin is the arachnoid cap cell. They constitute 13% to 18% of intracranial tumors and have a female predominance [39]. Rates of tumor recurrence have been estimated at 9% to 11% if the dural attachment is excised, at 19% to 22% if the dural attachment is left in place, and at almost 40% if the tumor is excised subtotally [40–43]. Incomplete tumor removal may be related to tumoral hemorrhage during surgery, particularly with hypervascular meningiomas. Angiography allows the arterial supply to the tumor to be determined. It shows the site of dural attachment; the presence

Box 1. Hypervascular central nervous system tumors

Intra-axial
Hemangioblastomas
Metastatic tumors
Glioblastomas multiforme

Extra-axial
Meningiomas
Hemangiopericytomas
Juvenile nasopharyngeal angiofibromas
Paragangliomas
Schwannomas
Hemangioendotheliomas

Skull tumors
Aneurysmal bone cysts
Hemangiomas
Ewing's sarcomas
Mesenchymal chondrosarcomas

of displacement; or the degree of encasement of key vascular structures, including the dural venous sinuses. It also helps to determine the vascularity of a tumor.

The vascular supply of meningiomas is twofold. Arterial feeders to the pedicle at the site of attachment and center of the tumor typically arise from branches of the ECA and supply the tumor radially to produce the characteristic "sunburst" appearance on angiography. The apex of the sunburst is usually the site of dural attachment. In most cases, pial and cortical arteries supply the capsule, and this contribution increases as the tumor enlarges. Dural pedicle feeders from the ECA include the middle meningeal artery, accessory meningeal artery, neuromeningeal branch of the ascending pharyngeal artery, and stylomastoid branch of the occipital artery. The dural supply from the ICA is usually from the ethmoidal, cavernous, clival, or tentorial branches. Depending on the location of the meningioma, the primary supply to the meningioma may be from the ICA, ECA, or both. Meningiomas supplied solely by the ICA include diaphragmatic or tuberculum sellar lesions.

Anterior fossa lesions are supplied by the ECA and ICA. High-convexity and parasagittal lesions are supplied by the middle meningeal artery and the artery of the falx cerebri. All parasagittal lesions must be examined for contributions from the contralateral middle meningeal artery. Frontal convexity or frontal falcine tumors are supplied by a combination of the meningeal branches of the ethmoidal artery and anterior falcine branches. Bilateral anterior and posterior ethmoidal arteries usually supply olfactory groove meningiomas. As a result, the distal internal maxillary branches and the middle meningeal artery must be evaluated.

Middle fossa tumors are supplied by branches from the ECA, including the artery of the foramen rotundum, vidian arteries, and ascending pharyngeal artery. In particular, meningiomas involving the sphenoid wing are supplied by the recurrent meningeal branch of the ophthalmic artery or branches of the middle meningeal artery. Parasellar tumors are frequently fed by branches of the petrous, cavernous, and supraclinoid segments of the ICA; the artery of the foramen rotundum; the artery of the foramen ovale; and the neuromeningeal branch of the ascending pharyngeal artery.

Table 2
Barrow Neurological Institute series of embolized central nervous system tumors (1995–present)

Tumors	Number
Meningiomas	
Olfactory groove	1
Parasagittal	2
Tentorial	2
Convexity	5
Sphenoid wing	1
Atypical	1
Juvenile nasopharyngeal angiofibromas	11
Hemangioblastomas	4
Paragangliomas	
Glomus tympanicum	1
Glomus jugulare	7
Glomus vagale	1
Carotid body tumor	1
Hemangiopericytomas	1
Others (14)	
Angiosarcoma	1
Vestibular schwannoma	1
12th nerve schwannoma	1
Ewing sarcoma	1
Hemangioma	1
Metastatic renal cell (cranial)	1
Aneurysmal bone cyst (spinal)	1
Plasmacytoma (spinal)	2
Giant cell tumor (spinal)	1
Spinal metastasis	3
Schwannoma (spine)	1

Posterior fossa meningiomas are primarily supplied by the posterior meningeal artery, the middle meningeal artery, and the accessory meningeal artery. The tentorial branch of the meningohypophyseal trunk, the inferolateral trunk, the middle meningeal artery, and the accessory meningeal artery can all supply tentorial meningiomas. These branches also may supply the third through sixth cranial nerves. Consequently, provocative testing may be beneficial. Petroclival meningiomas are supplied by the petrosal, petrosquamosal, and occipital branches of the middle meningeal artery; the transmastoid branches of the occipital and posterior auricular arteries; the subarcuate branch of the anterior inferior cerebellar artery (AICA); and neuromeningeal branches of the ascending pharyngeal artery. The posterior meningeal artery arising from the vertebral artery or branches of the ascending pharyngeal artery [1] supply meningiomas involving the foramen magnum. Posterior fossa tumors share their blood supply with the lower cranial nerves. This point must be recalled when embolizing these tumors. Also, EC-IC anastomoses, specifically between branches of the posterior auricular or occipital artery and the vertebral artery in the high cervical spinolaminar region, may be present.

Angiography is instrumental in determining the patency of the major dural venous sinuses. Meningiomas can invade and occlude a major sinus. Preoperative magnetic resonance venography or angiography can verify invasion, occlusion, and collateral venous drainage and thereby facilitate surgical decision making. If gross total resection is the goal, preexisting occlusion of a sinus allows more aggressive tumor resection by opening the sinus or resecting the involved segment.

In 1973, Manelfe et al [44] first described the preoperative embolization of meningiomas. Transcatheter embolization has been advocated to reduce the vascularity of tumors, to facilitate necrosis of the dural attachment site, to mitigate tumoral hemorrhage, and to facilitate tumor resection [2,19,45,46].

The most commonly used embolisate for meningiomas is PVA. Particles in the range of 150 to 350 μm are preferred because they can penetrate deeply into the tumor substance. If reflux into the parent artery occurs, embolization should be discontinued. Ideally, the postembolization angiographic goal is obliteration of the tumor blush on injection of the ECA. If embolization obliterates the feeding arteries but the tumor blush remains, the tumor is likely to remain hypervascular.

The presence of estrogen and progesterone receptors in many meningiomas introduces the attractive concept of ligand-specific selectivity to preoperative embolization. A report by Suzuki and Komatsu [47] using estrogen to embolize dural AVMs and meningiomas suggests that estrogen or progestins may be used as embolisates for tumors. Although the mechanism of action is unclear, estrogen is thought to injure the vascular endothelium and to increase vascular permeability.

Most meningiomas do not require preoperative embolization because the tumor can be devascularized during surgical resection as a first step. Embolization is valuable for large hypervascular skull base meningiomas with an arterial supply that is not readily accessible surgically [48]. Embolization should be considered for giant meningiomas (Fig. 1), meningiomas involving the skull base and middle cranial fossa, falcine or parasagittal meningiomas, and meningiomas in the pineal region. In patients with skull base meningiomas, the vascular pedicle is seldom encountered until a significant portion of the tumor has been resected, making embolization more imperative. To forestall tumor progression, embolization may be considered for patients who are poor surgical candidates.

Embolization of deep arterial feeders, such as the meningohypophyseal trunk and inferolateral trunk, is technically challenging, because their caliber is small and their angle of origin is acute. The introduction of variable stiffness and hydrophilic microcatheters and microwires has permitted selective microcatheterization of these vessels, however. Hirohata et al [49] described seven patients with large petroclival meningiomas who underwent preoperative embolization with 150- to 250-μm particulates. Branches of the meningohypophyseal trunk and inferolateral trunk (lateral clival, posterior branch, and tentorial branch), which provided the primary blood supply, were catheterized successfully. They did not use lidocaine because of the high reported rates of false-positive and false-negative results and for fear of introducing an epileptogenic agent into the distal territory [50,51]. All tumors were subtotally or completely resected; blood loss was 500 mL or less. Robinson et al [51] described five patients with skull base meningiomas who underwent successful preoperative embolization of the

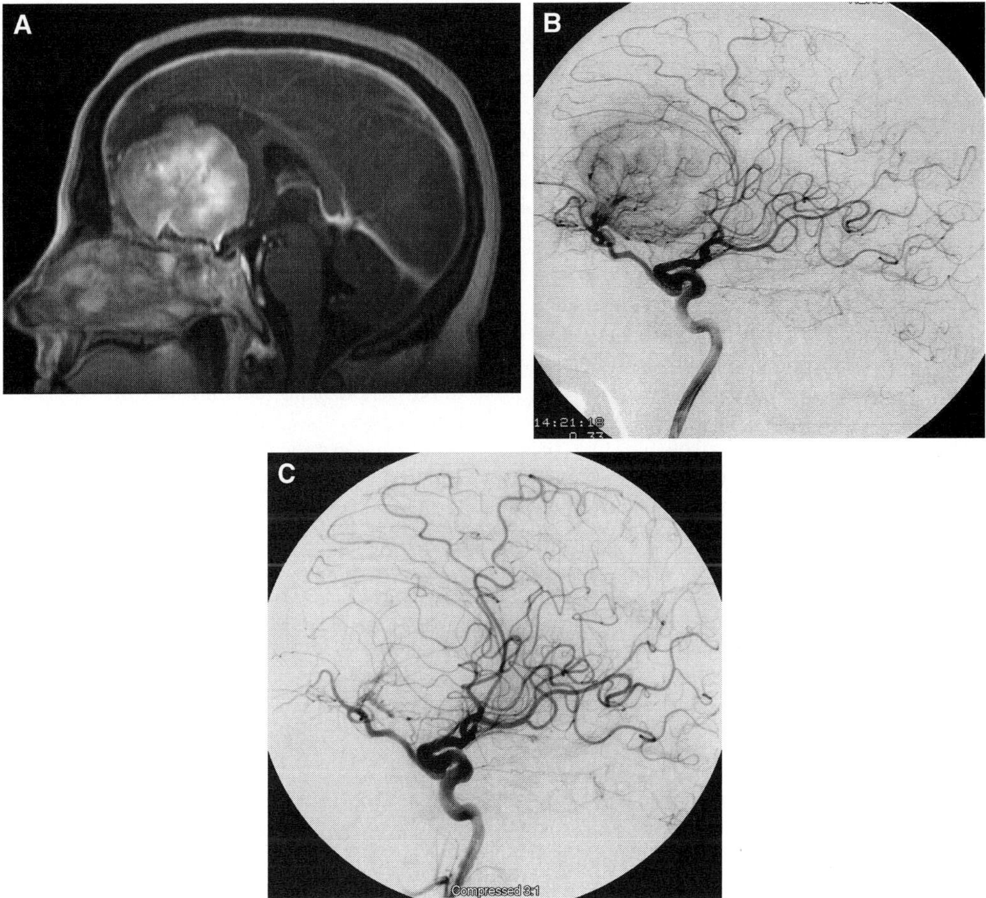

Fig. 1. (*A*) Sagittal MRI shows a giant anterior skull base meningioma. (*B*) Lateral internal carotid artery angiographic injection shows the "sunburst" pattern of arterial supply. Ethmoidal branches arising from the ophthalmic artery feed this giant tumor. (*C*) The vascularity is markedly reduced after glue embolization.

meningohypophyseal trunk and inferolateral trunk with particulate embolisates. No patient suffered complications, and the tumor blush was obliterated in 80% to 100% of the cases. The inferolateral trunk, however, must be embolized with caution because it can collateralize with the ophthalmic artery via the deep recurrent ophthalmic artery. Embolization of the inferolateral trunk is thus associated with the risk of blindness.

Pial and ophthalmic arteries supplying meningiomas are difficult to embolize, and the risk-benefit ratio often precludes an attempt. Kaji et al [52] described two cases in which distal cortical branches of the ICA were successfully and safely embolized with Gelfoam before surgical resection. They emphasized that embolization of the pial supply should be attempted only under the following conditions: the tumor is supplied solely by the ICA, the tumor is located in a noneloquent region of the brain, the patient has a negative Amytal test result, superselective microcatheterization is performed with the catheter abutting the tumor, and particles are used rather than acrylic glue.

Pineal region meningiomas are typically supplied by meningeal branches of the ECA, the tentorial artery, the medial and lateral posterior choroidal branches, the posterior pericallosal artery, small branches of the posterior cerebral artery, and branches of the superior vermian and superior cerebellar arteries (SCAs). Meningeal branches may arise from the vertebral artery and PICAs. Sagoh et al [53] successfully resected a pineal region meningioma after embolizing bilateral middle meningeal arteries with estrogen-alcohol and PVA. Postembolization MRI showed intratumoral necrosis.

Optic nerve meningiomas are seldom amenable to embolization because they are supplied by branches of the ophthalmic artery that concurrently supply the nerve. Terada et al [54] embolized five hypervascular meningiomas fed primarily by branches of the ophthalmic artery. One patient was blind before embolization, and another patient suffered a visual field deficit after embolization. They contended that this technique is feasible if the microcatheter is distal to the origin of the central retinal artery and emphasized that reflux into this artery must be avoided.

Bendszus et al [55] prospectively studied the effects of preoperative embolization on the excision of meningiomas at two similar centers. Thirty patients each were enrolled in the embolization and nonembolized groups. One patient in the embolization group suffered a permanent complication (thromboembolic occlusion of the central retinal artery). Overall, there was no significant difference in intraoperative blood loss. Only the subgroup of patients who underwent complete embolization without residual tumor blush had significantly less intraoperative blood loss. These investigators concluded that the value of nonselective preoperative embolization of meningiomas may be limited, especially given the time, expense, and complications associated with embolization.

A retrospective study from our institution examined the utility and risk-benefit profile of 33 appropriately matched embolized and 193 nonembolized meningiomas. Costs of treatment for the two groups were also compared. Preoperative embolization significantly reduced the intraoperative blood loss and need for transfusions associated with large meningiomas. There were no differences between the two groups in terms of cost, length of hospital stay, and rates of major or minor complications. Therefore, embolization may be beneficial for large meningiomas.

Bendszus et al [56] prospectively followed seven patients who underwent embolization with trisacryl gelatin microspheres (100–300 μm) alone without surgery. At a mean radiographic follow-up of 20 months, the tumors of six of the seven patients were smaller than before treatment. The reduction was most pronounced 6 months after treatment. They contended that embolization alone may be an option for patients who are poor surgical candidates. The drawback of this treatment modality is the lack of histologic verification of the diagnosis. Long-term follow-up is also required to determine the efficacy of treatment.

Complications

The overall risk associated with the embolization of meningiomas is low [19,57]. Minor complications include painful trismus, facial pain, or both and may occur in as many as 20% to 30% of patients [19]. Treatment of these complications includes corticosteroids and analgesic medications. In most patients, symptoms resolve within 2 to 3 days.

Major complications include stroke, blindness, hemorrhage, and cranial nerve palsies. Stroke or blindness is rare but can be the result of unappreciated EC-IC collaterals or can be caused by reflux of embolic material. These complications can be avoided by thorough angiographic evaluation, including a superselective examination to delineate anastomoses between the meningeal vessels and the ICA, vertebral artery, or ophthalmic artery.

Seventh cranial nerve palsy results from inadvertent embolization of the petrous branches of the middle meningeal artery, which supplies posterior parasellar and posterior fossa lesions. Lower cranial nerves are at risk when clival or petroclival meningiomas supplied by branches of the ascending pharyngeal artery are to be embolized. The risk of cranial nerve palsies can be mitigated by superselective catheterization of the external branches until the catheter tip is wedged within the vessel supplying the tumor. Cranial nerve damage is also less likely with particle embolization, specifically when larger particulates are used. Using particulates larger than 150 μm is thought to prevent inadvertent embolization of the vaso vasorum supplying the cranial nerves. Probst et al [14] reported cranial nerve deficits in 2 of 80 patients undergoing embolization, which were temporary in 1 patient and permanent in the other.

Hieshima et al [58] reported no permanent neurologic complications in 11 patients undergoing embolization for a meningioma. Richter and Schachenmayr [2] described 5 patients with transient neurologic deficits and no permanent deficits in 31 patients whose meningiomas were embolized. In a series of 51 patients who underwent embolization, Macpherson [46] described 8 patients who experienced scalp necrosis or temporary hemiparesis. Rosen et al [59] embolized skull base meningiomas in 167 patients, an ostensibly high-risk group for embolization or surgery. Transient neurologic deficit occurred in 12.6%, and 9% had permanent neurologic deficits. In their experience, embolization of the meningohypophyseal trunk, ascending pharyngeal artery, and middle meningeal artery was associated with a high risk of transient and permanent neurologic deficits. Swelling after embolization was readily controlled with intravenous steroids. If swelling persists, emergent surgical resection must be considered. Patients with skull base meningiomas frequently have baseline cranial nerve dysfunction. In this subgroup of patients, embolization may exacerbate this dysfunction, and this possibility should be highlighted during preoperative counseling [59]. Two patients developed monocular blindness after embolization, and neither patient was embolized via the ophthalmic artery.

Subarachnoid, subdural, peritumoral, or intratumoral hemorrhages have followed the embolization of meningiomas [60–64]. Hemorrhage may be caused by wire perforation or sudden dynamic changes in intracranial blood flow as a result of the embolization [60]. After reviewing the literature on the postembolization risks of intratumoral hemorrhage, Kallmes et al [65] were unable to discern a correlation between particle size and risk of hemorrhage. They found seven cases of hemorrhage into a meningioma. Eliminating the supply from the ECA to tumors with a significant ICA supply has been reported to increase blood flow from the ICA, exacerbating mass effect and intratumoral hemorrhage [48,66]. This potential complication must be considered when tumors have a significant ICA supply. Intratumoral hemorrhage also may be more common in tumors with cystic components or large necrotic areas than in homogeneous lesions [64]. Barr et al [67] described an iatrogenic carotid-cavernous sinus fistula that presumably resulted from microwire perforation of a meningohypophyseal artery supplying a skull base meningioma. The fistula was treated with transarterial coil embolization of the venous pouch. Given the risk profile, they concluded that skull base meningiomas must not be embolized indiscriminately.

Scalp necrosis can also follow embolization and surgical resection. Adler et al [68] described severe scalp necrosis treated with a vascularized free tissue transfer. Chan and Thompson [69] and Adler et al [68] emphasized the need to base the scalp flap on at least one patent supplying artery to prevent this complication. They also recommended maintaining the superficial temporal artery as a potential donor vessel for a free tissue transfer. Scalp necrosis is rare when larger particulates are used as the embolisate.

A potential concern is that embolized meningiomas may be overgraded on histologic examination because of the embolization-induced necrosis and reactive changes [69,70]. Ng et al [70] suggested that embolization-induced necrosis is characterized by a punched-out outline with confluent areas of necrosis. Embolized meningiomas lack the overall background of anaplasia associated with atypical or aggressive meningiomas. Perry et al [71] examined 64 embolized meningiomas and concluded that these morphologic changes are uncommon and that current grading schemes rarely overgrade these tumors. They found a higher proportion of atypical meningiomas in patients undergoing embolization but attributed it to selection bias rather than to the effects of embolization.

Hemangioblastomas

Hemangioblastomas constitute 1.1% to 2% of craniospinal tumors [72]. They most frequently occur within the cerebellar hemispheres and rarely at the vermis, cerebellopontine angle, or brain stem. Although most of these lesions are sporadic, approximately 20% are associated with von Hippel-Lindau (VHL) disease. VHL disease is transmitted in an autosomal dominant fashion with incomplete penetrance. Multiple hemangioblastomas are the norm in patients with this disease. The tumors are hypervascular, which makes their resection exceedingly difficult, particularly in eloquent areas. Severe intraoperative hemorrhage is a significant contributor to the morbidity and mortality rates associated with the resection of hemangioblastomas [73]. Before the advent of microsurgical techniques, morbidity and mortality rates approached 50% [74].

On angiography, the blood supply is typically via the PICA and, less commonly, via the AICA or branches of the SCA branches. Pontomedullary hemangioblastomas can recruit supply from the SCA. Branches of the vertebral artery or anterior spinal artery may supply cervicomedullary lesions. Dural branches of the vertebral artery, such as the posterior meningeal artery, may supply superficial lesions. The caliber of feeding arteries can exceed that of the basilar artery.

The criteria for embolizing hemangioblastomas include large tumors with well-defined arterial feeders that are not readily accessible surgically (Fig. 2). Preoperative embolization has been advocated for lesions larger than 3 cm [75]. The risk of embolization is high with hemangioblastomas, because the feeding arteries are often pial vessels (ie, branches of the PICA or AICA). Embolization should be performed with the microcatheter tip placed beyond the normal branches. The embolisate of choice is PVA or NBCA.

Tampieri et al [76] treated two patients with large hemangioblastomas, one spinal and one involving the posterior fossa, with preoperative embolization. Both lesions were then resected with blood loss of less than 100 mL. Eskridge et al [77] treated nine patients with craniospinal hemangioblastomas with PVA embolisate and incurred no permanent complications. One patient developed malignant posterior fossa edema associated with hydrocephalus after treatment, however. They advocated perioperative steroids, intensive care unit observation, and surgical resection within 48 to 72 hours because of the potential for recanalization of feeding arteries after embolization with PVA. The surgeons believed that embolization facilitated tumor manipulation and surgical resection.

Conway et al [78] described 4 of 40 patients with hemangioblastomas who underwent preoperative embolization. In a patient with a sacral

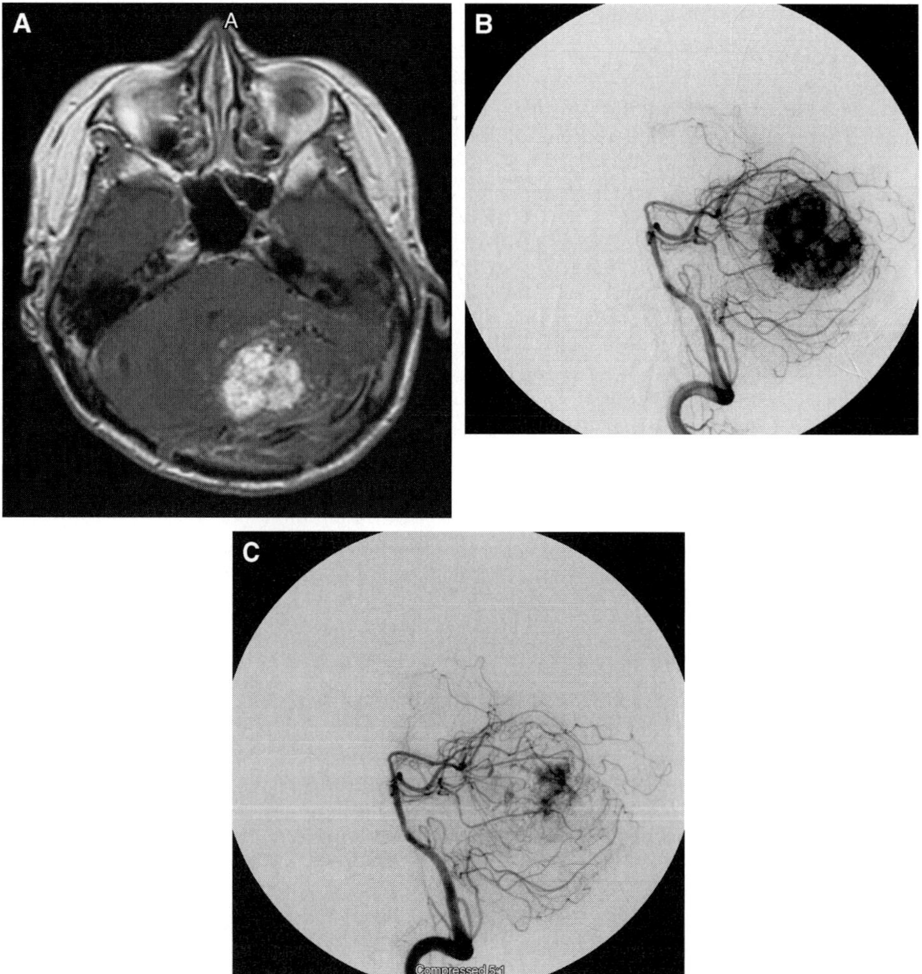

Fig. 2. (*A*) Axial postcontrast MRI shows an intensely enhancing posterior fossa mass. (*B*) The vertebral artery injection shows the dense vascularity of a hemangioblastoma. (*C*) The deep arterial supply is obliterated with glue embolization.

hemangioblastoma, embolization alone was sufficient to arrest progression of the patient's symptoms. One patient suffered a lateral medullary infarction after embolization of a medullary hemangioblastoma. These investigators recommended reserving embolization for tumors with large surgically inaccessible feeders.

Lee et al [79] treated 4 of 14 patients with spinal cord hemangioblastomas with embolization and surgical resection. Complete resection was achieved in all four cases. Subjectively, the surgeon reported significantly less blood loss in the embolized patients. Contraindications to embolization included supply to the hemangioblastoma from the artery of Adamkiewicz and a surgically accessible arterial supply. Four patients were treated before the advent of spinal embolization techniques. Tumor feeders emanating from the anterior spinal axis should not be embolized because of the risk of occluding the anterior spinal artery.

Hemangiopericytomas

Meningeal hemangiopericytomas are aggressive tumors originating from the contractile pericytes of Zimmerman, which envelop capillaries. They are rare, accounting for less than 1% of all CNS tumors [80]. They occur equally in both genders and are an affliction of middle age. They are associated with a high risk for recurrence and carry metastatic potential [81].

These tumors are quite vascular, and intraoperative bleeding can be significant. Hemorrhage is the most common cause of surgical morbidity and mortality as well as the primary reason for subtotal resection [78,90]. Embolization of these tumors must be aggressive, and the use of ethanol as well as direct surgical puncture should be considered (Fig. 3).

Several reports have described the utility of embolization in mitigating surgical blood loss [82–84]. Embolization of these tumors is exceptionally difficult because they parasitize the cortical vessels [79,81]. Reported complications include permanent Horner's syndrome [82]. Embolization alone typically provides insufficient tumor control or cure.

Muraszko et al [85] treated four patients with hemangiopericytomas of the spine with embolization and surgical resection. They advocated embolization to reduce the vascularity of the tumor. They caution that preoperative deficits may worsen, likely because the tumor swells after embolization. They therefore recommend urgent surgical resection after embolization.

Paragangliomas

Paragangliomas are typically benign slow-growing neoplasms that arise from neural crest paraganglion cells. In the head and neck, they occur in the temporal bone (glomus tympanicum and glomus jugulare; Fig. 4), the carotid bifurcation (glomus caroticum), and the upper parapharyngeal space (glomus vagale; Fig. 5). On extremely rare occasions, paragangliomas can be found within the spinal canal [86].

Approximately 4% of paragangliomas have documented catecholamine secretion [87–90]. This behavior can cause a pheochromocytoma-type syndrome associated with broad fluctuations in blood pressure or marked hypertension. If catecholamine secretion is documented, the patient must be pretreated with α- and β-blockade before embolization and surgical resection. The most common presenting symptoms include progressive unilateral hearing loss and pulsatile tinnitus.

Angiography must define the intracranial and extracranial arterial supply to the tumor as well as the involvement of the dural venous sinus. The patency of both transverse-sigmoid systems must be evaluated to determine if the involved sinus can be sacrificed without causing intracranial venous hypertension. The primary blood supply is from branches of the ascending pharyngeal artery. Temporal glomus tumors often recruit their blood supply from petrous branches of the ICA (eg, vidian artery) and from cavernous-carotid branches (clival branch of the meningohypophyseal trunk). Glomus tympanicum are usually small lesions that can be resected with conventional tympanoplasty techniques without preoperative embolization.

Glomus jugulare lesions, particularly those with an intracranial extension, require preoperative embolization [91]. Preoperative embolization of these tumors helps to reduce intraoperative blood loss, increases the extent of tumor resection, and decreases the length of surgery [92–95]. Reduced intraoperative bleeding permits more meticulous dissection of the crucial neurovascular structures at the skull base. Most glomus jugulare tumors tend to have a multicompartmentalized arterial supply. For embolization to be effective, each compartment should be catheterized selectively and embolized. The inferomedial compartment is supplied by the ascending pharyngeal

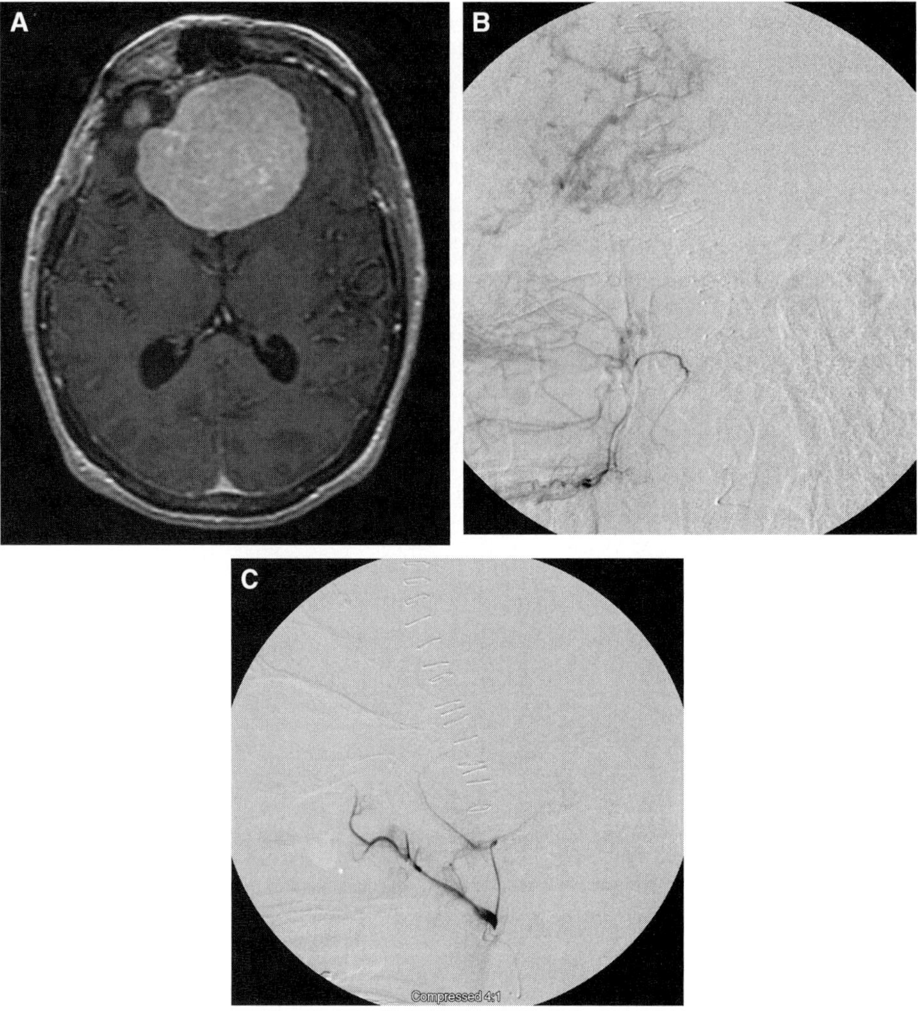

Fig. 3. (*A*) Axial postcontrast T1-weighted MRI shows a giant anterior skull base hemangiopericytoma. (*B*) Superselective injection of the internal maxillary artery shows a prominent tumor blush. (*C*) No tumor blush is seen after embolization with particulates (polyvinyl alcohol).

artery. The posterolateral compartment is supplied by the stylomastoid branch of the occipital or posterior auricular artery. The anterior compartment is supplied by branches of the internal maxillary artery and ICA (caroticotympanic artery), and the superior compartment is supplied by branches of the middle meningeal artery. Superselective microcatheterization can help to define this anatomy and to identify EC-IC anastomoses [96]. For tumors with significant supply from the ICA and those that encase the ICA, balloon test occlusion with preoperative sacrifice of the ICA is an option. Cohen et al [97] reported a case in which the tumor was devascularized and the ICA was preserved by using a covered stent placed within the petrous ICA.

Carotid body tumors occur sporadically, and bilateral tumors occur in 5% of cases. These lesions typically manifest in the fourth to sixth decades of life as a painless enlarging neck mass. Local mass effect, however, can cause dysphagia, hoarseness, stridor, tongue paresis, and vertigo. Continued growth leads to involvement of the ICA, ECA, and vagus and hypoglossal nerves. Pharyngeal compression with skull base and intracranial extension also occurs. Malignancy, as defined by distant metastatic spread, occurs in 2% to 6% of lesions [98–100]. Surgical excision can be

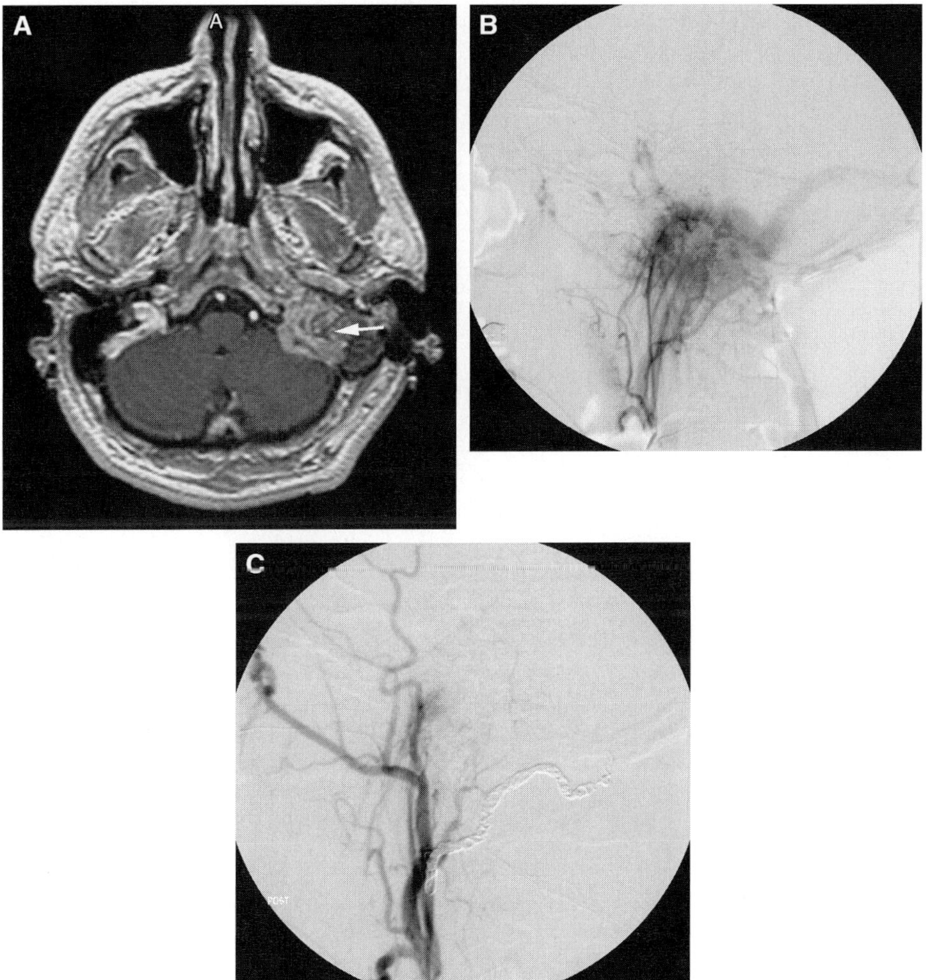

Fig. 4. (*A*) Axial postcontrast MRI shows an extensive left glomus jugulare tumor (*arrow*). (*B*) This tumor has a profound vascular supply derived from multiple branches of the external carotid artery. (*C*) The vascularity of the tumor is reduced drastically after glue and coil embolization.

challenging, because the tumors are hypervascular and they can involve the cranial nerves extensively.

LaMuraglia et al [101] embolized 11 patients with carotid body tumors before surgery. Tumors were supplied via the ascending pharyngeal artery, ascending cervical branches of the thyrocervical trunk, and vertebral artery. One patient suffered transient aphasia that resolved within 24 hours. Embolization significantly decreased intraoperative bleeding compared with nonembolized lesions. These investigators recommended preoperative embolization for tumors larger than 3 cm, followed by surgical resection within a few days. Embolization can be difficult because of the tumor's location at the carotid bifurcation. Therefore, they advocated temporary balloon occlusion with hypotensive challenge if the carotid artery is extensively involved. Borges et al [102] described 2 patients whose large carotid body tumors were completely resected with minimal blood loss after preoperative embolization with PVA.

Complications

Similar to embolization of other intracranial tumors, most severe complications are related to delivery of the embolisate into the intracranial circulation via reflux or through EC-IC collaterals. Palsy of the lower cranial nerves (IX–XII) can

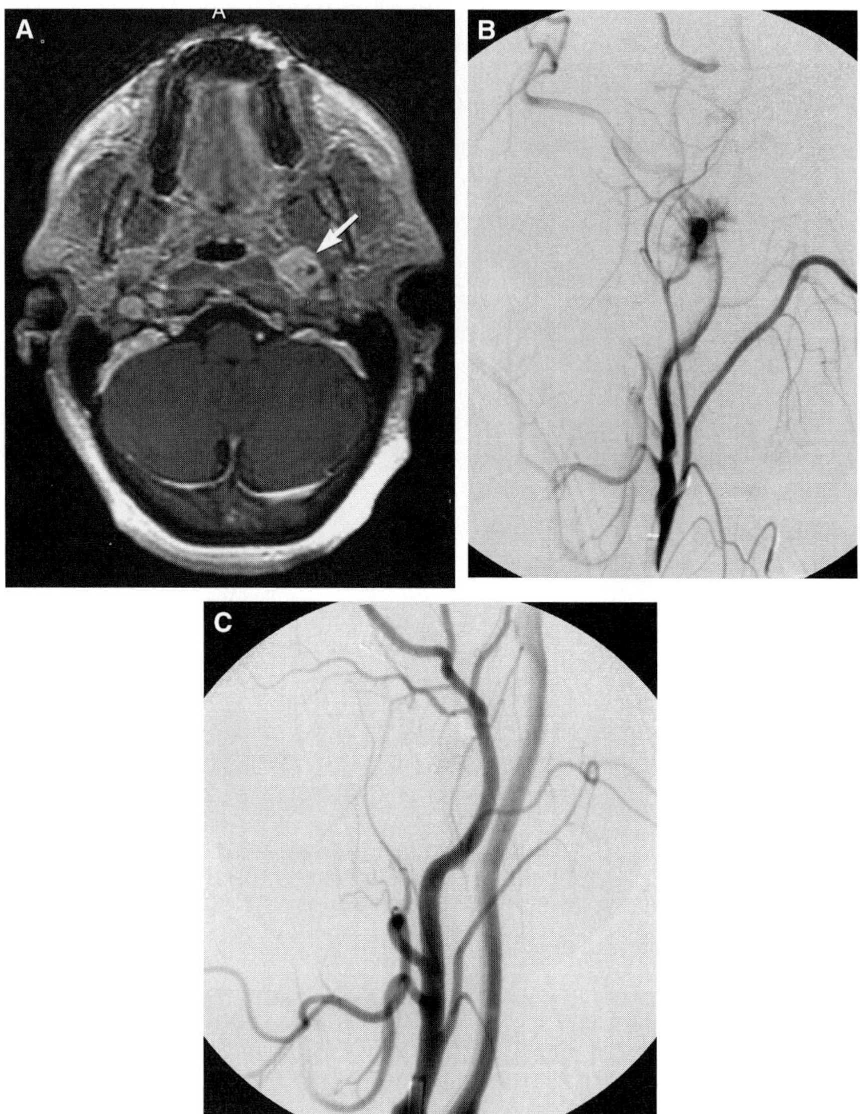

Fig. 5. (*A*) Axial postcontrast MRI shows an enhancing tumor consistent with a glomus vagale in the left carotid sheath (*arrow*). (*B*) The predominant blood supply is from a branch of the ascending pharyngeal artery. (*C*) No residual supply to the tumor is seen after glue embolization.

follow embolization of the vaso vasorum supplying these nerves. In an early report, Pandya et al [103] described a herniation syndrome that followed direct puncture and Gelfoam embolization of a glomus jugulare tumor. They theorized that significant tumor infarction exacerbated posterior fossa edema. Marangos and Schumacher [104] and Herdman et al [105] described two cases of facial palsy after embolization of a glomus jugulare tumor. One patient had recovered completely 1 year after treatment, and the other had improved significantly.

The facial nerve typically receives its blood supply from the stylomastoid artery and from petrosal branches of the middle meningeal or accessory meningeal artery. When the tumor has occluded the stylomastoid artery and the meningeal contribution to the nerve is small, facial nerve paresis is to be expected. Recovery of function is the rule after embolization with PVA, because the embolized vessels eventually recanalize. When a permanent embolisate, such as glue, is used, a provocative test should be considered before proceeding.

Juvenile nasopharyngeal angiofibromas

Juvenile nasopharyngeal angiofibromas are highly vascular benign neoplasms that account for 0.5% of all head and neck neoplasms [106]. These tumors originate within the superior posterior margin of the sphenopalatine foramen. They almost exclusively afflict adolescent boys; the mean age at diagnosis is 14 years. Although benign, juvenile nasopharyngeal angiofibromas are locally invasive and exhibit high rates of recurrence after subtotal resection [107,108]. The most common presenting symptoms include nasal obstruction or epistaxis.

On nasopharyngeal examination, a pink-blue nodular mass is seen in the oropharynx. Angiography shows multiple tortuous vessels, with a dense homogeneous blush during the capillary phase. Prominent draining veins become apparent immediately. These tumors are supplied by branches of the ipsilateral internal maxillary artery (Fig. 6). The ascending pharyngeal artery is involved in as many as one third of the cases [109]. Bilateral carotid angiography is vital, because these tumors, particularly if they have an intracranial extension, often recruit their blood supply from the ophthalmic artery, contralateral internal maxillary artery, and branches of the ICA.

Preoperative embolization is considered crucial for reducing the intraoperative blood loss associated with these tumors. The aim of embolization is to occlude the small distal vessels within the tumor and not simply to obstruct the feeding arteries. In an early study, Roberson et al [109] showed that, on average, preoperative embolization reduced intraoperative blood loss from 2400 to 800 mL. Siniluoto et al [110] demonstrated significantly less blood loss, improved extent of resection, and fewer recurrences in embolized patients compared with nonembolized patients. Their sample comprised only 10 patients, however. Several other studies have reported the safety and efficacy of embolization followed by surgical resection [5,111].

Complications

Complications reported to follow embolization of juvenile nasopharyngeal angiofibromas include fever and local pain. Postembolization fever should not postpone resection. Bradycardia may follow embolization of the internal maxillary or ascending pharyngeal arteries. Intracranial embolization is usually caused by unrecognized EC-IC collaterals or reflux of embolisate. Gay et al [112] have described postoperative palatal necrosis and an oronasal fistula after staged embolization and transpalatal resection of a juvenile nasopharyngeal angiofibroma. They believe that this complication is potentiated by embolization but maintain that embolization is still warranted for these tumors.

Miscellaneous

Aneurysmal bone cysts are benign nonneoplastic lesions primarily afflicting individuals younger than 20 years of age. Although the metaphyses of long bones are the primary sites of origin, the skull is affected in 2.5% to 6% of cases [113]. CT and MRI show multiple loculations within the lesion, with peripheral sclerosis. Angiography shows a tumor blush most prominent on the outer aspect of the lesion, which is typically vascular. The core of the lesion is often avascular.

Treatment options include surgical excision or curettage, radiotherapy, cryosurgery, and embolization. The treatment of choice is curative surgical excision. Sheikh [113] reviewed the literature on the management paradigms used to treat cranial aneurysmal bone cysts. Embolization may be used to devascularize the tumor before surgery or as the only treatment modality in surgically inaccessible lesions. Ikeda et al [114] described regression of an aneurysmal bone cyst after continuous embolization with estrogen for 9 days.

Bingaman et al [115] embolized an intracranial extraskeletal mesenchymal chondrosarcoma that became symptomatic with headache, nausea, and vomiting. The lesion was located extra-axially in the right frontal region and was prominently supplied from bilateral branches of the ECA. Branches of the right middle meningeal artery were embolized. The authors stressed the importance of gross total resection and close follow-up of this potentially aggressive tumor.

Avellino et al [116] described a Masson's vegetant intravascular hemangioendothelioma involving the cerebellopontine angle and middle cranial fossa. The lesion had recurred despite embolization followed by surgical resection on two separate occasions. This exceptionally

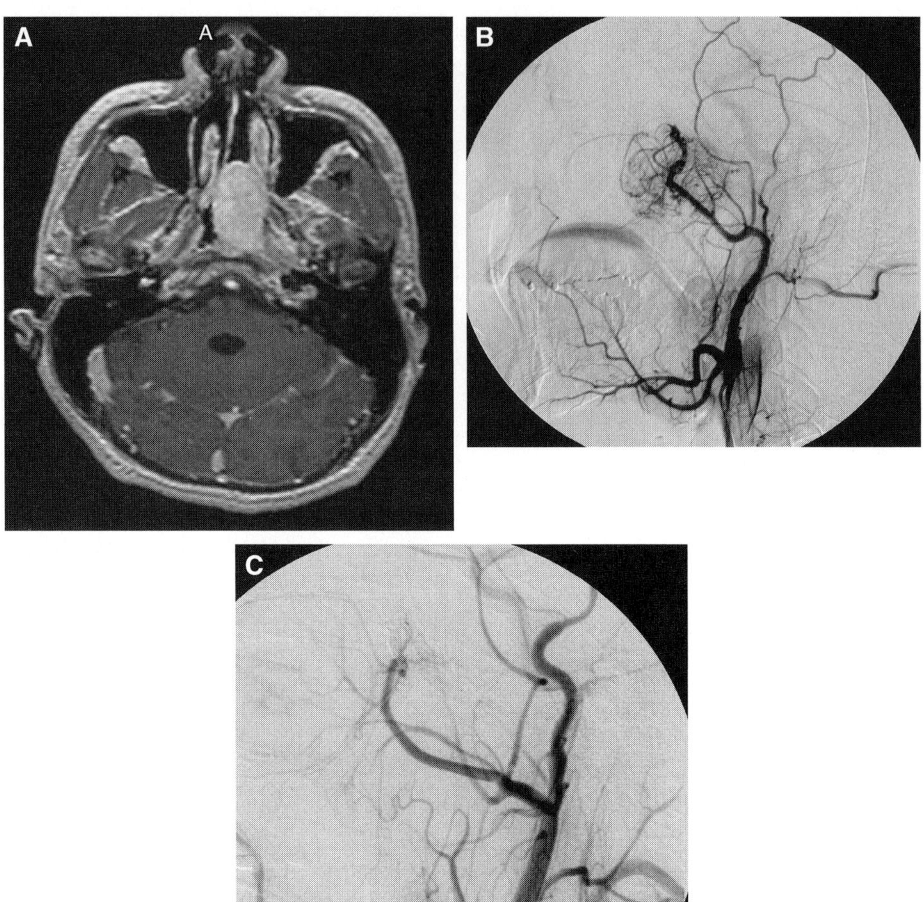

Fig. 6. (*A*) Axial MRI shows a 27-year-old man with a large juvenile nasopharyngeal angiofibroma. (*B*) The distal branches of the internal maxillary artery luxuriously supply the tumor. (*C*) Postembolization angiogram shows no residual arterial supply to this hypervascular tumor.

vascular lesion was supplied by the AICA, meningohypophyseal artery, and occipital arteries. Embolization of the left occipital artery with PVA particles at the patient's initial presentation was successful. When the tumor recurred, multiple branches of the ECA and the left meningohypophyseal artery were contributing significant blood supply. The branches of the ECA were embolized with PVA. The patient tolerated balloon test occlusion and underwent permanent balloon occlusion of the left ICA.

Summary

Preoperative embolization plays a vital role in the management of giant or skull base meningiomas and hypervascular tumors, such as hemangioblastomas, hemangiopericytomas, juvenile nasopharyngeal angiofibromas, and paragangliomas. Recent advances in microcatheter technology, microembolisates, and neurophysiologic monitoring have improved the safety of preoperative embolization. Sound endovascular principles and techniques are paramount to prevent major complications, such as stroke, blindness, or cranial neuropathy, however. Preoperative embolization of tumors has become a requisite tool for the neurosurgical team and represents a signifiant improvement in patient care.

References

[1] Choi IS, Tantivatana J. Neuroendovascular management of intracranial and spinal tumors. Neurosurg Clin N Am 2000;11:167–85.

[2] Richter HP, Schachenmayr W. Preoperative embolization of intracranial meningiomas. Neurosurgery 1983;13:261–8.
[3] Jungreis CA. Skull-base tumors: ethanol embolization of the cavernous carotid artery. Radiology 1991;181:741–3.
[4] Theron J, Cosgrove R, Melanson D, et al. Embolization with temporary balloon occlusion of the internal carotid or vertebral arteries. Neuroradiology 1986;28:246–53.
[5] Garcia-Cervigon E, Bien S, Rufenacht D, et al. Preoperative embolization of naso-pharyngeal angiofibromas. Report of 58 cases. Neuroradiology 1988; 30:556–60.
[6] Lefkowitz M, Giannotta SL, Hieshima G, et al. Embolization of neurosurgical lesions involving the ophthalmic artery. Neurosurgery 1998;43: 1298–303.
[7] Casasco A, Herbreteau D, Houdart E, et al. Devascularization of craniofacial tumors by percutaneous tumor puncture. AJNR Am J Neuroradiol 1994;15:1233–9.
[8] George B, Casasco A, Deffrennes D, et al. Intratumoral embolization of intracranial and extracranial tumors: technical note. Neurosurgery 1994;35: 771–3.
[9] Terada T, Nakamura Y, Tsuura M, et al. MRI changes in embolized meningiomas. Neuroradiology 1992;34:162–7.
[10] Bendszus M, Warmuth-Metz M, Klein R, et al. Sequential MRI and MR spectroscopy in embolized meningiomas: correlation with surgical and histopathological findings. Neuroradiology 2002;44: 77–82.
[11] Wakhloo AK, Juengling FD, Van VV, et al. Extended preoperative polyvinyl alcohol microembolization of intracranial meningiomas: assessment of two embolization techniques. AJNR Am J Neuroradiol 1993;14:571–82.
[12] Grand C, Bank WO, Baleriaux D, et al. Gadolinium-enhanced MR in the evaluation of preoperative meningioma embolization. AJNR Am J Neuroradiol 1993;14:563–9.
[13] Ahuja A, Gibbons KJ. Endovascular therapy of central nervous system tumors. Neurosurg Clin N Am 1994;5:541–54.
[14] Probst EN, Grzyska U, Westphal M, et al. Preoperative embolization of intracranial meningiomas with a fibrin glue preparation. AJNR Am J Neuroradiol 1999;20:1695–702.
[15] Rodesch G, Lasjaunias P. Embolization and meningiomas. In: Al-Mefty O, editor. Meningiomas. New York: Raven Press; 1991. p. 285–97.
[16] Desai R, Bruce J. Meningiomas of the cranial base. J Neurooncol 1994;20:255–79.
[17] Nelson PK, Setton A, Choi IS, et al. Current status of interventional neuroradiology in the management of meningiomas. Neurosurg Clin N Am 1994;5:235–59.
[18] Kai Y, Hamada J, Morioka M, et al. Appropriate interval between embolization and surgery in patients with meningioma. AJNR Am J Neuroradiol 2002;23:139–42.
[19] Manelfe C, Lasjaunias P, Ruscalleda J. Preoperative embolization of intracranial meningiomas. AJNR Am J Neuroradiol 1986;7:963–72.
[20] Flandroy P, Grandfils C, Collignon J, et al. (D, L) polylactide microspheres as embolic agent. A preliminary study. Neuroradiology 1990;32: 311–5.
[21] Kumar AJ, Kaufman SL, Patt J, et al. Preoperative embolization of hypervascular head and neck neoplasms using microfibrillar collagen. AJNR Am J Neuroradiol 1982;3:163–8.
[22] Latshaw RF, Pearlman RL, Schaitkin BM, et al. Intraarterial ethanol as a long-term occlusive agent in renal, hepatic, and gastrosplenic arteries of pigs. Cardiovasc Intervent Radiol 1985;8:24–30.
[23] Berenstein A, Graeb DA. Convenient preparation of ready-to-use particles in polyvinyl alcohol foam suspension for embolization. Radiology 1982;145:846.
[24] Herrera M, Rysavy J, Kotula F, et al. Ivalon shavings: technical considerations of a new embolic agent. Radiology 1982;144:638–40.
[25] Szwarc IA, Carrasco CH, Wallace S, et al. Radiopaque suspension of polyvinyl alcohol foam for embolization. AJR Am J Roentgenol 1986;146: 591–2.
[26] Kunstlinger F, Brunelle F, Chaumont P, et al. Vascular occlusive agents. AJR Am J Roentgenol 1981; 136:151–6.
[27] Inci S, Ozcan OE, Benli K, et al. Microsurgical removal of a free segment of microcatheter in the anterior circulation as a complication of embolization. Surg Neurol 1996;46:562–6.
[28] Hamada J, Kai Y, Nagahiro S, et al. Embolization with cellulose porous beads, II: clinical trial. AJNR Am J Neuroradiol 1996;17:1901–6.
[29] Bendszus M, Klein R, Burger R, et al. Efficacy of trisacryl gelatin microspheres versus polyvinyl alcohol particles in the preoperative embolization of meningiomas. AJNR Am J Neuroradiol 2000; 21:255–61.
[30] Ellman BA, Green CE, Eigenbrodt E, et al. Renal infarction with absolute ethanol. Invest Radiol 1980;15:318–22.
[31] Horowitz M, Whisnant RE, Jungreis C, et al. Temporary balloon occlusion and ethanol injection for preoperative embolization of carotid-body tumor. Ear Nose Throat J 2002;81:536–8, 540, 542.
[32] Lonser RR, Heiss JD, Oldfield EH. Tumor devascularization by intratumoral ethanol injection during surgery. Technical note. J Neurosurg 1998;88: 923–4.
[33] Kasuya H, Shimizu T, Sasahara A, et al. Phenytoin as a liquid material for embolisation of tumours. Neuroradiology 1999;41:320–3.

[34] Kubo M, Kuwayama N, Hirashima Y, et al. Hydroxyapatite ceramics as a particulate embolic material: report of the clinical experience. AJNR Am J Neuroradiol 2003;24:1545–7.

[35] American Society of Interventional and Therapeutic Neuroradiology. Head, neck, and brain tumor embolization. AJNR Am J Neuroradiol 2001; 22(Suppl):S14–5.

[36] Horowitz MB, Carrau R, Crammond D, et al. Risks of tumor embolization in the presence of an unrecognized patent foramen ovale: case report. AJNR Am J Neuroradiol 2002;23:982–4.

[37] Eskridge JM. Interventional neuroradiology. Radiology 1989;172:991–1006.

[38] Horton JA, Kerber CW. Lidocaine injection into external carotid branches: provocative test to preserve cranial nerve function in therapeutic embolization. AJNR Am J Neuroradiol 1986;7:105–8.

[39] Russell DS, Rubinstein LJ. Tumours of meninges and of related tissues. In: Pathology of tumors of the nervous system. 4th edition. Baltimore: Williams & Wilkins; 1977. p. 62–100.

[40] Adegbite AB, Khan MI, Paine KW, et al. The recurrence of intracranial meningiomas after surgical treatment. J Neurosurg 1983;58:51–6.

[41] Chan RC, Thompson GB. Morbidity, mortality, and quality of life following surgery for intracranial meningiomas. A retrospective study in 257 cases. J Neurosurg 1984;60:52–60.

[42] Jaaskelainen J. Seemingly complete removal of histologically benign intracranial meningioma: late recurrence rate and factors predicting recurrence in 657 patients. A multivariate analysis. Surg Neurol 1986;26:461–9.

[43] Simpson D. The recurrence of intracranial meningiomas after surgical treatment. J Neurochem 1957;20:22–39.

[44] Manelfe C, Guiraud B, David J, et al. Embolization by catheterization of intracranial meningiomas [in French]. Rev Neurol (Paris) 1973;128:339–51.

[45] Black PM. Meningiomas. Neurosurgery 1993;32: 643–57.

[46] Macpherson P. The value of pre-operative embolisation of meningioma estimated subjectively and objectively. Neuroradiology 1991;33:334–7.

[47] Suzuki J, Komatsu S. New embolization method using estrogen for dural arteriovenous malformation and meningioma. Surg Neurol 1981;16: 438–42.

[48] Gruber A, Killer M, Mazal P, et al. Preoperative embolization of intracranial meningiomas: a 17-years single center experience. Minim Invasive Neurosurg 2000;43:18–29.

[49] Hirohata M, Abe T, Morimitsu H, et al. Preoperative selective internal carotid artery dural branch embolisation for petroclival meningiomas. Neuroradiology 2003;45:656–60.

[50] Halbach VV, Higashida RT, Hieshima GB, et al. Embolization of branches arising from the cavernous portion of the internal carotid artery. AJNR Am J Neuroradiol 1989;10:143–50.

[51] Robinson DH, Song JK, Eskridge JM. Embolization of meningohypophyseal and inferolateral branches of the cavernous internal carotid artery. AJNR Am J Neuroradiol 1999;20:1061–7.

[52] Kaji T, Hama Y, Iwasaki Y, et al. Preoperative embolization of meningiomas with pial supply: successful treatment of two cases. Surg Neurol 1999; 52:270–3.

[53] Sagoh M, Onozuka S, Murakami H, et al. Successful removal of meningioma of the pineal region after embolization. Neurol Med Chir (Tokyo) 1997; 37:852–5.

[54] Terada T, Kinoshita Y, Yokote H, et al. Preoperative embolization of meningiomas fed by ophthalmic branch arteries. Surg Neurol 1996;45:161–6.

[55] Bendszus M, Rao G, Burger R, et al. Is there a benefit of preoperative meningioma embolization? Neurosurgery 2000;47:1306–11.

[56] Bendszus M, Martin-Schrader I, Schlake HP, et al. Embolisation of intracranial meningiomas without subsequent surgery. Neuroradiology 2003;45: 451–5.

[57] Ahuja A, Gibbons KJ, Hopkins LN. Endovascular techniques to treat brain tumors. In: Youman's neurological surgery. 4th edition. Philadelphia: WB Saunders; 1996. p. 2826–40.

[58] Hieshima GB, Everhart FR, Mehringer CM, et al. Preoperative embolization of meningiomas. Surg Neurol 1980;14:119–27.

[59] Rosen CL, Ammerman JM, Sekhar LN, et al. Outcome analysis of preoperative embolization in cranial base surgery. Acta Neurochir (Wien) 2002;144: 1157–64.

[60] Hayashi T, Shojima K, Utsunomiya H, et al. Subarachnoid hemorrhage after preoperative embolization of a cystic meningioma. Surg Neurol 1987; 27:295–300.

[61] Motozaki T, Otuka S, Sato S, et al. Preoperative embolization with Gelfoam powder for intracranial meningioma causing unusual peritumoral hemorrhage–with reference to the mechanism of hemorrhage [in Japanese]. No Shinkei Geka 1987;15: 95–101.

[62] Suyama T, Tamaki N, Fujiwara K, et al. Peritumoral and intratumoral hemorrhage after gelatin sponge embolization of malignant meningioma: case report. Neurosurgery 1987;21:944–6.

[63] Watanabe K, Matsumura K, Matsuda M, et al. Meningioma with intratumoral and subdural hemorrhage as an immediate complication of therapeutic embolization. Case report [in Japanese]. Neurol Med Chir (Tokyo) 1986;26:904–7.

[64] Yu SC, Boet R, Wong GK, et al. Postembolization hemorrhage of a large and necrotic meningioma. AJNR Am J Neuroradiol 2004;25:506–8.

[65] Kallmes DF, Evans AJ, Kaptain GJ, et al. Hemorrhagic complications in embolization of a meningi-

oma: case report and review of the literature. Neuroradiology 1997;39:877–80.

[66] Teasdale E, Patterson J, McLellan D, et al. Subselective preoperative embolization for meningiomas. A radiological and pathological assessment. J Neurosurg 1984;60:506–11.

[67] Barr JD, Mathis JM, Horton JA. Iatrogenic carotid-cavernous fistula occurring after embolization of a cavernous sinus meningioma. AJNR Am J Neuroradiol 1995;16:483–5.

[68] Adler JR, Upton J, Wallman J, et al. Management and prevention of necrosis of the scalp after embolization and surgery for meningioma. Surg Neurol 1986;25:357–60.

[69] Chan RC, Thompson GB. Ischemic necrosis of the scalp after preoperative embolization of meningeal tumors. Neurosurgery 1984;15:76–81.

[70] Ng HK, Poon WS, Goh K, et al. Histopathology of post-embolized meningiomas. Am J Surg Pathol 1996;20:1224–30.

[71] Perry A, Chicoine MR, Filiput E, et al. Clinicopathologic assessment and grading of embolized meningiomas: a correlative study of 64 patients. Cancer 2001;92:701–11.

[72] Russell DS, Rubinstein LJ. Tumours and hamartomas of the blood-vessels. In: Pathology of tumors of the nervous system. 4th edition. Baltimore: Williams & Wilkins; 1977. p. 127–45.

[73] Djindjian M. Successful removal of a brainstem hemangioblastoma. Surg Neurol 1986;25:97–100.

[74] Sanford RA, Smith RA. Hemangioblastoma of the cervicomedullary junction. Report of three cases. J Neurosurg 1986;64:317–21.

[75] Wang C, Zhang J, Liu A, et al. Surgical management of medullary hemangioblastoma. Report of 47 cases. Surg Neurol 2001;56:218–26.

[76] Tampieri D, Leblanc R, TerBrugge K. Preoperative embolization of brain and spinal hemangioblastomas. Neurosurgery 1993;33:502–5.

[77] Eskridge JM, McAuliffe W, Harris B, et al. Preoperative endovascular embolization of craniospinal hemangioblastomas. AJNR Am J Neuroradiol 1996;17:525–31.

[78] Conway JE, Chou D, Clatterbuck RE, et al. Hemangioblastomas of the central nervous system in von Hippel-Lindau syndrome and sporadic disease. Neurosurgery 2001;48:55–62.

[79] Lee DK, Choe WJ, Chung CK, et al. Spinal cord hemangioblastoma: surgical strategy and clinical outcome. J Neurooncol 2003;61:27–34.

[80] Guthrie BL, Ebersold MJ, Scheithauer BW, et al. Meningeal hemangiopericytoma: histopathological features, treatment, and long-term follow-up of 44 cases. Neurosurgery 1989;25:514–22.

[81] Pandey M, Kothari KC, Patel DD. Haemangiopericytoma: current status, diagnosis and management. Eur J Surg Oncol 1997;23:282–5.

[82] Jaaskelainen J, Servo A, Haltia M, et al. Intracranial hemangiopericytoma: radiology, surgery, radiotherapy, and outcome in 21 patients. Surg Neurol 1985;23:227–36.

[83] Cizmeli MO, Ilgit ET, Ulug H, et al. A giant paraspinal hemangiopericytoma and its preoperative embolization. Neuroradiology 1992;34:81–3.

[84] Payne BR, Prasad D, Steiner M, et al. Gamma surgery for hemangiopericytomas. Acta Neurochir (Wien) 2000;142:527–36.

[85] Muraszko KM, Antunes JL, Hilal SK, et al. Hemangiopericytomas of the spine. Neurosurgery 1982;10:473–9.

[86] Solymosi L, Ferbert A. A case of spinal paraganglioma. Neuroradiology 1985;27:217–9.

[87] Azzarelli B, Felten S, Muller J, et al. Dopamine in paragangliomas of the glomus jugulare. Laryngoscope 1988;98:573–8.

[88] Blumenfeld JD, Cohen N, Laragh JH, et al. Hypertension and catecholamine biosynthesis associated with a glomus jugulare tumor. N Engl J Med 1992;327:894–5.

[89] Farrior J. Surgical management of glomus tumors: endocrine-active tumors of the skull base. South Med J 1988;81:1121–6.

[90] Nelson MD, Kendall BE. Intracranial catecholamine secreting paragangliomas. Neuroradiology 1987;29:277–82.

[91] George B. Jugulare foramen paragangliomas. Acta Neurochir (Wien) 1992;118:20–6.

[92] Hilal SK, Michelsen JW. Therapeutic percutaneous embolization for extra-axial vascular lesions of the head, neck, and spine. J Neurosurg 1975;43: 275–87.

[93] Murphy TP, Brackmann DE. Effects of preoperative embolization on glomus jugulare tumors. Laryngoscope 1989;99:1244–7.

[94] Tikkakoski T, Luotonen J, Leinonen S, et al. Preoperative embolization in the management of neck paragangliomas. Laryngoscope 1997;107: 821–6.

[95] Young NM, Wiet RJ, Russell EJ, et al. Superselective embolization of glomus jugulare tumors. Ann Otol Rhinol Laryngol 1988;97:613–20.

[96] Djindjian R. Super-selective arteriography of branches of the external carotid artery. Surg Neurol 1976;5:133–42.

[97] Cohen JE, Ferrario A, Ceratto R, et al. Covered stent as an innovative tool for tumor devascularization and endovascular arterial reconstruction. Neurol Res 2003;25:169–72.

[98] Hodge KM, Byers RM, Peters LJ. Paragangliomas of the head and neck. Arch Otolaryngol Head Neck Surg 1988;114:872–7.

[99] Lack EE, Cubilla AL, Woodruff JM, et al. Paragangliomas of the head and neck region: a clinical study of 69 patients. Cancer 1977;39: 397–409.

[100] Meyer FB, Sundt TM Jr, Pearson BW. Carotid body tumors: a subject review and suggested surgical approach. J Neurosurg 1986;64:377–85.

[101] LaMuraglia GM, Fabian RL, Brewster DC, et al. The current surgical management of carotid body paragangliomas. J Vasc Surg 1992;15:1038–44.

[102] Borges LF, Heros RC, DeBrun G. Carotid body tumors managed with preoperative embolization. Report of two cases. J Neurosurg 1983;59: 867–70.

[103] Pandya SK, Nagpal RD, Desai AP, et al. Death following external carotid artery embolization for a functioning glomus jugulare chemodectoma. Case report. J Neurosurg 1978;48:1030–4.

[104] Marangos N, Schumacher M. Facial palsy after glomus jugulare tumour embolization. J Laryngol Otol 1999;113:268–70.

[105] Herdman RC, Gillespie JE, Ramsden RT. Facial palsy after glomus tumour embolization. J Laryngol Otol 1993;107:963–6.

[106] Magit AE. Tumors of the nose, paranasal sinuses, and nasopharynx. In: Bluestone CD, Stool SE, Kenna MA, editors. Pediatric otolaryngology. 3rd edition. Philadelphia: WB Saunders; 2004. p. 893–904.

[107] Bryan RN, Sessions RB, Horowitz BL. Radiographic management of juvenile angiofibromas. AJNR Am J Neuroradiol 1981;2:157–66.

[108] McCombe A, Lund VJ, Howard DJ. Recurrence in juvenile angiofibroma. Rhinology 1990;28: 97–102.

[109] Roberson GH, Price AC, Davis JM, et al. Therapeutic embolization of juvenile angiofibroma. AJR Am J Roentgenol 1979;133:657–63.

[110] Siniluoto TM, Luotonen JP, Tikkakoski TA, et al. Value of pre-operative embolization in surgery for nasopharyngeal angiofibroma. J Laryngol Otol 1993;107:514–21.

[111] Pletcher JD, Newton TH, Dedo HH, et al. Preoperative embolization of juvenile angiofibromas of the nasopharynx. Ann Otol Rhinol Laryngol 1975;84: 740–6.

[112] Gay I, Elidan J, Gordon R. Oronasal fistula—a possible complication of preoperative embolization in the management of juvenile nasopharyngeal angiofibroma. J Laryngol Otol 1983;97:651–6.

[113] Sheikh BY. Cranial aneurysmal bone cyst with special emphasis on endovascular management. Acta Neurochir (Wien) 1999;141:601–10.

[114] Ikeda H, Niizuma H, Yoshimoto T. Aneurysmal bone cyst of the skull. Surg Neurol 1986;25: 145–8.

[115] Bingaman KD, Alleyne CH Jr, Olson JJ. Intracranial extraskeletal mesenchymal chondrosarcoma: case report. Neurosurgery 2000;46:207–11.

[116] Avellino AM, Grant GA, Harris AB, et al. Recurrent intracranial Masson's vegetant intravascular hemangioendothelioma. Case report and review of the literature. J Neurosurg 1999;91:308–12.

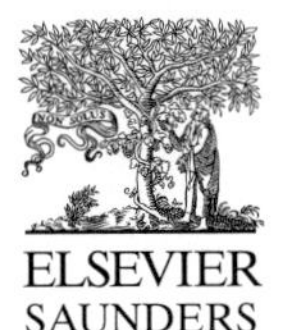

ELSEVIER
SAUNDERS

Neurosurg Clin N Am 16 (2005) 433–444

NEUROSURGERY
CLINICS
OF NORTH AMERICA

Endovascular Treatment of Acute Stroke

Mark R. Harrigan, MD[a], Lee R. Guterman, PhD, MD[b,*]

[a]*Division of Neurosurgery, Department of Surgery, The University of Alabama at Birmingham, 510 20th Street South, Room 1005, Birmingham, AL 35294, USA*

[b]*Department of Neurosurgery and Toshiba Stroke Research Center School of Medicine and Biomedical Sciences, State University of New York at Buffalo, 3 Gates Circle, Buffalo, NY 14209–1194, USA*

Stroke is a major cause of death and disability. In the United States, it is the third-leading cause of death, exceeded only by heart disease and cancer, and is a major cause of disability [1]. Approximately 700,000 strokes occur annually at a cost of $51.2 billion. Approximately 88% of strokes are ischemic, resulting from occlusion of a cervical or intracranial artery. Embolic strokes account for 24% of all strokes.

The last decade has seen the emergence of techniques to reopen occluded arteries in patients with acute ischemic stroke. Intravenous thrombolysis for acute stroke attained prominence with the results of the National Institute of Neurological Disorders and Stroke (NINDS) study [2], which demonstrated the efficacy of intravenous thrombolysis and led to the only US Food and Drug Administration (FDA)–approved treatment for acute stroke. Endovascular techniques applying intra-arterial pharmacologic and mechanical thrombolysis have also emerged as effective treatment options for selected patients with acute ischemic stroke. A recent consensus statement from the Brain Attack Coalition on recommendations for comprehensive stroke centers includes the presence of an endovascular team [3].

In this article, the authors focus on the endovascular treatment of acute stroke. Clinical experience with intravenous thrombolysis is summarized, followed by a discussion of intra-arterial pharmacologic and mechanical thrombolysis. Patient selection and technique for intra-arterial thrombolysis are also presented.

* Corresponding author.

Thrombolytic agents

Several thrombolytic agents have been introduced (Table 1). Most act by converting plasminogen to plasmin. Plasmin then cleaves the fibrin meshwork of the clot, leading to lysis. The first-generation agents urokinase and streptokinase are not fibrin (ie, clot) specific. Urokinase, a naturally occurring serine protease with low antigenicity, was withdrawn from the market in the United States for several years but has recently been reintroduced. Streptokinase, an activator of plasminogen but not an enzyme despite the name, has limited usefulness, because many patients have preformed antistreptococcal antibodies and have the potential for an anaphylactic reaction to this agent. The second-generation agents are fibrin specific and include prourokinase (also known as pro-urokinase, pro-UK, or saruplase) and alteplase. They have the disadvantage of lowering levels of fibrinogen and plasminogen, leading to an increased risk of hemorrhagic complications. Prourokinase is a precursor of urokinase and is activated at the thrombus surface to urokinase by fibrin-bound plasmin, resulting in superior fibrin specificity and lytic efficacy compared with urokinase. Prourokinase has the distinction of being the agent used in the Prolyse in Acute Cerebral Thromboembolism (PROACT) trials [4,5] but is not currently available for clinical use. Tissue plasminogen activator (t-PA) is currently the only agent approved by the FDA specifically for intravenous thrombolysis for ischemic stroke. The third-generation thrombolytic agents offer the theoretic advantages of longer half-lives and greater penetration into the thrombus matrix compared with the second-generation agents and

doi:10.1016/j.nec.2004.08.009

neurosurgery.theclinics.com

Table 1
Thrombolytic agents

	Half-life (minutes)	Intra-arterial dose	Description
First generation			
Urokinase	14–20	500,000–1,000,000 U	Serine protease
Streptokinase	18–23	NA	Protein isolated from group C β-hemolytic streptococci
Second generation			
Prourokinase	20	6–9 mg	Proenzyme precursor of urokinase
Alteplase	3–5	5–40 mg	Serine protease
Third generation			
Tenecteplase	17	NA	t-PA mutant
Reteplase	15–18	4–8 U	Deletion mutant of t-PA

Abbreviations: NA, not available; t-PA, recombinant tissue plasminogen activator.

include reteplase and tenecteplase. Reteplase is a deletion mutant in which the finger, epidermal growth factor, and kringle-1 domains have been deleted from the wild-type t-PA molecule. Tenecteplase is also a t-PA mutant.

Three main thrombolytic agents are currently available in the United States: alteplase (Activase; Genentech, San Francisco, California), urokinase (Abbokinase; Abbott Laboratories, Abbott Park, Illinois), and reteplase (Retavase; Centocor, Malvern, Pennsylvania). Five milligrams of alteplase is considered equivalent to 1 U of reteplase. Although each agent has its own theoretic advantages, a direct comparison of the effectiveness of these agents in acute stroke is lacking. In a recent retrospective comparison of t-PA with urokinase for intra-arterial thrombolysis, no differences in recanalization rates were found with respect to thrombolytic agent or dosage [6]. Thrombolytic reversal can be undertaken by administering fresh-frozen plasma in the event of a hemorrhagic complication.

In contrast to thrombolytic agents that act on plasminogen, ancrod, a protease derived from Malaysian pit viper venom, produces a rapid decrease in serum fibrinogen by accelerating cleavage of the fibrinogen A-chain [7]. Reducing serum fibrinogen levels produces anticoagulation by depleting the substrate needed for thrombus formation. Depletion of fibrinogen also reduces blood viscosity [8].

Intravenous thrombolysis

Several major phase III clinical trials of intravenous thrombolysis for acute stroke have been reported. Clinical results and symptomatic intracranial hemorrhage (ICH) rates have been variable, reflecting the differing time to treatment and thrombolytic doses used. In the NINDS trial, patients received 0.9 mg/kg of intravenous t-PA (maximal dose of 90 mg) within 3 hours of stroke onset [2]. At 3 months, these patients were approximately 30% more likely to have minimal or no disability than those receiving placebo. Symptomatic ICH occurred within 36 hours after treatment in 6.4% of patients given t-PA compared with 0.4% of those given placebo; however, mortality rates in the two groups were not significantly different. A subgroup analysis of the NINDS trial results found that t-PA efficacy is independent of stroke severity or subtype [9]. In the European Cooperative Acute Stroke Study (ECASS) I and II, patients received treatment with intravenous t-PA up to 6 hours after stroke onset [10,11]. In ECASS I, although there was no significant difference in outcomes between patients given t-PA (1.1 mg/kg) compared with those receiving placebo, the incidence of symptomatic ICH was 19.8% in the treatment group compared with 6.5% in the placebo group [10]. In ECASS II, the treatment group received t-PA (0.9 mg/kg) [11]. Although there was also no significant difference in outcomes, the incidence of symptomatic ICH was 8.85% in the treatment group versus 3.4% in the placebo group. In the Alteplase Thrombolysis for Acute Noninterventional Therapy in Ischemic Stroke Study, patients were treated with intravenous t-PA (0.9 mg/kg) 3 to 5 hours after symptom onset [12]. No significant differences in outcomes were observed, but the incidence of symptomatic ICH was 7.0% in the treatment group compared with 1.1% in the placebo group. In the Stroke Treatment with Ancrod Trial, patients were treated with ancrod as a continuous 72-hour intravenous infusion beginning within 3 hours of stroke onset, followed by infusions lasting approximately 1 hour at 96 and 120 hours [13]. The regimen was designed to decrease plasma fibrinogen levels to a range of

1.18 to 2.03 μmol/L. Patients in the treatment group achieved a significantly greater rate of favorable functional status than those in the placebo group (42.2% versus 34.4%). Mortality was not significantly different, although there was a trend toward a higher incidence of symptomatic ICH in the treatment group (5.2% versus 2.0%; $P = 0.06$).

In 1996, the FDA approved the use of intravenous recombinant t-PA in patients who present within 3 hours of the onset of acute ischemic stroke. In recent years, the use of intravenous t-PA for patients presenting within 3 hours after acute stroke has become widespread, with approval in Canada, South America, Australia, and the European Union [14]. Intravenous thrombolysis has numerous limitations, however. As few as 1% to 6% of patients with acute stroke meet the rigid time constraint and other criteria for intravenous thrombolysis [15,16]. Several randomized trials have failed to demonstrate a significant benefit for intravenous thrombolysis initiated beyond 3 hours after stroke onset [11,12,17,18]. Moreover, intravenous thrombolysis carries a significant risk of symptomatic ICH.

Endovascular thrombolysis

Rationale

Intravenous thrombolysis is most successful in the treatment of mild or moderate strokes caused by small thrombi occlusion of second-degree vessels [9,19]. Recanalization strategies for large-vessel occlusions are needed. Intra-arterial thrombolysis offers potential advantages over intravenous thrombolysis. Angiography permits precise diagnosis and exclusion of patients in whom spontaneous recanalization has occurred. During intra-arterial thrombolysis, pharmacologic as well as mechanical means can be applied to achieve recanalization rates superior to those obtained with intravenous thrombolysis. In addition, a smaller dose of thrombolytic agent can be administered intra-arterially, thus minimizing the risk of hemorrhagic complications. Disadvantages of intra-arterial thrombolysis (compared with intravenous thrombolysis) include increased cost, possible delay in treatment, and risk and discomfort associated with cerebral angiography and neuroendovascular procedures.

Pharmacologic intra-arterial thrombolysis

Early experience with intra-arterial thrombolysis resulted in widely variable recanalization rates ranging from 45% to 90% [20–23]. This variability was attributable to differing thrombolytic agents and dosing regimens as well as to the different vessels treated. For instance, in a retrospective study of intra-arterial urokinase, recanalization rates for occlusions of the internal carotid artery, basilar artery, and anterior cerebral artery were found inferior to those for occlusion of the middle cerebral artery (MCA) [24].

The PROACT I and II studies were the first randomized, double-blind, multicenter trials to evaluate intra-arterial thrombolysis in patients with acute stroke [4,5]. Recanalization rates were graded according to the Thrombolysis in Myocardial Infarction (TIMI) system (Table 2) [25]. In PROACT I, intra-arterial recombinant prourokinase or placebo, 6 mg, was administered to patients with MCA occlusion (TIMI grade 0 or 1 occlusion of the M1 or M2 segment of the MCA) within 6 hours after symptom onset [4]. End points were recanalization efficacy and the rate of ICH causing neurologic deterioration within 24 hours of treatment. Fifty-four patients received recombinant prourokinase (n = 40) or placebo (n = 14) and were treated a median of 5.5 hours after symptom onset. The recombinant prourokinase or placebo was infused into the thrombus over the course of 120 minutes. All patients received one of two intravenous heparin regimens: high-dose (100-U/kg bolus plus continuous infusion of 1000 U/h for 4 hours) or low-dose (2000-U bolus plus continuous infusion of 500 U/h for 4 hours). The patients were treated a median of 5.5 hours after symptom onset. The recanalization rate (TIMI grade 2 or 3) was significantly higher in the recombinant prourokinase group (82% in those who received high-dose

Table 2
Thrombolysis in myocardial infarction scale

Grade	Definition
0	No flow
1	Some penetration past the site of occlusion but no flow distal to occlusion
2	Distal perfusion but delayed filling in distal vessels
3	Distal perfusion with adequate perfusion of distal vessels

From Chesebro JH, Knatterud G, Roberts R, et al. Thrombolysis in Myocardial Infarction (TIMI) Trial, Phase I: a comparison between intravenous tissue plasminogen activator and intravenous streptokinase. Clinical findings through hospital discharge. Circulation 1987;76(1):142–54; with permission.

heparin and 40% in those who received low-dose heparin) than in the placebo group (14%). Hemorrhagic transformation causing neurologic deterioration during the first 24 hours after treatment occurred in 15.4% of patients receiving recombinant prourokinase versus 7.1% of those receiving placebo. The rates of recanalization and hemorrhagic complications were directly related to the heparin dose.

In the PROACT II trial, neurologic disability at 90 days (assessed using the modified Rankin Scale score) was the primary outcome measure [5]. The rate of MCA recanalization, frequency of ICH with neurologic deterioration, and rate of mortality were secondary outcomes. Similar entrance criteria were used, but the recombinant prourokinase dose was increased to 9 mg. A total of 180 patients were randomized to receive either intra-arterial recombinant prourokinase plus heparin (n = 121) or heparin alone (n = 59). All patients received heparin (2000-U bolus and a 500-U/h infusion for 4 hours beginning at the time of angiography). At the 90-day follow-up evaluation, 40% of patients receiving recombinant prourokinase and 25% of those receiving heparin alone had a modified Rankin Scale score of 2 or less ($P = 0.04$). The recanalization rate (TIMI grade 2 or 3) was 66% for the recombinant prourokinase group and 18% for the heparin-only group ($P < 0.001$). ICH with neurologic deterioration within 24 hours occurred in 10% of patients receiving recombinant prourokinase and in 2% of control patients ($P = 0.06$).

Combination intravenous and intra-arterial thrombolysis

An alternative strategy for acute stroke therapy is a combination of intravenous thrombolysis with intra-arterial thrombolysis [26–29]. This approach seeks to combine the advantage of early initiation of therapy with intravenous administration with the precision and greater lytic potential of intra-arterial therapy. Several series and a randomized pilot study have demonstrated the feasibility of "bridging" from reduced-dose intravenous thrombolysis to selective intra-arterial thrombolysis. Ernst and colleagues [26] reported a series of 20 patients treated with intravenous t-PA (0.6 mg/kg), followed by intra-arterial administration of t-PA (maximum dose of 0.3 mg/kg). The median baseline National Institutes of Health Stroke Scale (NIHSS) score was 21 (range: 11–31). Ten (50%) patients recovered to a modified Rankin Scale score of 0 or 1, and 1 (5%) patient developed a symptomatic ICH. Suarez et al [29] reported a series in which 24 patients received intravenous t-PA (0.6 mg/kg), followed by intra-arterial urokinase (up to 750,000 U) or t-PA (maximum dose of 0.3 mg/kg). Complete recanalization was achieved in 9 (38%) patients, 19 (79%) patients had a Barthel Index score of greater than or equal to 95% at 3 months, and none of the patients had symptomatic ICH. The Emergency Management of Stroke Bridging Trial was a phase I, randomized, controlled study of combination intravenous and intra-arterial thrombolysis [28]. Thirty-five patients received either intravenous t-PA (0.6 mg/kg) or intravenous placebo, followed by intra-arterial administration of t-PA (maximum dose of 20 mg). Complete recanalization was obtained in 6 (55%) of 11 patients in the intravenous–intra-arterial therapy group versus 1 (10%) of 10 patients in the intravenous-placebo group. Although only one symptomatic ICH occurred (in an intravenous placebo patient), 2 intravenous–intra-arterial patients had life-threatening nonintracranial hemorrhagic complications. There were no significant differences in 90-day outcomes in the treatment groups as measured by a variety of scales. Larger trials are needed to assess the effectiveness of combination therapy.

Another approach to combination therapy uses glycoprotein (GP) IIb-IIIa receptor antagonists, such as tirofiban and abciximab. Platelet activation and accumulation during and after thrombolysis can lead to vessel reocclusion, which can occur in up to 8% of cases [30]. The platelet GP IIb-IIIa receptor promotes thrombosis by forming stable fibrin bonds between activated platelets. The GP IIb-IIIa antagonists selectively inhibit the platelet integrin $\alpha_{IIb}\beta_{III}$ fibrinogen receptor and thereby inhibit adenosine diphosphate–induced platelet aggregation. In a preliminary clinical study, significantly better outcomes (in terms of Rankin Scale scores) were achieved with intravenously administered low-dose t-PA in combination with parenterally administered tirofiban than with standard-dose intravenous t-PA (0.9 mg/kg) alone [31]. In a pilot study of 10 patients with acute ischemic stroke who were treated with intra-arterial urokinase plus abciximab, the recanalization rate (TIMI grade 2 or 3) was 90%, which was significantly better than the rate experienced by an earlier series of patients at the same center receiving intra-arterial urokinase alone (43.8%) [32]. The mean dose of urokinase required for recanalization was significantly lower in the group receiving abciximab (418,000 versus 828,000 U), and there were no significant differences in the rate of symptomatic ICH.

Mechanical thrombolysis

Mechanical thrombolysis can have a role in acute stroke treatment for several reasons. Mechanical disruption of the thrombus can increase the effectiveness of thrombolytic agents and reduce the total dose and time required for vessel recanalization. Animal studies have demonstrated that mechanical clot disruption increases the surface area of clot exposed to the thrombolytic agent, thereby enhancing the drug's effectiveness [33,34]. In those situations in which an underlying atheroma is associated with the vessel occlusion, angioplasty can widen the lumen of the affected portion of the vessel and increase flow, thereby reducing the risk of reocclusion caused by sluggish flow. Mechanical thrombolysis can also be a useful adjunct in cases in which the clot burden is too great for pharmacologic thrombolysis alone, such as carotid bifurcation ("T") occlusions [35]. In addition, other means are required to dislodge calcified atheromatous debris and other embolic materials that are resistant to thrombolytic agents. Further advantages associated with mechanical thrombolysis are the potential to extend the treatment window for thrombolysis and avoidance of thrombolytic drugs in patients for whom thrombolytic drugs are contraindicated.

A variety of devices and techniques are currently available for use in mechanical thrombolysis. The Amplatz Goose-Neck Microsnare (Microvena, White Bear Lake, Minnesota) is a fine wire snare that can be passed through a microcatheter into the thrombus. Passage of the snare through the thrombus can break up the clot and increase the surface area of the thrombus exposed to thrombolytic drug. In a series of five patients in whom intra-arterial pharmacologic thrombolysis failed to result in vessel recanalization, snares were used to obtain complete recanalization in three patients and partial recanalization in two others [36]. Suction thrombectomy is a technique that is useful for aspiration of large vessel occlusions, such as thrombus within the internal carotid artery, provided that the catheter tip can be positioned within the thrombus. In a series of three patients with occlusions of the internal carotid artery, suction thrombectomy led to recanalization in all cases [37]. The In-Time retrieval device (Boston Scientific, Fremont, California) is an expandable wire mesh that can be passed through a microcatheter to engage and retrieve or fragment clot. Balloon angioplasty can be useful in occlusions with underlying stenosis caused by atherosclerosis or a dissection. Angioplasty can also be useful in the treatment of proximal or middle basilar artery thrombosis, which tends to be the result of thrombosis superimposed on atherosclerotic lesions in contrast to distal basilar occlusions, which tend to be embolic [38]. In this setting, angioplasty can be used to reduce the risk of rethrombosis [39]. Several authors have reported favorable results with "rescue angioplasty," in which angioplasty is used to obtain recanalization in vessel occlusions that are resistant to thrombolytic agents alone. Two retrospective series have reported recanalization using angioplasty in a total of 10 of 16 occluded arteries that were resistant to pharmacologic thrombolysis [40,41].

A common strategy is to combine pharmacologic thrombolysis with clot fragmentation. In an early report, Barnwell et al [42] described a series of 13 patients in whom intra-arterial urokinase infusion was used in conjunction with mechanical thrombolysis. Disruption of the clot was achieved by frequent passage of a microcatheter through the clot matrix. Recanalization was obtained in 10 (77%) patients, with significant neurologic improvement (greater than four-point decrease in NIHSS score) occurring in 9 (69%). Mechanical thrombolysis can supplement low-dose pharmacologic thrombolysis, serving to reduce the incidence of symptomatic ICH while obtaining recanalization rates comparable to those with higher dose thrombolytic regimens. In a series of 19 patients with acute stroke, Qureshi and colleagues [43] used intra-arterial infusion of reteplase (maximum dose of 4 U) supplemented as needed with angioplasty (for proximal occlusions, such as in the cervical internal carotid artery) or snare manipulation (for distal occlusions, such as those in the MCA). Complete recanalization was obtained in 12 (63%) patients, and no symptomatic ICHs were observed.

Several devices for mechanical thrombolysis are currently undergoing evaluation. The Concentric Thrombus Retriever System (Concentric Medical, Mountain View, California) uses a fine wire retrieval device that can be placed within a thrombus by passage through a microcatheter. The retrieval device has a corkscrew shape and is designed to firmly engage the clot for removal.

The Concentric guide catheter is equipped with a balloon at the tip that can temporarily arrest flow in the carotid artery during retraction of the retrieval device and removal of the clot. This device is being tested in the Mechanical Embolus Removal in Cerebral Ischemia trial in patients with acute stroke ineligible for treatment with intravenous t-PA or presenting within 3 to 8 hours after symptom onset. The Neuronet Endovascular Snare (Guidant Corp., Indianapolis, Indiana) is a snare device with a basket shape for use in acute stroke, and it is being used in the Neuronet Evaluation in Embolic stroke Disease trial in Europe.

The AngioJet (Possis Medical, Minneapolis, Minnesota) is a mechanical thrombectomy catheter that uses several high-pressure saline jets to break up clot and aspirate debris simultaneously. This device has received FDA approval for use in coronary arteries and the periphery; a version modified for use in cerebral vessels is being tested in the Thrombectomy in Middle Cerebral Artery Embolism trial.

The EKOS Ultrasound Thrombolytic Infusion Catheter (EKOS Corp., Bothell, Washington) combines low-energy ultrasound with infusion of a thrombolytic agent. Preliminary clinical trial data demonstrated a recanalization rate (TIMI grade 2 or 3) of 57% in patients with MCA or carotid "T" occlusions [44]. The Endovascular Photo Acoustic Recanalization (EPAR) system (EndoVasix, Belmont, California) uses a fiberoptic laser to break up clot. In a pilot study of the EPAR system in patients with acute stroke, the recanalization rate (TIMI grade 2 or 3) was 48%, although two vessel perforations occurred during the placement of the catheter [45]. The LaTIS laser device (LaTIS, Coon Rapids, Minnesota) also uses laser energy to dissolve clots and is undergoing testing in a phase I trial at two centers in the United States.

Patient selection

The clinical criteria for enrollment in the PROACT studies can serve as guidelines for patient selection for endovascular therapy of acute stroke. The leading factor in patient selection is time from symptom onset, generally within 6 hours for anterior circulation occlusions. In PROACT II, the typical interval from initiation of intra-arterial infusion of thrombolytic drug to completion of recanalization was 90 to 120 minutes; therefore, the 6-hour treatment window may be viewed as an 8-hour recanalization window [5]. Thus, for situations in which recanalization can be accomplished more rapidly than in the PROACT trials, such as with mechanical thrombolysis, the time window for recanalization may be extended to 8 hours. For patients with basilar artery occlusions, intra-arterial thrombolysis can be undertaken up to 24 hours after symptom onset [46,47]. Additional clinical inclusion criteria for PROACT II were a minimal NIHSS score of 4, except for isolated aphasia or hemianopia, and age ranging from 18 to 85 years. Angiographic findings were graded according to the TIMI scale (see Table 2). The TIMI scale is limited by not considering occlusion location or collateral circulation; Qureshi [48] introduced an alternative classification scheme for acute ischemic stroke that incorporates these angiographic findings (Table 3). Only patients with angiographic evidence of complete occlusion (TIMI grade 0) or contrast penetration with minimal perfusion (TIMI grade 1) were included. Exclusion criteria for PROACT II are listed in Box 1. The strict exclusion criteria for PROACT II were developed for a randomized controlled trial and can serve as relative exclusion criteria for the management of the care of individual patients who are not enrolled in a study.

Radiographic evaluation

Brain imaging is required before an intervention for acute stroke is performed. CT scanning is the most important brain imaging modality for this purpose, permitting rapid evaluation for the presence of ICH as well as early signs of infarction and thrombus within intracranial vessels. CT perfusion cerebral blood flow imaging can be done at the same time as the initial screening CT scan and can provide useful information that can guide intervention (Fig. 1A–C) [49,50]. CT perfusion imaging is a recent addition to CT technology and is now widely available as a software package included with most high-speed spiral CT scanners. CT perfusion uses a single dose of intravenous contrast in combination with rapid scanning during the passage of the contrast through the intracranial vessels to measure cerebral blood flow, cerebral blood volume, and time-to-peak or mean transit time. Acquisition and processing of the data take only several minutes. Quantitative color-coded maps of the brain can identify regions of ischemia and vascular territories affected by the stroke. CT perfusion maps can also be used to

Table 3
Qureshi grading system for acute ischemic stroke

Grade 0	No occlusion		
Grade 1	MCA occlusion (M3 segment)	ACA occlusion (A2 or distal segments)	1 BA/VA branch occlusion
Grade 2	MCA occlusion (M2 segment)	ACA occlusion (A1 and A2 segments)	≥2 BA/VA branch occlusions
Grade 3	MCA occlusion (M1 segment)		
3A	Lenticulostriate arteries spared and/or leptomeningeal collaterals visualized		
3B	No sparing of lenticulostriate arteries or leptomeningeal collaterals visualized		
Grade 4	ICA occlusion (collaterals present)		BA occlusion (partial filling direct or via collaterals)
4A	Collaterals fill MCA		Anterograde filling*
4B	Collaterals fill ACA		Retrograde filling*
Grade 5	ICA occlusion (no collaterals)		BA occlusion (complete)

Abbreviations: ACA, anterior cerebral artery; BA, basilar artery; ICA, internal carotid artery; MCA, middle cerebral artery; VA, vertebral artery; *, the predominant pattern of filling.

From Qureshi AI. New grading system for angiographic evaluation of arterial occlusions and recanalization response to intra-arterial thrombolysis in acute ischemic stroke. Neurosurgery 2002;50(6):1405–15; with permission.

identify patients who would not be good candidates for endovascular intervention, such as those with lacunar strokes and those without arterial occlusions, which account for up to 25% [51] and 29% [52] of patients with acute stroke, respectively. In addition, CT perfusion imaging can provide prognostic information, because patients with profound widespread ischemia can be expected to have a poorer outcome than those with borderline ischemia [53].

MRI can also have a role in the evaluation of patients with acute stroke. MRI has superior anatomic resolution when compared with CT and is also capable of identifying brain tissue with or at risk of ischemia. Perfusion-weighted MRI allows visualization of areas of diminished blood flow. Diffusion-weighted MRI demonstrates regions of restricted water movement that are associated with bioenergetic failure. Used together, perfusion- and diffusion-weighted MRI can identify tissue that is at risk of infarction but amenable to salvage with revascularization [54]. The primary disadvantage of MRI in the evaluation of acute stroke is the time required to obtain the study. Therefore, care must be taken not to allow the use of MRI to delay rapid intervention.

Technique

The technique of intra-arterial thrombolysis for acute stroke varies slightly from institution to institution. The following is a general outline of the steps taken at our center. A representative case is illustrated in Fig. 1. After a rapid but thorough evaluation in the emergency room, the patient is brought to the angiography suite. Local anesthesia with mild sedation is adequate for approximately one half of patients; those with mental status changes or aphasia as a result of dominant hemisphere lesions are often unable to cooperate and are best managed under general anesthesia. To save time, patients requiring general anesthesia are usually intubated in the emergency room.

In the angiography suite, a 6-French guide catheter is placed in the femoral artery and a loading dose of intravenous heparin is given (3–5 U/kg) to achieve an activated coagulation time of at least 250 seconds. A focused diagnostic angiogram is performed, beginning with the aortic arch to identify a common carotid or vertebral artery occlusion. Selective angiography of the common carotid or vertebral artery is then performed, including cervical and intracranial imaging. Once an arterial occlusion has been identified, a guide catheter is placed in the cervical vessel as close to the skull base as possible. Our preference is to place a 6-French Envoy guide catheter (Cordis, Miami Lakes, Florida) in the distal cervical internal carotid artery or vertebral artery. Using a road-mapping technique, a microcatheter is then guided over a microwire into the region of occlusion. A microcatheter that is large enough to accommodate a snare (eg, Prowler-Plus microcatheter; Cordis) should be selected should a snare become necessary. The microwire and then the microcatheter are gently advanced through the lumen of the occluded vessel for a distance likely to

Box 1. Exclusion criteria for PROACT II

- NIHSS score greater than 30
- Coma
- Rapidly improving neurologic signs
- Stroke within the previous 6 weeks
- Seizures at onset of presenting stroke
- Clinical presentation suggestive of subarachnoid hemorrhage
- Previous ICH, neoplasm, or subarachnoid hemorrhage
- Septic embolism
- Suspected lacunar stroke
- Surgery, biopsy of a parenchymal organ, trauma with internal injuries, or lumbar puncture within 30 days
- Head trauma within 90 days
- Active or recent hemorrhage within 30 days
- Known hemorrhagic diathesis, baseline international normalized ratio greater than 1.7, activated partial thromboplastin time greater than 1.5 times normal, or baseline platelet count less than 100×10^9 L
- Known sensitivity to contrast agents
- Uncontrolled hypertension defined by blood pressure greater than or equal to 180 mm Hg systolic or greater than or equal to 100 mm Hg diastolic on three separate occasions at least 10 minutes apart or requiring intravenous therapy
- CT evidence of hemorrhage, intracranial tumors except for small meningiomas, significant mass effect from the infarction, and acute hypodense parenchymal lesion or effacement of cerebral sulci in more than one third of the MCA territory
- Angiographic evidence of arterial dissection, arterial stenosis precluding safe passage of a microcatheter into the MCA, nonatherosclerotic arteriopathy, no visible occlusion, or occlusion of an artery other than the M1 or M2 segment of the MCA

From Furlan A, Higashida R, Wechsler L, et al. Intra-arterial prourokinase for acute ischemic stroke. The PROACT II study: a randomized controlled trial. Prolyse in Acute Cerebral Thromboembolism. JAMA 1999; 282(21):2003–11; with permission.

be distal to the embolus or thrombus. This point is typically at the next branch point of the occluded vessel. (For instance, in MCA strokes involving occlusion of the M1 division, the embolus is often lodged in the vessel at the MCA bifurcation.) The microwire is then withdrawn, and a microcatheter angiogram is obtained to clarify the extent and position of the occlusion. The microcatheter is then drawn back into the occluded portion of the vessel, and the thrombolytic agent is injected through the microcatheter. Our preference is to administer urokinase in doses of 125,000 U to a maximum of 750,000 to 1,000,000 U. After each dose is given, the microcatheter is gradually withdrawn through the area of occlusion so as to distribute the thrombolytic agent within the clot. A guide catheter angiogram is obtained after each dose of the agent is administered to track progress of the thrombolysis and to monitor for vessel perforation by checking for contrast extravasation. The procedure is complete once recanalization of the vessel has been obtained or when the maximum dose of the thrombolytic agent has been administered and all other maneuvers, such as mechanical thrombolysis, have been undertaken. A head CT scan is obtained to check for ICH, and the patient is admitted to the intensive care unit.

Mechanical thrombolysis can be useful for situations in which pharmacologic thrombolysis alone does not lead to recanalization. Our preference is to begin by readvancing the microcatheter and microwire past the region of occlusion and then to advance a 2- or 4-mm Amplatz Goose-Neck Microsnare through the microcatheter into the vessel just distal to the occlusion. The microcatheter and snare are then withdrawn through the embolus or thrombus in back-and-forth movements to macerate the clot and increase the surface area available for pharmacologic thrombolysis. Another device that is useful to help break up clot is the In-Time retrieval device. Angioplasty using a coronary artery balloon can also help to break up debris.

Suction thrombectomy is a technique that is useful when the amount of thrombus (the "clot burden") is large, such as in occlusions of the distal internal carotid artery. A 7-French catheter must be positioned immediately proximal to the thrombus, and aggressive suction is undertaken through the catheter with a 60-mL syringe.

For those cases in which an arterial dissection is located at the origin of the vessel occlusion, placement of a stent is usually required. In the cervical carotid system, acute dissections can be

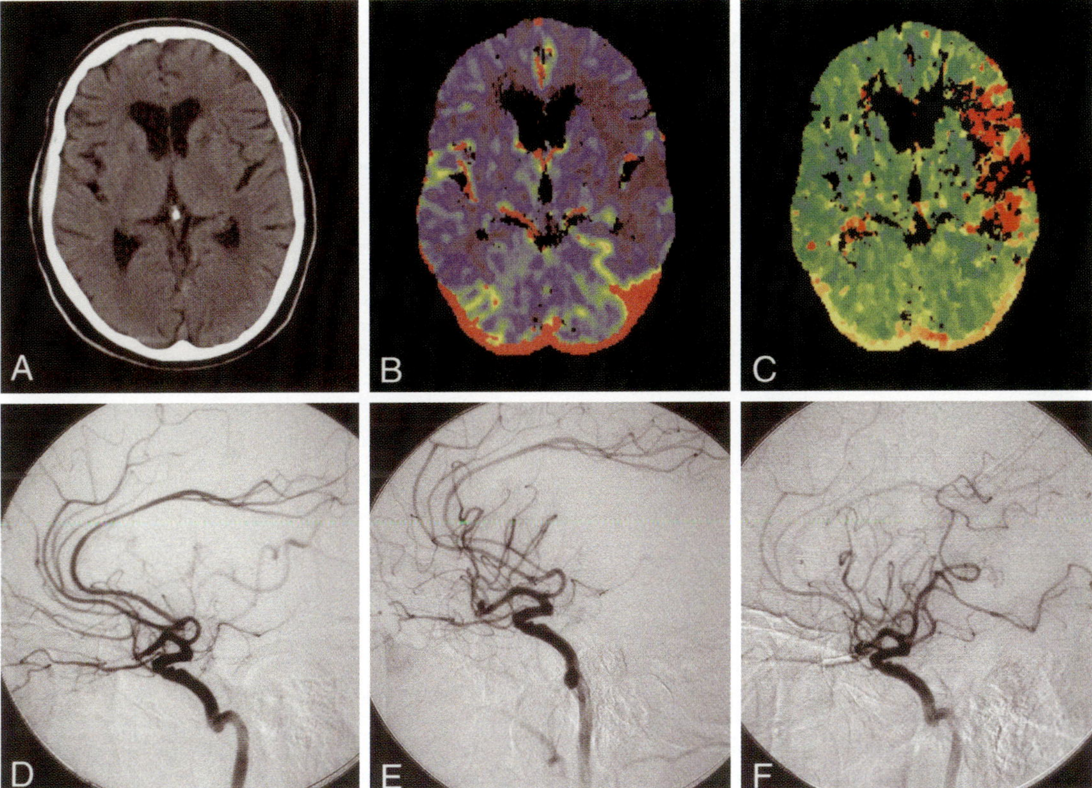

Fig. 1. An 87-year-old man with acute right hemiparesis and aphasia. The initial National Institutes of Health Stroke Scale score was 12. (*A*) Initial CT scan. A CT perfusion study was obtained when the patient developed mental status changes; cerebral blood flow (CBF) (*B*) and time-to-peak (TTP) (*C*). Reduced perfusion in the left middle cerebral artery (MCA) territory is indicated by diminished CBF and extended TTP. (*D*) Angiogram showing an occlusion of the M1 segment of the left MCA. Angiograms were done after intra-arterial infusion of urokinase (750,000 U) and recanalization of the superior division (*E*) and inferior division (*F*) of the left MCA. The patient's neurologic examination returned to normal during the procedure. A CT perfusion study done after the intervention showed normal CBF and TTP in the left MCA territory.

treated by deployment of a self-expanding Wallstent (Boston Scientific), followed by poststent deployment angioplasty. Intracranial vessel dissections usually require deployment of a balloon-mounted coronary stent, such as the Bx Velocity (Cordis). When a stent is deployed during the treatment of an acute stroke, care must be taken to provide an adequate antiplatelet regimen to prevent acute thrombosis within the freshly placed stent. A loading dose of clopidogrel (300 mg) and aspirin (325 mg) is given orally or via nasogastric tube during or immediately after the case. To provide antiplatelet coverage during the interval before the enteric medications can take effect, an intravenous infusion of a GP IIb-IIIa inhibitor is begun at the time of stent placement and continued for 24 hours.

Summary

Acute ischemic stroke is a major public health threat. Intravenous thrombolysis has been shown in several randomized clinical trials to improve outcomes in selected patients, and intravenous t-PA is currently approved by the FDA for patients presenting within 3 hours of symptom onset. Three generations of thrombolytic agents have been introduced. Intra-arterial thrombolysis offers several potential advantages over intravenous thrombolysis for acute stroke, such as precise diagnosis and the opportunity to reduce the overall dose of thrombolytic agent used, and thus lowers the chance of ICH. The PROACT trials showed that intra-arterial thrombolysis can improve recanalization rates and outcomes in patients presenting with MCA occlusions up to 6 hours after symptom onset. Alternative strategies for endovascular treatment of acute stroke include combination intravenous–intra-arterial administration of thrombolytic agents, use of GP IIb-IIIa antagonists, and mechanical thrombolysis. Options for mechanical thrombolysis include microsnares, the In-Time thrombus retrieval device, angioplasty, and suction thrombectomy. Several investigational devices are undergoing clinical evaluation. The PROACT enrollment criteria can serve as guidelines for patient selection. Radiographic evaluation of acute stroke patients begins with imaging to exclude the presence of ICH; recent developments in CT and MRI perfusion promise to permit identification of patients who will benefit from thrombolysis with greater precision.

References

[1] American Heart Association. Heart disease and stroke statistics—2004 update. Available: http://www.americanheart.org/presenter.jhtml?identifier=1200026. Accessed February 16, 2004.

[2] The National Institute of Neurological Disorders and Stroke rt-PA Stroke Study Group. Tissue plasminogen activator for acute ischemic stroke. N Engl J Med 1995;333(24):1581–7.

[3] Alberts MJ, Hademenos G, Latchaw RE, et al. Recommendations for the establishment of primary stroke centers. Brain Attack Coalition. JAMA 2000;283:3102–9.

[4] del Zoppo GJ, Higashida RT, Furlan AJ, Pessin MS, Rowley HA, Gent M. PROACT: a phase II randomized trial of recombinant pro-urokinase by direct arterial delivery in acute middle cerebral artery stroke. PROACT Investigators. Prolyse in Acute Cerebral Thromboembolism. Stroke 1998;29(1):4–11.

[5] Furlan A, Higashida R, Wechsler L, et al. Intra-arterial prourokinase for acute ischemic stroke. The PROACT II study: a randomized controlled trial. Prolyse in Acute Cerebral Thromboembolism. JAMA 1999;282(21):2003–11.

[6] Eckert B, Kucinski T, Neumaier-Probst E, Fiehler J, Rother J, Zeumer H. Local intra-arterial fibrinolysis in acute hemispheric stroke: effect of occlusion type and fibrinolytic agent on recanalization success and neurological outcome. Cerebrovasc Dis 2003;15(4):258–63.

[7] Ewart MR, Hatton MW, Basford JM, Dodgson KS. The proteolytic action of Arvin on human fibrinogen. Biochem J 1970;118(4):603–9.

[8] Ehrly AM. Influence of Arwin on the flow properties of blood. Biorheology 1973;10(3):453–6.

[9] Generalized efficacy of t-PA for acute stroke. Subgroup analysis of the NINDS t-PA Stroke Trial. Stroke 1997;28(11):2119–25.

[10] Hacke W, Kaste M, Fieschi C, et al. Intravenous thrombolysis with recombinant tissue plasminogen activator for acute hemispheric stroke. The European Cooperative Acute Stroke Study (ECASS). JAMA 1995;274(13):1017–25.

[11] Hacke W, Kaste M, Fieschi C, et al. Randomised double-blind placebo-controlled trial of thrombolytic therapy with intravenous alteplase in acute ischaemic stroke (ECASS II). Second European-Australasian Acute Stroke Study Investigators. Lancet 1998;352(9136):1245–51.

[12] Clark WM, Wissman S, Albers GW, Jhamandas JH, Madden KP, Hamilton S. Recombinant tissue-type plasminogen activator (Alteplase) for ischemic stroke 3 to 5 hours after symptom onset. The ATLANTIS Study: a randomized controlled trial. Alteplase Thrombolysis for Acute Noninterventional Therapy in Ischemic Stroke. JAMA 1999;282(21):2019–26.

[13] Sherman DG, Atkinson RP, Chippendale T, et al. Intravenous ancrod for treatment of acute ischemic stroke: the STAT study: a randomized controlled trial. Stroke Treatment with Ancrod Trial. JAMA 2000;283(18):2395–403.

[14] Lindsberg PJ, Kaste M. Thrombolysis for acute stroke. Curr Opin Neurol 2003;16(1):73–80.

[15] Chiu D, Krieger D, Villar-Cordova C, et al. Intravenous tissue plasminogen activator for acute ischemic stroke: feasibility, safety, and efficacy in the first year of clinical practice. Stroke 1998;29(1):18–22.

[16] Katzan IL, Furlan AJ, Lloyd LE, et al. Use of tissue-type plasminogen activator for acute ischemic stroke: the Cleveland area experience. JAMA 2000;283(9):1151–8.

[17] Randomised controlled trial of streptokinase, aspirin, and combination of both in treatment of acute ischaemic stroke. Multicentre Acute Stroke Trial—Italy (MAST-I) Group. Lancet 1995;346(8989):1509–14.

[18] Donnan GA, Davis SM, Chambers BR, et al. Streptokinase for acute ischemic stroke with relationship to time of administration: Australian Streptokinase (ASK) Trial Study Group. JAMA 1996;276(12):961–6.

[19] del Zoppo GJ, Poeck K, Pessin MS, et al. Recombinant tissue plasminogen activator in acute thrombotic and embolic stroke. Ann Neurol 1992;32(1):78–86.

[20] Ezura M, Kagawa S. Selective and superselective infusion of urokinase for embolic stroke. Surg Neurol 1992;38(5):353–8.

[21] Mori E, Tabuchi M, Yoshida T, Yamadori A. Intracarotid urokinase with thromboembolic occlusion of the middle cerebral artery. Stroke 1988;19(7):802–12.

[22] Ueda T, Hatakeyama T, Kohno K, Kumon Y, Sakaki S. Endovascular treatment for acute thrombotic

occlusion of the middle cerebral artery: local intra-arterial thrombolysis combined with percutaneous transluminal angioplasty. Neuroradiology 1997;39(2):99–104.

[23] Zeumer H, Freitag HJ, Zanella F, Thie A, Arning C. Local intra-arterial fibrinolytic therapy in patients with stroke: urokinase versus recombinant tissue plasminogen activator (r-TPA). Neuroradiology 1993;35(2):159–62.

[24] Ueda T, Sakaki S, Kumon Y, Ohta S. Multivariable analysis of predictive factors related to outcome at 6 months after intra-arterial thrombolysis for acute ischemic stroke. Stroke 1999;30(11):2360–5.

[25] Chesebro JH, Knatterud G, Roberts R, et al. Thrombolysis in Myocardial Infarction (TIMI) Trial, Phase I: a comparison between intravenous tissue plasminogen activator and intravenous streptokinase. Clinical findings through hospital discharge. Circulation 1987;76(1):142–54.

[26] Ernst R, Pancioli A, Tomsick T, et al. Combined intravenous and intra-arterial recombinant tissue plasminogen activator in acute ischemic stroke. Stroke 2000;31(11):2552–7.

[27] Hill MD, Barber PA, Demchuk AM, et al. Acute intravenous–intra-arterial revascularization therapy for severe ischemic stroke. Stroke 2002;33(1): 279–82.

[28] Lewandowski CA, Frankel M, Tomsick TA, et al. Combined intravenous and intra-arterial r-TPA versus intra-arterial therapy of acute ischemic stroke: Emergency Management of Stroke (EMS) Bridging Trial. Stroke 1999;30(12):2598–605.

[29] Suarez JI, Zaidat OO, Sunshine JL, Tarr R, Selman WR, Landis DM. Endovascular administration after intravenous infusion of thrombolytic agents for the treatment of patients with acute ischemic strokes. Neurosurgery 2002;50(2):251–60.

[30] Ueda T, Hatakeyama T, Kumon Y, Sakaki S, Uraoka T. Evaluation of risk of hemorrhagic transformation in local intra-arterial thrombolysis in acute ischemic stroke by initial SPECT. Stroke 1994; 25(2):298–303.

[31] Seitz RJ, Hamzavi M, Junghans U, Ringleb PA, Schranz C, Siebler M. Thrombolysis with recombinant tissue plasminogen activator and tirofiban in stroke: preliminary observations. Stroke 2003; 34(8):1932–5.

[32] Lee DH, Jo KD, Kim HG, et al. Local intraarterial urokinase thrombolysis of acute ischemic stroke with or without intravenous abciximab: a pilot study. J Vasc Interv Radiol 2002;13(8):769–74.

[33] Larsson J, Carlson J, Olsson SB. Ultrasound enhanced thrombolysis in experimental retinal vein occlusion in the rabbit. Br J Ophthalmol 1998; 82(12):1438–40.

[34] Shangguan HQ, Gregory KW, Casperson LW, Prahl SA. Enhanced laser thrombolysis with photomechanical drug delivery: an in vitro study. Lasers Surg Med 1998;23(3):151–60.

[35] Arnold M, Nedeltchev K, Mattle HP, et al. Intraarterial thrombolysis in 24 consecutive patients with internal carotid artery T occlusions. J Neurol Neurosurg Psychiatry 2003;74(6):739–42.

[36] Kerber CW, Barr JD, Berger RM, Chopko BW. Snare retrieval of intracranial thrombus in patients with acute stroke. J Vasc Interv Radiol 2002; 13(12):1269–74.

[37] Lutsep HL, Clark WM, Nesbit GM, Kuether TA, Barnwell SL. Intraarterial suction thrombectomy in acute stroke. AJNR Am J Neuroradiol 2002; 23(5):783–6.

[38] Cross DT III, Moran CJ, Akins PT, Angtuaco EE, Derdeyn CP, Diringer MN. Collateral circulation and outcome after basilar artery thrombolysis. AJNR Am J Neuroradiol 1998;19(8):1557–63.

[39] Nakayama T, Tanaka K, Kaneko M, Yokoyama T, Uemura K. Thrombolysis and angioplasty for acute occlusion of intracranial vertebrobasilar arteries. Report of three cases. J Neurosurg 1998;88(5): 919–22.

[40] Mori T, Kazita K, Mima T, Mori K. Balloon angioplasty for embolic total occlusion of the middle cerebral artery and ipsilateral carotid stenting in an acute stroke stage. AJNR Am J Neuroradiol 1999;20(8): 1462–4.

[41] Ringer AJ, Qureshi AI, Fessler RD, Guterman LR, Hopkins LN. Angioplasty of intracranial occlusion resistant to thrombolysis in acute ischemic stroke. Neurosurgery 2001;48(6):1282–90.

[42] Barnwell SL, Clark WM, Nguyen TT, O'Neill OR, Wynn ML, Coull BM. Safety and efficacy of delayed intraarterial urokinase therapy with mechanical clot disruption for thromboembolic stroke. AJNR Am J Neuroradiol 1994;15(10):1817–22.

[43] Qureshi AI, Siddiqui AM, Suri MF, et al. Aggressive mechanical clot disruption and low-dose intra-arterial third-generation thrombolytic agent for ischemic stroke: a prospective study. Neurosurgery 2002;51(5):1319–29.

[44] Mahon B, Nesbit G, Barnwell S, et al. North American clinical experience with the EKOS ultrasound thrombolytic drug infusion catheter for treatment of embolic stroke. Presented at the American Society of Neuroradiology 39th Annual Meeting. Boston, April 23–27, 2001.

[45] Lutsep H, Campbell M, Clark W. EPAR therapy system for treatment of acute stroke: safety study results [abstract]. Stroke 2001;32:319b.

[46] Brandt T, von Kummer R, Muller-Kuppers M, Hacke W. Thrombolytic therapy of acute basilar artery occlusion. Variables affecting recanalization and outcome. Stroke 1996;27(5):875–81.

[47] Kirton A, Wong JH, Mah J, et al. Successful endovascular therapy for acute basilar thrombosis in an adolescent. Pediatrics 2003;112(3 Part 1): e248–51.

[48] Qureshi AI. New grading system for angiographic evaluation of arterial occlusions and recanalization

response to intra-arterial thrombolysis in acute ischemic stroke. Neurosurgery 2002;50(6):1405–15.

[49] Mayer TE, Hamann GF, Baranczyk J, et al. Dynamic CT perfusion imaging of acute stroke. AJNR Am J Neuroradiol 2000;21(8):1441–9.

[50] Reichenbach JR, Rother J, Jonetz-Mentzel L, et al. Acute stroke evaluated by time-to-peak mapping during initial and early follow-up perfusion CT studies. AJNR Am J Neuroradiol 1999;20(10):1842–50.

[51] Chamorro A, Sacco RL, Mohr JP, et al. Clinical-computed tomographic correlations of lacunar infarction in the Stroke Data Bank. Stroke 1991; 22(2):175–81.

[52] Derex L, Tomsick TA, Brott TG, et al. Outcome of stroke patients without angiographically revealed arterial occlusion within four hours of symptom onset. AJNR Am J Neuroradiol 2001;22(4):685–90.

[53] Wintermark M, Reichhart M, Thiran JP, et al. Prognostic accuracy of cerebral blood flow measurement by perfusion computed tomography, at the time of emergency room admission, in acute stroke patients. Ann Neurol 2002;51(4):417–32.

[54] Neumann-Haefelin T, Wittsack HJ, Wenserski F, et al. Diffusion- and perfusion-weighted MRI. The DWI/PWI mismatch region in acute stroke. Stroke 1999;30(8):1591–7.

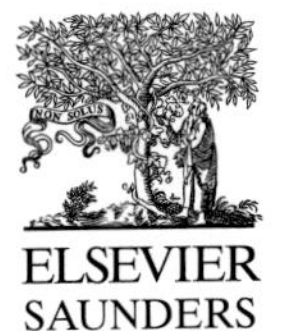
ELSEVIER
SAUNDERS

Neurosurg Clin N Am 16 (2005) 445–449

NEUROSURGERY
CLINICS
OF NORTH AMERICA

Training Standards in Endovascular Neurosurgery

Jay U. Howington, MD[a], L. Nelson Hopkins, MD, FACS[a,*], David G. Piepgras, MD[b], Robert E. Harbaugh, MD[c]

[a]*Department of Neurosurgery and Toshiba Stroke Research Center, School of Medicine and Biomedical Sciences, State University of New York at Buffalo, 3 Gates Circle, Buffalo, NY 14209, USA*

[b]*Department of Neurologic Surgery, Mayo Clinic, 200 First Street SW, Rochester, MN 55905, USA*

[c]*Department of Neurosurgery, Penn State University College of Medicine, Milton S. Hershey Medical Center, 500 University Drive, Hershey, PA 17033, USA*

The fact that interventional neuroradiology, endovascular neurosurgery, and endovascular surgical neuroradiology refer to the same subspecialty is a testament to the diversity seen among its practitioners. The group that practices these techniques includes neurosurgeons, neuroradiologists, neurologists, and, sometimes, cardiologists; the single attribute that all have in common is wielding a catheter to treat vascular lesions affecting the central nervous system (CNS). Neuroendovascular therapy began as a hybrid of traditional neurosurgical and neuroradiologic approaches and has become an established medical subspecialty with program requirements for residency education set forth by the Accreditation Council for Graduate Medical Education (ACGME) [1]. Behind the development of these educational standards exists a cooperative effort between neurosurgeons and neuroradiologists that is now exemplified by the combining of the meetings held annually by the respective groups. The Joint Section on Cerebrovascular Surgery of the American Association of Neurological Surgeons and Congress of Neurological Surgeons (CV Section) and the American Society of Interventional and Therapeutic Neuroradiology (ASITN) have joined together to advance the treatment of cerebrovascular diseases as well as to facilitate the standardization of the training curriculum. By virtue of their training and experience, neurosurgeons have had a superior understanding of the pathophysiology of CNS diseases, the indications and contraindications for treatment alternatives, and the clinical management of affected patients, whereas neuroradiologists have had better expertise in diagnostic neuroimaging, endovascular skills, and an increased awareness of available materials used for interventional procedures. The result of a nearly two decade–long collaborative effort between these specialists has been the production of new practitioners from both disciplines who possess expertise in the clinical and radiologic arenas. The requirements from the ACGME [1], along with the training standard guidelines recommended by the Executive Committees of the CV Section and the ASITN [2,3], seek to solidify the position of the endovascular neurosurgeon as a true hybrid of surgery and radiology.

Endovascular neurosurgery is a subspecialty that uses radiologic imaging, endovascular techniques, and clinical expertise to diagnose and treat those diseases that affect the CNS vasculature. Although one can narrow down the goal of training to the mastery of these three areas, there are many other aspects that such a curriculum must encompass. An effective curriculum must include training in the following areas: (1) the neurologic examination of patients; (2) the clinical signs and symptoms and neuroimaging manifestations of different neurovascular diseases; (3) the pathophysiology and natural history of these diseases; (4) the therapeutic avenues available for management of the different vascular diseases that affect the CNS as well as the indications and contraindications for each option; (5) the technical aspects of endovascular procedures; (6) the

* Corresponding author.

1042-3680/05/$ - see front matter
doi:10.1016/j.nec.2004.08.008

neurosurgery.theclinics.com

periprocedural management of patients treated with endovascular techniques, including neurointensive care; (7) a fundamental understanding of radiation physics, biology, and safety; and (8) an avenue for clinical or basic science research that will expand the current endovascular neurosurgical knowledge base.

The ACGME guidelines call for a fellowship in this subspecialty to be jointly administered by ACGME-accredited programs in neurological surgery, diagnostic radiology, and neuroradiology that are present at the same institution. Exceptions are subject to approval by the Residency Review Committees (RRCs) for neurological surgery and diagnostic radiology. The subspecialty program in endovascular neurosurgery should not adversely affect the educational experience of the institution's neuroradiology and neurosurgery residents. The program director of an endovascular neurosurgery fellowship must be certified by the American Board of Radiology or the American Board of Neurological Surgery or possess the equivalent qualifications as determined by the RRC. The faculty must also include at least one other full-time member with the same qualifications as the program director.

Prerequisites

The approved ACGME training requirements currently stipulate for 1 year of graduate medical education in endovascular neurosurgery. Because of variations in prefellowship training programs, some common prerequisites are essential to produce practitioners with mastery in all areas of the subspecialty. The CV Section and the ASITN recommend a full year of diagnostic neuroradiology training that provides adequate exposure to catheter techniques. For those trainees who do not come from a radiology training program, this training should be provided by the institution sponsoring the endovascular neurosurgery program. It is desirable, however, that this training also be obtained through an ACGME-accredited neuroradiology program at the prospective fellow's home institution and enfolded into the residency elective time. Within the prerequisite training, it is recommended that the trainees perform at least 100 diagnostic cerebral angiograms during the 12-month period. The importance of this prerequisite experience cannot be overemphasized inasmuch as cervicocerebral angiography is technically challenging and the organ supplied is uniquely vulnerable to vascular insults. Another requirement is that there must be adequate exposure to neurointensive patient care and neurosurgical techniques in the management of cerebrovascular diseases. For those residents who do not come from a neurosurgery training program, this requirement is satisfied by 3 months of clinical experience in an ACGME-accredited neurologic surgery training program. With a firm foundation in the fundamentals of neuroradiology and neurointensive care, the trainee is better able to increase his or her expertise in the final 12 months.

Training curriculum

As with any other training program, an endovascular neurosurgery fellowship must provide sufficient exposure to the full spectrum of diseases one can expect to encounter in practice as well as the many different endovascular procedures used to treat these diseases. Trainees should have the opportunity to perform periprocedural examinations of patients, evaluate preliminary diagnostic studies, and formulate treatment plans. Mandatory for effective training is the opportunity for trainees to perform diagnostic and interventional procedures and generate procedural reports that include and adhere to Current Procedural Terminology coding. In addition, the trainee should participate in the postprocedural management, which should include critical care and short- and long-term follow-up care. This continuity of care ensures that the trainee is familiar with the varied outcomes of these procedures and their delayed sequelae.

Along with clinical training, the ACGME specifically lists the following as areas that should be covered in the endovascular neurosurgery curriculum: (1) anatomic and physiologic basic knowledge; (2) technical aspects of endovascular neurosurgery; (3) applicable pharmacology; (4) the coagulation cascade; (5) vascular diseases affecting the CNS; (6) tumors of the head, neck, spine, and CNS; (7) revascularization for occlusive diseases; (8) embolization for hemorrhage; (9) invasive functional testing; and (10) balloon test occlusions [1]. To facilitate education, conferences should be held on a routine basis and should include but not be limited to journal clubs, anatomy and pathology reviews, morbidity and mortality reviews, and interdepartmental meetings with neurosurgeons and neuroradiologists. Of major importance for training is the access to a patient population large enough to provide case material that encompasses the entire range of neurovascular diseases. In addition to the 100 diagnostic angiograms recommended by the CV Section and the ASITN, we think that trainees should perform at least 100 interventional procedures, including embolization of aneurysms, arteriovenous malformations, and tumors; the treatment of intracranial and extracranial occlusive vascular disease; and the performance of invasive functional testing. These cases should be recorded in a log that is certified by the program director at the completion of the training.

As part of the training curriculum for endovascular neurosurgery, the need for additional training in cervical carotid angioplasty and stent placement (CAS) has been recognized [2,3]. A collaborative panel comprising members of the ASITN, American Society of Neuroradiology, and Society of Interventional Radiology recently published guidelines for CAS [4,5]. Although these guidelines have not been officially adopted by the ACGME, they do constitute the recommendations of a group of leading practitioners who seek to establish criteria for competent performance of CAS. Such guidelines are important, given the growing prevalence of this procedure and the numerous different specialties seeking to perform it. This diverse group includes cardiologists, vascular surgeons, interventional radiologists, neurosurgeons, neurologists, and interventional neuroradiologists. Aside from possessing the fundamental knowledge and skills for the appropriate application and performance of CAS, the operator, according to these guidelines, must have met certain prerequisites. These include the performance of at least 100 diagnostic cervicocerebral angiograms as the primary operator and 10 consecutive CAS procedures under the supervision of an on-site qualified physician. A satisfactory training alternative for an individual with existing catheter skills would be experience with a minimum of 25 non-carotid stent procedures and attendance at an Accreditation Council for Continuing Medical Education–sponsored program providing at least 16 category I credits and hands-on training in CAS, followed by completion of at least 4 successful and uncomplicated CAS procedures as principal operator under the supervision of an on-site qualified physician. The purpose of these guidelines is to ensure that those individuals who perform this procedure do so after demonstrating appropriate awareness of the indications, contraindications, risks, benefits, and technical requirements of CAS.

Equipment and facilities

To evaluate and treat patients with cerebrovascular disease adequately, the imaging and procedure areas and equipment must be up to date and available for the performance of all endovascular neurosurgical procedures. The ACGME training requirements provide recommendations regarding this ancillary equipment and space. Physiologic monitoring and resuscitative equipment should be present in the room where these procedures are performed. In addition to biplanar fluoroscopy with live digital subtraction roadmapping capability, ancillary imaging equipment (eg, MRI scanner, CT scanner, perfusion analysis software, intra- and extracranial ultrasound) is mandatory. There must also be adequate space and facilities for the storage of the materials used in endovascular procedures and film display and interpretation as well as for consultation with other physicians. It is highly desirable that the training program be hospital based to provide the appropriate inpatient, outpatient, emergency, and intensive care facilities necessary for comprehensive endovascular neurosurgical care.

As with training programs in other disciplines, the curriculum for endovascular neurosurgical training must foster an environment in which the trainees have ample opportunity to participate in the development of new knowledge. The members of the teaching staff, who are responsible for establishing and maintaining such an environment, should be involved in a broad spectrum of scholarly activities, including conferences, active participation in professional societies, active clinical and scientific research projects, and support for trainee participation in these endeavors.

Program director

The program director should evaluate the progress of each trainee on a semiannual basis, and this evaluation should focus on the knowledge, skills, and professionalism of the trainee. The results of this evaluation must be made available to the trainee in a timely fashion and be maintained as part of the training institution's permanent record of each trainee's progress. It is expected that as trainees expand their knowledge and skills, they will be advanced to positions of increased responsibility by the program director. The evaluation process must also include an evaluation of the teaching staff by the trainee.

This evaluation should also be performed on a semiannual basis and include an assessment of the teaching staff's teaching abilities, commitment to the educational program, clinical knowledge, technical skills, and scholarly activity. At the end of the training program, a final written evaluation for each trainee should be completed, including a review of the trainee's performance as well as verification that the trainee has demonstrated sufficient professional ability to practice endovascular neurosurgery in a competent and independent fashion. Evaluations of the trainees and teaching staff must be reviewed on a regular basis by the program director and the institutional review committee to ensure the educational effectiveness of the program.

In-residency experience

During their training, residents in neurosurgery receive some exposure to most, if not all, areas of neurosurgical subspecialization. Endovascular neurosurgery should be no different. As with the other areas of subspecialization, a brief clinical rotation should not count as part of fellowship training. Some neurosurgical training programs have chosen to use elective time for residents to undergo enfolded "fellowship" training in certain disciplines. Although this may be appropriate for the prerequisite training, the authors think that the defined fellowship in endovascular neurosurgery should occur on completion of the required neurosurgery training. As with other subspecialty areas in neurosurgery, the diagnosis and management of complex cerebrovascular diseases require the professional and emotional maturity that is developed over the years of residency training, including the duties and responsibilities that come with serving as the chief resident. Individuals who have not completed the residency may lack this maturity, resulting in a suboptimal experience for the individual, the training program, and, most importantly, the patient.

American Association of Neurological Surgeons Endovascular Task Force

Two of the authors (R.E. Harbaugh, L.N. Hopkins) cochaired an American Association of Neurological Surgeons Endovascular Task Force charged with generating ideas for promoting the number of endovascular neurosurgeons and ensuring that endovascular surgery becomes a mainstream discipline within neurosurgery. An abbreviated summary of the Endovascular Neurosurgery Task Force report is as follows:

1. An accelerated pathway for training in endovascular neurosurgery to allow practitioners to perform a limited scope of endovascular procedures should be considered.
2. Neurosurgical residents should have opportunities for exposure to and training in endovascular neurosurgical techniques during the residency.
3. Cerebrovascular neurosurgeons as well as endovascular neurosurgeons and interventional neuroradiologists should continue to collaborate within their own institutions and through common forums to promote in a mutual fashion their science, patient care, and training of future practitioners from both disciplines.

Summary

Endovascular neurosurgery/interventional neuroradiology/endovascular surgical neuroradiology is a rapidly evolving subspecialty that incorporates the knowledge and skills from neurosurgery and neuroradiology. The CV Section and ASITN have worked together extensively to establish a training curriculum that allows for the diverse backgrounds of potential trainees. The ACGME has recognized this curriculum and has adopted it as the standard for training program accreditation. Nevertheless, we should be cognizant of the fact that as the field of neuroendovascular therapy evolves, last year's solutions may prove to be this year's problems. It may be time for neurosurgeons to consider training in endovascular neurosurgery in the same way that we train neurosurgeons in every other neurosurgical discipline.

References

[1] Program requirements for residency education in endovascular surgical neuroradiology. Accreditation Council for Graduate Medical Education. Available at: http://www.acgme.org/downloads/RRC_progReq/422pr403.pdf. Accessed March 20, 2004.

[2] Higashida RT, Hopkins LN, Berenstein A, Halbach VV, Kerber C. Program requirements for residency/fellowship education in neuroendovascular surgery/

interventional neuroradiology: a special report on graduate medical education. AJNR Am J Neuroradiol 2000;21(6):1153–9.

[3] Program requirements for residency/fellowship education in neuroendovascular surgery/interventional neuroradiology: special report on graduate medical education: a joint statement by the American Society of Interventional and Therapeutic Neuroradiology, Congress of Neurological Surgeons, and American Association of Neurological Surgeons, American Society of Neuroradiology. Neurosurgery 2000; 46(6):1486–97.

[4] Barr JD, Connors JJ III, Sacks D, et al. Quality improvement guidelines for the performance of cervical carotid angioplasty and stent placement. J Vasc Interv Radiol 2003;14(9 Part 2):S321–35.

[5] Barr JD, Connors JJ III, Sacks D, et al. Quality improvement guidelines for the performance of cervical carotid angioplasty and stent placement. AJNR Am J Neuroradiol 2003;24(10):2020–34.

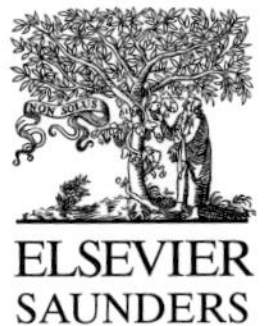

ELSEVIER
SAUNDERS

Neurosurg Clin N Am 16 (2005) 451–461

NEUROSURGERY
CLINICS
OF NORTH AMERICA

Index

Note: Page numbers of article titles are in **bold face** type.

A

1042-3680/05/$ - see front matter
doi:10.1016/S1042-3680(05)00010-0

B

C

D

J

L

M

N

O

P

R

S

T

U

V

W

Changing Your Address?

Make sure your subscription changes too! When you notify us of your new address, you can help make our job easier by including an exact copy of your Clinics label number with your old address (see illustration below.) This number identifies you to our computer system and will speed the processing of your address change. Please be sure this label number accompanies your old address and your corrected address—you can send an old Clinics label with your number on it or just copy it exactly and send it to the address listed below.

We appreciate your help in our attempt to give you continuous coverage. Thank you.

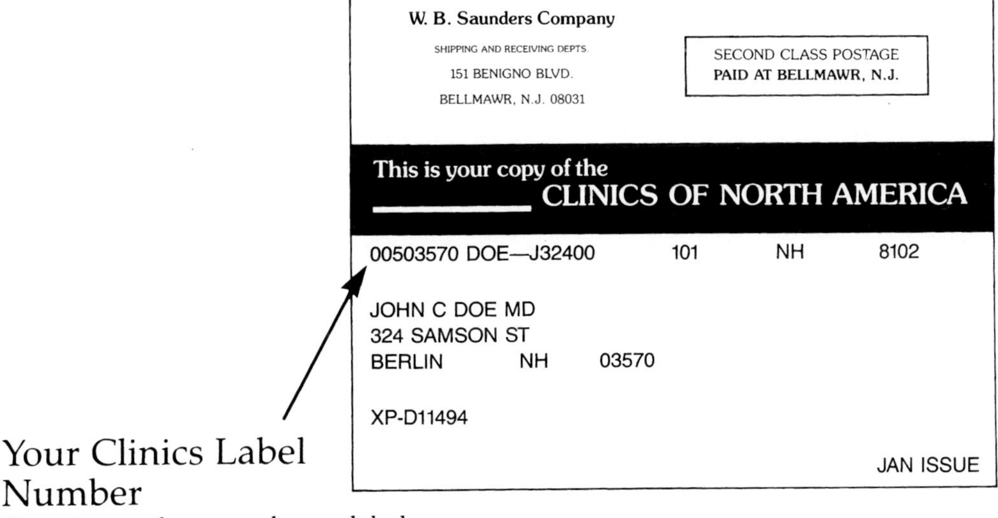

Your Clinics Label Number

Copy it exactly or send your label along with your address to:
W.B. Saunders Company, Customer Service
Orlando, FL 32887-4800
Call Toll Free 1-800-654-2452

Please allow four to six weeks for delivery of new subscriptions and for processing address changes.